JOSLIN

A Pioneer in Diabetes Care

S K Sinha

JOSLIN - A Pioneer in Diabetes Care

S K Sinha

ISBN: 978–0–6489470–0–4 (paperback)
ISBN: 978-0-6489470-1-1 (ebook)

Cover Design: Praveen Chandra
Book Design: Praveen Chandra

To my wife Lee

Contents

Preface

In late 1968 I learned that I had been awarded a fellowship for further studies on diabetes at the Joslin Clinic in Boston. When my wife and I travelled to Boston in June 1969 with our two daughters; one aged four years, and the other 18 months, the name Joslin represented an institution, not a man. I was unaware that the founder, Elliott Proctor Joslin had been born exactly 100 years earlier on June 6, 1869.

In retrospect, my first and only acquaintance with Joslin was in 1964 when I chanced upon his textbook on diabetes in the library of the hospital in Sydney where I was doing my "residency" after completing the medical course at the University of Sydney, Australia. The name of the author did not register! I vaguely recalled that it was a hardcover volume in green. I now realise that it was the ninth edition, published in 1952. In the final sixth year of my medical course, the lecture on diabetes – only one lecture – had occupied 30 min of the one hour devoted to "therapeutics of endocrine conditions." I have no recollection of what we were told about diabetes. However, I remember very clearly the lecturer. The urbane silver-haired Sir William Morrow, always immaculately dressed in bespoke three-piece suits, was Physician to Field Marshal Sir William Slim, the Governor- General of Australia.

It is a remarkable fact that Joslin worked till the last day of his life of 92 years. Our arrival, a mere seven years later coincided with celebrations at the Clinic of the centenary of his birth. Five of the original six colleagues who, together with the founder, were often referred to as "the original seven", were still active in clinical practice.

I learnt a great deal about Joslin from my conversations with this group as well as other members of the staff who had started working there at a later date. During a visit in 2014, I had the good fortune to speak to Donald Barnett. Apart from the pleasure of catching up with him – he had been a friend and guide during my time there – I was able to gain valuable insights into Joslin's life. Barnett, in his mid-80s in 2014, was still as mentally alert as ever, and graciously shared information from his recollections as well as from the numerous documents he had obtained from various members of the Joslin family.

The idea of embarking on this project arose after that visit to the Joslin Diabetes Centre in 2014. I was struck by the fact that although its founder, Dr Elliott P. Joslin, was held in great esteem by his medical colleagues as well as members of the public, not only in America but also in Canada, Britain, Europe and South America, no one had undertaken a study of the man and his work.

In a recent letter to me, Dr Donna Younger remarked that 2019 was "the 150th anniversary of Dr Joslin's birth".

I felt that the occasion was an appropriate time to complete my reflections on the life of this man whose remarkable contributions had influenced multitudes of men, women and children with diabetes. Joslin's attitudes and practices in his professional and personal life set a standard which many of his colleagues, especially those in his practice, tried to emulate. Many of his work practices however, were rules which he insisted, had to be followed by all members of his staff even if they were unhappy about doing so and grumbled about it – behind his back!

I am also confident that the scores of Joslin Fellows scattered around the world would echo my sentiments on the debt we owe to Elliott Proctor Joslin and the profound influence of the impressive men and women on the staff of The Joslin Clinic, the institution he established, on our professional development and experience, to say nothing of the lifelong associations and friendships forged as a result of our time there.

That two members of the staff from my time at the Joslin, namely Don Barnett and Donna Younger have been able to help me with my many enquiries, has been of incalculable assistance and a privilege.

Many men of influence have had friends or associates who have known them well enough to write of their lives.

Perhaps the best-known example of this is the biography, "The Life of Samuel Johnson, L.L.D." written in 1791 by James Boswell. It is well-known that Boswell had only met Johnson in 1763, and much of his first-hand knowledge of the well-known writer was from a three-month tour of the Scottish Highlands and the Hebrides jointly undertaken by the two of them.

Two medical biographies written in Joslin's time were the Pulitzer prize-winning study of William Osler by Harvey Cushing in 1920, and a biography of Cushing by John Fulton in 1946. In both instances the writers had worked with or known their subject through their association in the medical institutions where they had worked. Cushing had come to know Osler during his time at Johns Hopkins, and then had remained in contact for the rest of Osler's life. Fulton had known, and been a friend of Cushing in Johns Hopkins. They also shared a common interest in collecting books on medical history.

Several of Joslin's associates had known him for an even longer period– the first six physicians he employed had spent their entire professional lives working with, and for him.

Dr Howard F. Root (1890 – 1967), had died 2 years before I began my fellowship. He had joined Joslin as his first full-time assistant in September 1920. A Harvard graduate, he did his internship at Peter Bent Brigham in Boston (1919 – 1920) followed by a Fellowship at the Johns Hopkins Hospital in Baltimore. For nearly half a century Root was active in virtually every aspect of Joslin's work, including the day – to - day care of his patients in hospital. He also wrote several chapters in Joslin's textbook on diabetes.

Dr Priscilla White, in 1922 and Alexander Marble in 1923 were the next two to join Joslin.

1949 marked the beginning of the tenure of Robert F Bradley, a Board-Certified internist. He had been in the U.S. Navy before joining Joslin. Bradley was to play pivotal roles at the Joslin in years to come.

Leo P. Krall had worked at the New England Deaconess Hospital, and was recruited by Joslin in 1953, largely for his expertise demonstrated during the epidemiological studies on diabetes in Oxford (Massachusetts), Joslin's birthplace, in 1947.

The founder's eldest son, Allen Proctor Joslin who had joined his father's practice in 1934, completed "the original seven."

In all my conversations with each of the surviving "original seven", I sensed that the regard each had for their leader verged on reverence.

3

But unlike Osler and Cushing, Joslin did not have a "Boswell."

There are only two books on Joslin: the first, "Elliott Proctor Joslin. A Memoir 1869 to1962," was written by Anna C. Holt and published in 1969. This was to mark the Centenary of Joslin's birth. Holt, a librarian by profession had known Joslin for many years. Their fathers had known each other as both the Holt and the Joslin families were originally from Oxford. The slim volume of 67 pages, provides insights into his background and aspects of his professional life but there is little in-depth treatment of his major contributions such as the measures he employed, and advocated, to improve the treatment and care of patients with diabetes. In the preface to the book Holt said, "so much was crowded into the lifetime of this remarkable man that much more could and should be written, especially about his medical achievements during more than 63 years of practice."

Nearly 30 years later, in 1998, Dr Donald M. Barnett wrote the second book, "Elliott P Joslin, MD: A Centennial Portrait" to mark the Centenary of Joslin's practice.

The book starts at the beginning of Joslin's medical career in the fall of 1898 when he completed his internship at Massachusetts Gen Hospital and ends with his death in 1962. The work is remarkable for its lucidity. It is concise and conservative – almost understated – in its treatment of Joslin's many achievements. Having personally known Don Barnett and being familiar with his faultless command of English, I was not surprised by the quality of scholarship evident in the work. In spite of his admiration for Joslin, Barnett was able to produce a balanced account entirely free of hagiography.

Although the writer modestly refers to his work as an essay, the account is remarkable for its breadth including gems of personal insights gleaned from sources ranging from chance discoveries like a portrait of John Wesley (clearly valued, perhaps even an exemplar, though never mentioned by Joslin), to personal recollections as when Joslin's secretary grumbled–Barnett tactfully described it as "driven to distraction"–about Joslin's insistence on personally writing to every patient, including those who gave "even $.50" to one of Joslin's "appeals for donations to hospital, research laboratory, or camps for diabetic boys and girls." He draws attention to the importance of the many facets of Joslin's life which he considered important when reflecting on "his favourite people and important stations in his life."

In describing Joslin's professional life, Barnett described the history and evolution of the management of diabetes from the pre-insulin era to the advanced care made possible, firstly, and most dramatically by insulin followed by improvements in laboratory procedures and advances in treatment such as tablets for lowering blood glucose.

Remarkably, he accomplishes all this in less than 90 pages. Little wonder then that the reader feels tantalised and is left wanting.

Holt was a lifelong friend and later, an associate, especially in preparations of his medical writings. She was an unabashed admirer of Joslin and said so on more than one occasion. Having known Joslin for many years and having worked for him at different times, including at one stage as a governess of his children, she was clearly able to write about him, as she said, largely from "personal recollections." Her association with Joslin, she said, was from 1913 to 1962.

Barnett, very much "a people person," known and respected for his acute perception in assessing patients, held Joslin in high regard. Having joined the staff in 1960, he had known Joslin in the final two years of the founder's life. Barely a hint of criticism can be found in his account.

Neither work provides references, notes, or an index. Fortunately the Joslin archives headed by Don Barnett at the Joslin Diabetes Centre, provide a much needed source of information on Joslin. Barnett had voluntarily come out of retirement to do this. The archives proved to be invaluable as a resource for this work.

Much of the material from the archives was gathered during the visit in 2014. Without the generosity of the President of the Joslin Diabetes Centre in allowing me to access papers, letters, books and photographs held in the Marble Library, it would have been impossible to engage in this exercise.

This work is based on my personal recollections and the experiences and recollections of others. It is therefore, my interpretation and reporting of incidents and impressions from my time in Boston in 1969 and 1970 as well as over the succeeding years. After my wife and I, with our two daughters returned to Sydney, and I began my specialist practice with emphasis on diabetes and heart disease, my relationship with the Joslin Centre remained very much alive as I kept in touch with the Clinic throughout my professional life. Over the years, several members of the staff visited Sydney, often staying in our home.

On one occasion, an ex-Joslin Fellow, Prof Joseph Schipp, contacted me during a visit to Sydney at a time when I was giving public lectures on diabetes. I asked him if he would like to give a lecture to the lay audience. As was typical of the man, he agreed without hesitation. Walking on to the stage that evening, he said, "I want three people in the audience to tell me what they'd like to know." I still remember his succinct and practical advice on the three topics chosen; how to lose weight, the best treatment for low blood sugar reactions, and how to avoid gangrene. He finished by saying, "learn about diabetes, especially *your* diabetes." As will be seen in this book Schipp was repeating one of the lessons strongly impressed upon patients –and Fellows-by Joslin.

During my fellowship, I joined a group of some 12 men and women who had received grants to study there. They came from all corners of the globe: Germany, Switzerland, South America, Mexico, Canada, Philippines, India, as well as other parts of America. We kept in touch with each other over the years. Many including Drs.Muni Choodappa (Bangalore), Jean Philip Assals (Geneva), Eberhard Standl (Munich) Suresh Mehtalia (Bombay)and Charles "Bing" Brinegar Jr.(Loma Linda, California), went on to occupy senior positions as professors and/or Department Heads. Our time at the Joslin was a common topic of conversation whenever we met at international conferences on diabetes. My continuing friendship and contact with them, as well as collaboration with many of them in writing for medical textbooks and scientific journals, and presenting papers at scientific meetings, has been one of the joys and privileges of my professional life.

In the course of my preparations for this book, I was surprised to realise how much I was able to learn about the man by reading his letters to patients, his articles in medical journals, his books, and, more than any of these, his compassionate and thoughtful advice to patients contained in the instruction manuals he produced over a period spanning some 50 years. The manuals in particular provided hitherto unexpected insights into his personality.

Samuel Johnson, while working on the book "Lives of Poets" warned against being too exact in telling tales of those with living friends and relatives. "Rather to say nothing that is false than all that is true," he counselled.

Some current biographies include criticisms of their subject to present what is seen as a more "balanced" account – a "warts and all" approach, as it is often described.

My personal view is that one has to be careful not to give undue prominence to the negative aspects of a person's life when he is remembered for particular acts or contributions especially if these are his major achievements and the reason for writing about him in the first place.

Clearly, there are gaps in this account. One could argue that no biography is truly complete. Even an autobiography is sometimes criticised on the basis of lacking objectivity.

I was conscious of the silences in the Joslin story, silences which troubled me and continue to do so. I thought about, then dismissed an earlier plan to contact his descendants. In my experience, memories of one's ancestors tend to fade after two generations. My one regret is the paucity, no, the almost complete absence, of information on Joslin's wife. Phrases describing wives of impressive men, "behind every great man…" etc. are hackneyed but often relevant all the same.

Joslin mentioned his wife Elizabeth but once. "To my dear wife" appears as a dedication to her of the first edition of his textbook on diabetes. Clearly she had many responsibilities including bringing up three children and coping with his long hours at work, frequent absences to attend meetings, or speaking engagements, locally and internationally, in addition to entertaining visitors – expected and unexpected. Elizabeth

Joslin also attended to "social" correspondence such as thank-you letters. I was frustrated by my failure to discover any details of her health, which clearly deteriorated to the point of possible dementia in her final years. Donna Younger told me that when Joslin died his wife was unaware of the event. Yet in spite of their long years of a strong and loving partnership, all I was able to unearth was a copy of a handwritten letter he had written to her on her 80th birthday and a few photographs of them taken with their grandchildren towards the end of her life.

Apart from this, not a word. Details of the childhood and adolescence of his three children and details of his family-life including family holidays, the children's times at school, college, university, and their careers and marriages are also scant. I found this surprising, especially in the memoir written by Holt, who was clearly close to the Joslin family for most of her life. She had worked for him at home and in his practice when she was young and had retained a close contact in the years when she worked in the Harvard Medical School Library. She kept in touch with him even after her retirement and helped him with his writings in the final years of his life. Would it be mischievous to suggest that she wanted his approval for protecting the privacy of his family, even posthumously?

My first port of call during my visit in 2014, was Massachusetts Gen Hospital to meet its archivist, Jeff Mifflin. I found Jeff's quiet, courteous and patient demeanour, coupled with a remarkable memory for details, humbling and stimulating. It was following this time with him that I felt encouraged to contact librarians and archivists in other centres in the United States, mostly in Boston. I found them all to be extremely helpful. They are named in the acknowledgements at the back of this book, together with many other friends, associates and acquaintances. They have all been kind and unstintingly generous.

Twice I stopped working on this project, putting it down to various difficulties, only some of which were valid reasons for doing so. The materials sat in my study gathering dust for over two years. I had been disorganised in the way I had collected and stored the material without appreciating the actual amount of information accumulated through the generosity of virtually anyone I had approached. I had to admit that what I had, exceeded what I did not.

Even after stopping, I had no doubt that the Joslin story deserved to be told.

In all the years since my first contact with colleagues at the Joslin clinic the founder was always referred to as "Dr. Joslin," and in writings, by his initials, "EPJ." Formality was part of the conduct in the clinic, especially in the first half of the 20th century, particularly in New England. Donna Younger told me that even as late as 1960, when she occupied an office next to Joslin's and sometimes overheard his conversations, Joslin and his first assistant Howard Root, who had been working together for 40 years, still referred to each other as "Dr Joslin" and "Dr Root." I have taken the liberty of using the surname alone when referring to Dr Joslin in this work. Therefore the other Joslins have had their first names included.

The Indian leader, M. K. Gandhi, who was the same age as Joslin, and who Joslin admired, warned against disciples writing about their teacher. He said *"bhakti"* (devotion) is blind to shortcomings."

Until I arrived in Boston, I knew nothing of Joslin except that he had written a book on diabetes. Neither did I have any feelings of a personal association. Admittedly, after the time spent reading about him, if given the choice, I would undoubtedly have preferred to have known this exceptional man during his lifetime.

In conclusion, I return to the earlier quote of Samuel Johnson and express my sincere hope of "saying nothing that is false" even if the many gaps in the information presented, or other shortcomings in this account, fail to reveal "all that is true."

Sydney, 2019.

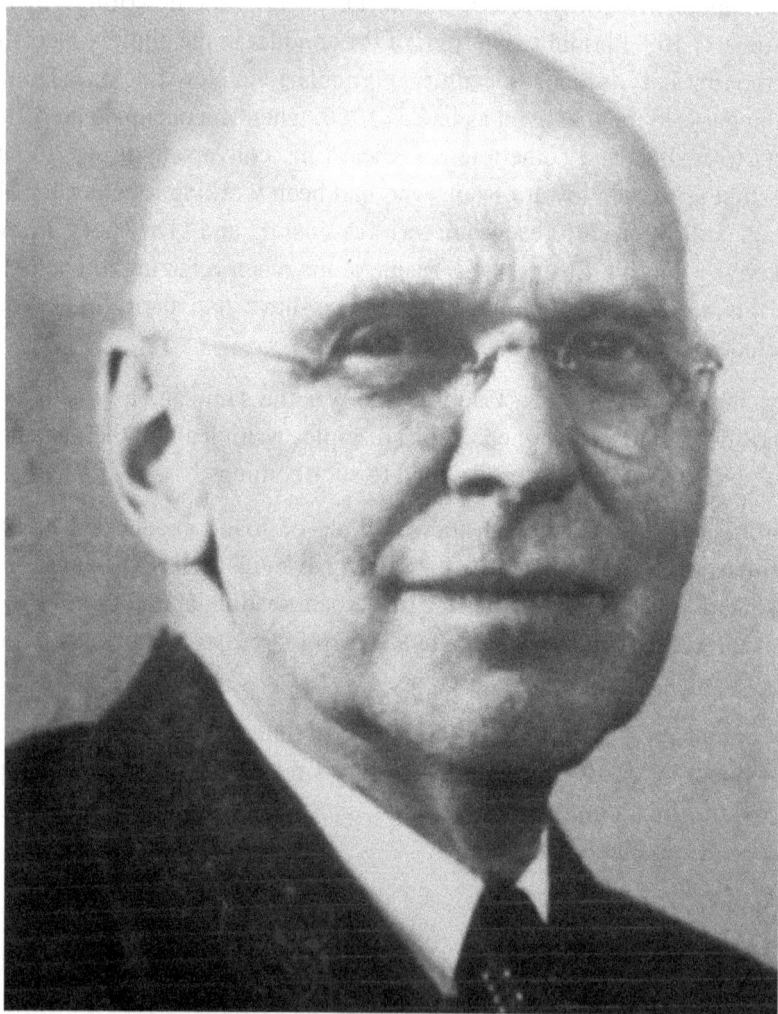

Elliott P Joslin (1869-1962)

Introduction – A Life That Cannot Be Forgotten

"To have lived through the changing panorama of medicine for 70 years, to have been an important figure in that changing panorama, to have served his fellow men, and to have won the gratitude and respect and affection of an uncounted multitude, is to have lived a life that cannot be forgotten."

Frederick M Meek

In 1916 the first textbook of diabetes in the English language was published in the United States. The writer was a 47-year-old physician from Boston. The book covered in detail the entire clinical spectrum of the condition as known at that time. Lucid in language and comprehensive in its coverage of not only the manifestations of diabetes but of the practical day-to-day management of the condition by the practising doctor and nurse, the initial run sold out within months. The book remains a standard textbook on the subject to this day, the last edition, fourteenth, published in 2014. It is remarkable that after his first book, the writer over the next forty years, although engaged in full-time medical practice, wrote revised editions at regular intervals. The tenth edition of the textbook was released in 1959 .The physician was then 90 years old and still engaged in caring for diabetic children and adults.

Already well known in Boston due to his popularity as a physician, the publication of the book spread his name throughout the United States, as well as in other English-speaking countries, especially Canada and Britain. Later, translations into other languages reached patients and doctors in countries where the predominant languages were Spanish, French and German.

To accompany each edition of the textbook, he also published manuals for patients. Invariably, the manuals outsold the textbook. Written to help with the day-to-day treatment of diabetics, the manuals are, in themselves, a study in the progress of the knowledge of the condition as a whole. The simplicity of the language to explain the physiological principles of diabetes enabled the patient and his carers to understand what and why treatment was necessary. The writer's capability in this educative process was one of his greatest gifts. In today's language he would be called a capable communicator, which he was, and more.

Important changes, especially advances in the treatment of diabetes, were quickly made available to the medical community in each new issue of his textbook. Within a year, at times the same year, a manual would be released. The writer included diabetics as part of the team treating the condition, and from the very beginning of his practice advocated the centrality of the patient in the treating team. That even young diabetics were encouraged to be part of the team managing their condition was repeatedly shown, even championed, in the manuals. To emphasise this on his colleagues in what at that time was a particularly conservative profession, this theme was repeated in the textbook as well. For added interest and emphasis he often added details of particular patients. To emphasise that his illustrations were based on actual patients, he included the case number from his patient ledger which he kept throughout his life to record details of every patient attending his practice. Often the textbook as well as the manual included photographs of patients.

The emphasis on the role of the patient in his or her own treatment of diabetes often obscured the writer's other achievements. Yet his determination to maintain this emphasis never faltered, as shown in the manual which accompanied the final edition of his textbook.

He was feted in the village where he was born. He was admired and respected in every circle in which he moved; the church, the schools, the college and university where he studied, the institutions he visited, and editors of the medical journals he supported including *The Boston Medical and Surgical Journal* which, later as *The New England Journal of Medicine*, went on to become a publication respected throughout the scientific world.

All this in addition to a prodigious output of writings on diabetes over a period of more than sixty years, were the result of the vision and efforts of one man. *Just one man.*

So who was this man and what drove him to pursue a career so strongly dominated by a desire, no, a determination, to study a single condition and to pioneer several aspects of its management which were to influence thousands of patients not only in his native country but throughout the world?

What challenges did he have to face and overcome to achieve this?

What were his individual personality traits, and who, and what, were the influences in his formative and later years to mould him into the person with the breadth of capability and vision to achieve so much?

He lived in an era of great thinkers, not only in the medical but also in the literary world. It was a time of the introduction of the ether anaesthetic for operations, and of using x-rays to check on bones and the lungs.

He lived in a time when specialisation was only a small part of a doctor's practice. Giants of the medical profession in the United States, especially in Boston, counted men like Oliver Wendell Holmes and John Collins Warren in their ranks of practising luminaries.

Yet this man, through his own initiative, and contrary to established practices followed by the rest of the medical profession at that time, managed to negotiate the tortuous path to forge a career in medicine unique for specialising not only in a single branch of medicine as was to happen in medical practice in the years that followed, but in fact narrowed it to the study of one single malady. In later years, terms such as "super specialist" or even later, "sub specialist", would come into everyday use.

This man was Elliott Proctor Joslin.

Characters

Elliott Proctor Joslin

Family:

Elizabeth Elliot Denny Joslin: wife

Mary Joslin, Allen Proctor Joslin, Elliott Proctor Joslin Jr: children

Allen Lafayette Joslin: father

Sarah Proctor Joslin: mother

Ada Luella Joslin: (half) sister

Homer Shumway Joslin: (half) brother

Orrin Franklin Joslin: uncle, older brother of Allen Lafayette Joslin.

John Proctor (of the 1692 notoriety)

Abel Waters Proctor: Joslin's maternal grandfather

Thomas Emerson Proctor senior: Joslin's maternal uncle

Ellen Osborne Proctor: Sarah Proctor's younger sister

Lucrecia Miller Shumway: Allen Joslin's first wife

Lauriston Shumway: Allen Joslin's first father-in-law

Childhood:

Dr Samuel Paine: village doctor

Dr Adams of Webster: treated Joslin for measles. An early inspiration

Ella Paine: village doctor's daughter and Joslin's Sunday School teacher

Early Educational Influences:

Russel Chittenden

Reginald Heber Fitz (Massachusetts General hospital)

Harvey Cushing

Francis Denny

Medical Practice:

Howard Root, Priscilla White, Alexander Marble, Allen Joslin, Robert Bradley, Leo Krall.

(These first six physicians were employed by Joslin as assistants and later as associates)

Francis Gano Benedict

Francis Madison Allen

European Contacts:

Naunyn

Minkowski

Von Noorden

Bouchardat

Younger Associates:

Anna C. Holt

Charles Best

Albert Renold

Patients:

Mary Higgins: The first diabetic seen by Joslin

Sarah Proctor Joslin: Joslin's mother, an "in-house" patient

George Fisher Baker: "The Sphinx of Wall Street"

George Richards Minot: Nobel Laureate Joslin's prize patient

Amelia Peabody: Sculptress, fellow gentleman - farmer and friend of Joslin

Part 1.
History and Ancestry

The Gallows of Salem an Inauspicious Beginning?

On the 19th of August 1692, in Salem, a small town in Massachusetts, John Proctor, the thrice-married father of 17, known for his robust physique and firm adherence to Puritan principles, was sent to the gallows.

His crime?

Supporting his wife who had been found guilty of witchcraft during the infamous Salem witch trials. Her sentence was suspended because she was expecting a child. Inexplicably, she escaped punishment, even though the death sentence for witchcraft was not abolished till 4 months after she had given birth.

The child she bore was a son, and even though she had remarried shortly after John Proctor was hanged – remember there were seventeen mouths to feed- she called him John Proctor 2nd, thus continuing the Proctor lineage.

One hundred and seventy seven years later, another Proctor woman was to give birth to a male child.

On 6 June 1869 Sarah Emerson Waters Proctor, the second wife of Allen Lafayette Joslin, a shoe store owner in Oxford, Massachusetts, produced the child who would be the first in his generation of the Joslins to carry the Proctor lineage.

They called him Elliott Proctor Joslin.

A Country Upbringing

Joslin was the youngest in a family of three children. Allen Lafayette Joslin had two children from a previous marriage. The eldest, a girl, Ada was 9 and the second, a son Homer was 7 years old. Joslin was the only surviving child of Allen Joslin's second wife, Sarah Proctor Joslin.

The families on both sides of Joslin's parents played important roles in his upbringing, especially in his formative years.

Also important was the influence of Joslin's birthplace, Oxford. A small town with a population of about 2000, it remained a focus for him throughout his life. Barnett attributes Joslin's fondness for agrarian metaphors to his early formative years in Oxford where farming, agriculture and cottage industries were the main enterprises.

The importance of the history of New England was stressed on the children of the Joslin family, especially by Joslin's mother. It is therefore pertinent to review some aspects of the history of the English settlers in the New World, especially their turbulent beginnings in an isolated village some 60 miles from Boston. This village later came to be known as Oxford.

Historical Background: Arrival of the English in the New World

The American flag is dominated by stars and stripes. 13 stripes occupy the largest area. The founding of the American nation began with the struggles of the original thirteen colonies represented by the stripes. Their story has never been forgotten.

"A country without memory is a country of mad men." George Santayana.

The earliest white settlement in the north-eastern United States dates back to the early to mid-1600s with the arrival of English settlers and French Huguenots. However, English explorers had ventured into the New World even earlier. One of the best known was John Smith who founded Jamestown. Smith is also credited with giving the name, New England to the north-eastern part of America.

The English presence in the New World can be traced to 10 April 1606, when King James 1st of England granted a charter to the London and Plymouth Virginia Company, to establish trading relationships in the New World. In actual fact, this was a licence to engage in aggressive land acquisition. The following year, 1607, John Smith, previously known for his acts of piracy, but at that time employed by the Plymouth Virginia Company, founded James Fort. This was the first permanent British settlement in North America. Later James Fort became known as Jamestown.

Smith carried out important explorations in North America, mainly Chesapeake Bay and Potomac and Rappahannock Rivers. Skilled in cartography, he made detailed and accurate maps of the area, including locations of various Indian villages. In 1608 he was elected President of the colony. He introduced regulations which brought about an orderly settlement by the English. One regulation which is often quoted included a clause "... He that will not work shall not eat." An effective administrator, Smith kept the Fort in good repair. He encouraged cultivation of the land and a reliable supply of safe drinking water by having a well dug. Trees were cut for clapboard which, together with other products such as pitch, tar, and soap, was shipped back to England.

Importantly, Smith also kept a well - drilled and equipped army which ensured peace, as Chief Powhaton, the leader of the predominant local tribe which Smith had defeated, feared English weapons. At the same time, the vanquished warrior harboured secret hopes that by maintaining cordial relations with the resident English administrator, he might acquire modern weapons with which he could subjugate other Indian tribes, thus increasing his own wealth and power.

Smith was recalled to London in 1615 and reassigned to different duties. He never returned to America. Relations between the local Indian tribes and the English were never maintained with the same care and diplomacy as in his time. Isolated incidents of thieving and looting led to a gradual deterioration of the comparatively harmonious working relationship established by the first president.

The violent confrontations which are part of Oxford's early history had their beginnings in several full-scale armed conflicts in the early years of the English presence in New England. Two of the most notable engagements were the Pequot War, 1636-1638, and King Philip's War, 1675–1678.

The Pequots, who were the dominant tribe at that time, having subjugated other tribes, engaged in armed conflict with colonists from Massachusetts Bay, Plymouth and Saybrook together with their native allies from the Narragansett and Mohegan tribes for over two years. Although they were defeated by the colonists, the resentment felt by the

Indians continued to simmer and an even more bloody conflict followed several decades later. This was King Philip's War.

Perhaps the most widely known and recorded, King Philip's War, which took place in the New England area, has been referred to as "the bloodiest war in American history on a per capita basis." It left 5000 inhabitants of New England dead, three quarters of that number being Indians. In terms of the percentage of the population killed, King Philip's War led to the death of twice as many soldiers as the American Civil War and seven times more than the American Revolution.

Led by their Chief Metacom, (dubbed Philip by the English), the settlers were confronted by skilled Indian warriors. Fierce and crafty himself, Metacom, who was worshipped by his soldiers, inflicted heavy losses on the intruders. It was only through a plot hatched by a wily English officer, who bribed an Indian warrior to betray his leader, that Metacom was ambushed and killed by the traitor. The English beheaded the Indian leader, whose body was then drawn and quartered. The captors celebrated their victory by triumphantly displaying his head on a stake in Plymouth. The lingering resentment caused by this incident would continue to reverberate through the Indian community, leading to an uneasy relationship between the indigenous people and the new settlers for decades to come.

New Settlers in New England and the Arrival of Joslin's Ancestors, the Proctors

The first European settlement in New England was a colony in Plymouth established by 100 Puritans who had travelled on the *Mayflower* from England, reaching the American shores on a very cold day on 11 November 1620. Although now known as the Pilgrim Fathers, at the time of their arrival, and indeed for the next 200 years, they were called Pilgrims or "old comers". It was during the Bicentennial Celebrations in 1820 that they were first referred to as "Pilgrim Fathers" in a speech by the well-known politician and orator Daniel Webster, and the term has persisted since.

In 1626, more English immigrants arrived and established another community, this time in Salem, a coastal city in Essex, Massachusetts. The Massachusetts Bay Colony was initially established around two natural harbours and in areas surrounding them in Salem and in Boston. It also included Connecticut, as it covered most of the New England area in the 1630s.

The first John Proctor and his wife Mary and their three year old son, also called John, had arrived in 1635.

Joslin's strongly Puritanical background can be traced to the very beginnings of the English settlement in New England. The largest group of settlers who arrived during this early period numbered some 20,000. They set about organising their day-to-day lives in their new home in a way which reflected their culture and religion. They elected governors and restricted the electorate to "free men" selected through a thorough examination of the religious views before formal admission to the local church. The Puritans were intolerant of other religious denominations, including Anglicans, Quakers and Baptists.

An important, perhaps the major reason for the decision of some groups of settlers like the pilgrims, to come to the New World was religious freedom. There were, however, other attractions as well, including the possibility of acquiring wealth, the adventure and excitement of exploring a new country, and the prospect of owning land. Thus it is easy to understand the broad mix of interests and priorities which motivated these newcomers to the New World.

Oxford, Its Early History

The history of Oxford has been an abiding interest for its citizens for over 300 years. Successive generations have celebrated its development in its 200- and 250- year anniversaries. The 100-year celebrations were overtaken by the events surrounding the First World War, 1914-18.

Oxford's earlier years, however, were marked by repeated and protracted disputes with the indigenous dwellers of the area.

First There Were Indians

The indigenous presence in the New World had been a fact of history from the time of Columbus's discovery in 1492. Whether or not the early settlers had expected to find natives inhabiting their new-found haven is not known. Or had they taken too literally the account of Columbus's assessment of the natives when, upon his return to Spain, he had reported to Queen Isabella that in his opinion it would not need more than fifty men to subjugate the indigenous dwellers?

The Massachusetts History Timeline dates the origins of Indians back to 10,000 BC, the Paleo Indian Era, when the earliest inhabitants dwelt in caves. They were nomadic hunters.

The modern occupation of this part of Massachusetts was by Nipmuc Indians whose current history dates from the early 1600s before the arrival of white settlers. Today's Oxford occupies the middle of the territory then known as Nipmuc or Nipmuck or Nepmug country. Within the territory close to the actual location of Oxford was a settlement originally called Mauchaug.

The nomadic lifestyle of the Indians had stood the test of time. When the new settlers arrived, the temporary dwellings of the Indians dotted the region. The camps were usually located on the plain, which, judging by the luxuriant vegetation, had rich soil, especially in the south-eastern region.

George F Daniels' book on the history of the town includes geographic and botanical details as existed towards the end of the 1800s.

"Its natural attributes are varied and rich, it is full of streams supporting a wide variety of fish, and it has natural ponds, hills, and meadows. There are cedar swamps which yield wood and timber useful for the construction of fences and production of clapboard, shingles and coopers' materials for making casks, buckets, and barrels as well as a special container called Hogshead, which was used to ship large quantities of tobacco from the colonies to England.Cedar swamps, useful for providing 'fencing stuff', and meadows were allotted to settlers."

The soil in the town area was rich enough to support grazing while the plains had a warm alluvial soil easily cultivated to produce farm products, including garden vegetables and grapes, strawberries, and other small fruit.

According to the beautifully descriptive report on this area of New England in 1890 by Nason and Varney, "nearly a third of the town area is forested mostly with oak, chestnut, pine and maple." The quality of its soil is praised again as supporting "numerous apple trees, and blueberries, huckleberries, strawberries and cranberries, being a source of more than usual profit."

The river flowing southward through the basin on which Oxford is situated was an integral part of its early history for both the Indians as well as the new settlers. It was an important route for travel and destination for fishing for the Nipmuck people who lived in the surrounding hills and rode through the plain to their hunting grounds. For the first settlers, the Huguenots, its left bank was favoured as the site on which they built their homes. It is called French River after the early settlers from France.

Harsh Realities: The Huguenot Experience in the New World

Although the English had come to New England earlier and, as already noted, had acquired land in Oxford, they did not physically occupy the territory. The first people to actually settle in Oxford were Huguenots who arrived in Oxford in the summer and autumn of the 1686. They had been driven out of France by the Edict of Nantes which revoked a previous royal decree granting them religious freedom. Their reputation for craftsmanship and industriousness was well-known. The English owners of the land in Oxford, keen to avail themselves of the opportunity to enlist the services of the talented newcomers, welcomed them with a generous offer. They arranged a grant of land for the Huguenots to build homes as well as other structures needed by their community. The original grant of 2500 acres was given to Gabriel Bannon. This parcel of land was situated in the eastern part of the town.

The newcomers who were deeply religious and skilled artisans had a

24

strong work ethic. They built a grist mill, a saw mill, a glove factory, a church and a fort, as well as a garrison house to live in.

After an initial period of harmonious relations with the local Indian tribe, the Nipmucs, the newcomers began to encounter increasing hostility. There were frequent skirmishes as the Indians continued to harass the new settlers, often setting fire to their farms and crops and stealing their stock and household goods.

The Johnson Massacre

In 1696 the Indians attacked the settlement and killed an owner John Johnson and three of his children. His wife, with a child in arms, was carried by a neighbour across the French River to a garrison in Worcester.

For the Huguenots, this was the last straw. The plantation was broken up and the French returned to Boston. After two further attempts at resettling failed, they returned the land granted to them by the owners and settled permanently in Boston.

Some of their descendants returned later or had remained in Oxford. Today they are known as "valuable citizens." Relics of their habitation in Oxford remain and are preserved for historical interest and significance. These include remains of fortifications, wells, trees and vines. The tragedy of the Johnson massacre has not been forgotten and there is a monument to record the tragic event.

An oak tree on the corner of Huguenot Road and Russell Lane has become a treasured landmark. It stands by an old Indian trail but now commands attention on its own merit. More than 400 years old, its trunk has a girth of over 25 feet. Just as the Indian trail no longer bears witness to the thundering hooves of the Indian warrior's steed, the majestic oak is no longer a guide to the modern traveller using "sat nav." Yet it still stands, a lasting reminder of the Huguenot presence in Oxford and, at least, a "photo opportunity" for the modern tourist.

English Settlers Arrive in Oxford

After the Huguenots left, 30 English families arrived in 1713 and their descendants established the town which remains their home to this day. Their early years, however, were challenging, not only through the difficulties of establishing themselves in an isolated environment but because access to and from Boston was limited to transport by horse or on foot. They were aware of the uneasy relationship and the difficulties with the Indians which had been experienced by the Huguenots.

Initially, the new arrivals were able to maintain good relations with the local Indian tribes. The natives taught them how to plant corn which became an important crop. They showed them the best fishing spots, and, in the forests, where to hunt beaver. They welcomed the newcomers to their feasts. Indeed, some scholars believe that a feast with the native tribe called Pokanokats in the fall of 1621 could be the basis of today's Thanksgiving celebrations.

However, the differences between the two peoples created obstacles to a lasting and durable coexistence. The natives, steeped in the ancient practices and traditions of their hunter-gatherer ancestors, could not reconcile their way of life and priorities with those of the newcomers who were products of the new pastoralist culture.

The sedentary urban lifestyle of the English was in stark contrast to that of the nomadic natives. For example, the Indians, with the change of seasons, were quite happy to pick up their wigwams and move to new locations, depending on their plans for hunting and fishing. They were alarmed and confused by the way the newcomers established themselves in the landscape which the indigenous population felt was their inheritance, passed on to them by their ancestors over thousands of years.

The settlers built timber houses, then surrounded them with fences. The fences had gates which could be locked. And finally, they erected an even stranger construction. Watchtowers were built to warn of an approaching enemy.

The English established farmlands with vastly different agricultural methods and farming techniques. Their tools, implements and machinery were more sophisticated than those used by the natives. But the natives had their own tools, made of stone as opposed to the Europeans' iron implements. Indians fashioned the tools which, over the years, had proved useful for their own purposes, and as far as they were concerned, their tools were perfectly adequate.

There was little change in their way of life after the European arrival. They followed their own customs and attitudes to coexistence with other tribes. Coexistence with the new arrivals, however, does not appear to have been in the Indian mindset at that time.

Clearly, neither the Indians nor the new settlers could reconcile themselves to the new realities. The Indians smarted at what they considered was usurpation of their territory. The new settlers, on the other hand, believed that land granted to them was theirs to use for the benefit of their families.

The English, with a strong work ethic, had little in common with the habits of the Indians in general and their work practices in particular. They were disparaging in their opinion of the natives, as illustrated by a quotation contained in George F Daniels' book attributed to a Miss Larned in her *History of Wyndham County*.

"They were subject clans of little spirit or distinctive character. Their number was small. A few families occupied favourite localities, while large sections (of land) were left vacant and desolate. Their dwellings were poor, their weapons and utensils rude and scanty. They raised corn and beans, and wove mats and baskets. Their lives were chiefly spent in hunting, fishing and idling."

Daniels also joined in, commenting, "Gaming, of which they were excessively fond, might be added." It is important to note that Daniels (1820–1897),a prominent member of the village community, was also known to Joslin's father, Allen Lafayette Joslin (1833–1911), both being involved in the leather industry, as well as other community activities in Oxford at that time. I make this point in order to draw attention to attitudes held by at least some of the citizens of Oxford towards the Indians at the time of Joslin's childhood.

The Joslin Family's Indian Connection

Indian tools are still found in parts of New England and many are preserved in museums. At least one such relic, a stone mortar, was treasured by the Joslins in Oxford for more than 100 years. Its story is part of the Joslin family history.

When Joslin's paternal grandfather Deakin Elliott Joslin and grandmother Almira Joslin lived in Thompson, a small village in Connecticut, their sons had, one day, brought home a stone mortar which they had found at the site of an old, long-disused Indian settlement. It was a common item in Indian camps where it was used for pounding maize and corn. When the boys were young and ran around barefoot, they had to wash their feet in the bowl before entering the house. When they moved to Oxford in the mid-1800s, the foot washing bowl was brought to their new home on Main Street. There the stone relic was used as a bird bath and also to wash the dog, Major.

Joslin regarded it as an important heirloom and persuaded his parents to let him take it to his country estate, Buffalo Hill.

It remained a treasured possession until the death of his much-loved sister Ada in 1941, when Joslin, in cooperation with another member of the congregation of their local church in Oxford, had the stone incorporated into a handsome and substantial stone pedestal with a carrying beam to serve as a baptismal font in memory of Ada Joslin.

The Oxford of Joslin's Childhood

At the time of Joslin's birth in 1869, Oxford was a thriving and prosperous community of merchants, farmers and landholders, but still very much a small village even though officially, having been incorporated, it rightly laid claims to being called a town.

Its community institutions were typical of the English way of life.

A post office first established in 1801 received mail once a week.

Transport to and from Worcester, initially by stagecoach, had been replaced by the Norwich Worcester Railroad in 1840. In 1868, a year before Joslin's birth, railroad had come to Oxford, facilitating the delivery of materials for manufacture and taking away the finished products. This had contributed greatly to the general prosperity of the community, and had made life much easier as far as travelling was concerned than had been possible when horses were the most popular mode of transport. (It also fitted in perfectly with the building plans of a certain aspiring shoe manufacturer called Allen Lafayette Joslin!)

The New Englanders clung to their Puritan faith, and churches were an integral part of the community from the very beginning. Joslin's strict adherence to Christian precepts defined his entire life, personally and professionally.

The first Meeting House had been completed by 1717. Initially it also doubled as the venue for town meetings.

The Congregational Church was built in 1829. Several others followed, including the Methodist, Baptist and Roman Catholic. The early Puritans, however, were not known for religious tolerance and remained absolutist in this regard.

Education was highly valued, second only to religious practice. Schools were established and laws made to ensure strict adherence to the provisions of the educational system. Universal public education had been enshrined in law as early as 1647, and every community of more than 50 households was required to maintain a master to teach reading and writing, while communities in excess of 100 households had to establish a grammar school, "the Masters thereof being able to instruct youth so far as they may be fitted for the universitie [sic]." There was a firm belief that intelligence and piety, harnessed with hard work and daring, if emphasised and inculcated in the young, would promote success in life. One need go no further than the subject of this book to see a life lived with unwavering adherence to these principles.

The first library was a collection of 10 books for the Congregational church. Several other libraries followed, usually through donations by individuals or businesses. The present library, built in 1903-4, is called the Landes Memorial Library in memory of the mother of the donor

Charles Landes. His mother was a descendant of the Rev. John Robinson, a minister to the Pilgrims when they were in Holland.

The more prominent citizens did more than their share to attend to the needs of the community. Thus men like Joslin's father Allen, a prominent and respected merchant, were chosen as leaders for community projects ranging from renovations needed for public buildings like churches to constructions of schools and improvement in the different industries like agriculture, as well as doing their duty as volunteer firefighters. Many also served as *"Selectmen"* who were empowered to ensure adherence to the law in various commercial activities such as the sale of liquor by licensees of taverns.

By the mid-1800s, when the Joslin family was well established in Oxford, it was no longer the frontier town of the days of the early settlement when the original English settlers of 1713 had travelled on horseback following Indian trails to reach their destination; when they had to fortify their new homes against Indian attacks, and when "it was not safe for a farmer to plough his field without a gun on his shoulder."

In the first hundred years agriculture had been the main industry. There were crops, and timber was plentiful. There were sawmills and grist mills. Millwrights were sought-after members of the community.

The second hundred years saw industrialisation come to Oxford. Farms still existed as recalled by Joslin when reminiscing about his childhood. However, manufacturing took hold; new shops and mills were built, wool carding machines, machinery for spinning cotton, grist mills and lumber mills, a dye house and manufacture of cotton and woollen goods, altered the face of the small town.

The year 1822 had seen the use of water power for manufacturing purposes. Hence the value of rapid-flowing streams and rivers. French River of Oxford was one such stream and several mills were built on its banks.

Oxford became known throughout New England for its school of artisans and millwrighting, fulling mills and shafts. It had the air of a prosperous community; the noise of machinery in the mills, the bustle of activity in the stores in the town, and a familiarity which exists within small populations, all invested Oxford with the qualities of a vibrant yet peaceful habitation which are hard to imagine today. Yet Oxford only had around 2000 people, even in the years when Joslin was at college in the final decade of the 1800s.

Main Street of Oxford

One interesting feature of many towns of that period was the prominence of the main thoroughfare in town. Probably continuing the tradition of prominent streets in their home country of England where they were often called High Street, some New England towns – Oxford included – called it Main Street.

In Oxford, Main Street was known for its length and breadth. Indeed, originally it had been planned in the hope that the impressive dimensions might sway the authorities to make Oxford the seat of local government. But when the time came for this, the town fathers rejected the proposal on the grounds that giving such importance to the town could "corrupt the morals of its youth".

In the early days Main Street was more than a thoroughfare. In fact, on one occasion it doubled as a local racecourse! According to an early issue of *The Worcester Gazette*, the first horse race to be run in Oxford had to be moved from the prearranged course just before it was due to start because of a sudden, heavy downpour. Consternation gripped the race organisers until the town physician commented that the only suitable, flat, straight stretch was the town's central road—which was commandeered forthwith!

Oxford's first horse race has therefore made it into the historical records of the town for two reasons – as has its Main Street!

Even as late as 1969 when Holt wrote her memoir of Joslin, Main Street had retained its charm. She commented that "the wide street bordered by stately old elm trees to this day bears the name "Main" street and preserves much of the charm and serenity of the time before the invasion

31

of the automobile and all the nuisances of high-speed, noise, confusion, and congestion of our present day life developed. Many of the spacious white houses with their lawns and shade trees continue to stand as reminders of an earlier period of more gracious and less harried living."

Among the family papers is a photograph of a portion of Main Street, on the back of which many years later Dr Joslin wrote: "This is the way Oxford looked when I was a boy, 1875. I remember well the house on the right where now the high school stands. George Lamb lived in it."

Joslin's Childhood Home on Main Street

Often the more prosperous citizens, especially merchants, aspired to build their homes on Main Street. During Joslin's childhood there were no more than half a dozen such houses on Main Street. Interestingly, one of them belonged to none other than the proprietor of the Joslin Shoe Store.

In 1866 Allen Joslin had built an imposing residence on Main Street, Oxford. More than 100 years later (1969), Holt described the building and its surrounds in admiring detail as …" One of the larger homes from this broad tree-shaded street, the square three-storey house with the mansard roof characteristic of this period of the Victorian era, still stands in the corner of Maple and Main Streets."

Joslin remembered his early years as happy ones, playing in and around the family home. "Of course I was spoiled," he remarked in an interview to a reporter from a Boston newspaper many years later.

I had managed to find a faded black-and-white newspaper photograph of the house published in the Boston Globe in the 1950s. Unfortunately, its age and limited facilities for reproduction did not permit me to get any more than a rough idea of its exterior.

It had not occurred to me to look for it online. When I did, I was surprised and delighted to discover that the house still exists and has been in continuous occupation more than 150 years. Judging by its appearance, it remains in good repair.

Its provenance is preserved and respected, further testimony to Oxford's awareness of, and pride in, its history. The information provided by the realtors in the district records it as having been the "home of Dr Elliott Proctor Joslin, famous for pioneering the treatment of diabetes."

It is an impressive building, even by today's standards. There are eight bedrooms—for the family of five.

Joslin had two other siblings but clearly there was accommodation for house-help as well as guests. Remember, it was 1867 when the young widower married a second time and brought his new bride to her impressive new home. Was the much sought-after new address, as well as the opulent abode, entirely Allen Joslin's idea? Or was there a not- so-subtle hint from the second father-in-law, perhaps even the prospective second wife, for her to be treated in a manner to which she was accustomed! The Proctors were known as having old money. Although Allen Joslin, after starting his own enterprise, was prosperous in his own right, he was not in the same league as the Proctors of Peabody.

I was interested in Don Barnett's view of the possible effect of Allen Joslin's second marriage on his commercial fortunes. In a conversation with me during my visit to Boston in 2014, he said that before the Proctor marriage, the Joslin business was hardly more than "just a small village shoe store." After the Proctor alliance however, Barnett felt that the Joslin concern "went gangbusters." In his book on Joslin, he wrote that after Joslin's mother's death in 1913, her legacy made Joslin, "a millionaire many times over by today's standards. Sarah Proctor Joslin, her sisters and one brother were heirs to a very large fortune derived from their father Abel's leather tanning trade."

Whatever the background, the house remained in the Joslin family till the end of the couple's lives and beyond. Allen Joslin lived there to the end of his life. After his death in 1911, the house was occupied by the older son, Homer Shumway Joslin. The first son, as was the custom in Puritan families, had joined the family business in 1881 and, even though his father remained the nominal head to the end of his life, the day- to- day running of the organisation had been left to the son for several years.

After his father's death, Joslin's mother had moved to their Beacon Street house in Boston. She lived there with her stepdaughter Ada to the end of her life. After the mother's death in 1913 Ada moved back to Oxford, but whether she lived in the house on Main Street or somewhere else is not known.

I was unable to discover further information on when the property was sold by the Joslins and how many owners it has had since then. Although listed on the site of at least one realtor, it was not for sale in mid—2019.

The Modern Oxford

The original town occupied a much larger area than today's Oxford. The original grant of land was a holding of 41,250 acres (65 mi.²), divided equally among five proprietors, three from London and two from Boston. Roughly rectangular, the northern and southern borders were each 10 miles long and the eastern and western sides 6 miles.

The original boundaries have been altered through the establishment of new towns: Leicester and Auburn to the north, Millbury and Sutton to the east, Douglas and Webster to the south, and Dudley and Charlton to the west. Today's Oxford is less than half its original size, with an area of 27.5 square miles.

This of course is not the only change visible in the Oxford of later years.

The Indian presence has been largely replaced by the Indian absence.

History, ancient as well as modern, repeatedly describes, and often dwells upon, differences between warring factions. Both parties fail, or refuse, to recognise their shared similarities. To this day, when we may consider ourselves to have relegated our hunter-gatherer heritage to ancient history, we still forage in the forests. We still hunt and gather at least some of our food, one obvious example being fishing, particularly in parts of the Pacific and Atlantic Oceans. Whaling continues in Antarctica despite ongoing controversy.

Sensitivities to racial diversity are now different from the time of Joslin's parents or indeed during Joslin's own lifetime. It would be interesting to see, or rather read, an account of the coming of the New Settlers into

Indian territory from an Indian viewpoint or written by a descendant of the Nipmucs.

Joslin's Ancestors

Both sides of Joslin's family, the Joslins and the Proctors, settled with their families in different parts of New England. The Proctors were one of the earliest settlers, and, as mentioned earlier, had arrived in 1635.

The Irish genealogist John Burke (1786–1848), mentions Egidius Josselyn, a nobleman from Brittany (France) emigrating to England at the time of Edward the Confessor (1003–1066). However, he stopped short of actually suggesting this as a possible link of the American Joslins to their English and French ancestors. Joslin himself did not mention France as the home of his ancestors. There is no record of his visiting any particular area of France from this viewpoint. He traced his ancestry on his mother's side and on more than one occasion mentioned his English ancestry. The Joslin archives contain a handwritten account by Joslin of his ancestry, but only in the Proctor family tree.

The Joslin ancestry in America began with Israel Joslin arriving in about 1718. He married Ruth Bayley and settled in Higham, Massachusetts. In 1725 they moved to Thompson, a small village in Connecticut.

Israel Joslin died in 1761, but his son, also called Israel, born on 30 September 1719, remained in Thompson. He had married a Sarah Brown. Their fourth child, Edward (1746–1822), married Elizabeth Alton. Edward Joslin is remembered for being a sergeant in the Revolutionary War.

Edward Joslin's son Jesse 1782–1848), married Sybil Bates.

Their son Elliot Joslin, (1807–1876), married Almira Davis (1811–1890).

Elliott Joslin and his wife Almira had four sons: Orrin Franklin, born 14 December,1831,AllenLafayette,30August,1833,Abner,29November,18 37, Howard, 1852, and a daughter Erma.

Thus five generations of the Joslin family had lived in Thompson, Connecticut before Orrin and Allen moved to Oxford. Both of them settled in Oxford, married local women and raised their families there.

Elliott and Almira Joslin's second son, Allen Lafayette Joslin, married twice.

From his second marriage to Sarah Ann Emerson Proctor he had one surviving child, a son whom they called Elliott Proctor Joslin.

Allen Lafayette Joslin (1833–1911)

The depressed economic conditions in Thompson, Connecticut led to the eldest two sons of the Joslin family leaving for Oxford in 1848 in order to find work. The 15-year-old Allen was noticed by a shoemaker called Loriston Shumway (1806–1884). In addition to owning a shoemaking business in town, Shumway had a shoemaking workshop at home. Allen Joslin was young, enthusiastic and hard-working. He picked up the basics of shoemaking quickly. He was popular with the Shumways and their children. It was a large family, for they had seven children including a vivacious 11-year-old daughter, Lucretia.

In 1857, the 24-year-old Allen Joslin had married the 20-year-old Lucretia Miller Shumway. They had two children: a daughter, Ada Louella, born in 1858 and a son, Homer Shumway, in 1862.

Loriston Shumway (1806–1884)

The Shumways were among the earliest settlers of Oxford. In the genealogy section of Daniels' book on the history of the town, the Shumway family features more prominently than most.

The family originated in France. The first, Peter Shumway, arrived in 1678. The name Shumway is probably derived from Chamois or Charmois. Their American name is one instance of the alteration of the French to the American spelling and pronunciation, being documented in Daniels' *History of Oxford*. A letter written by William H Shumway

Esq. who was a lawyer at Syracuse, New York in May 1871, is quoted as saying:

"I understand from an attaché of Joseph Bonaparte that our name Shumway is a corruption of Chamois, a person bearing it was Compte De Chamois, a member of the court of Louis XIV." Another account spoke of probably the same attaché commenting that the Americans could not pronounce the French name correctly and Shumway was simply a distortion of the French version.

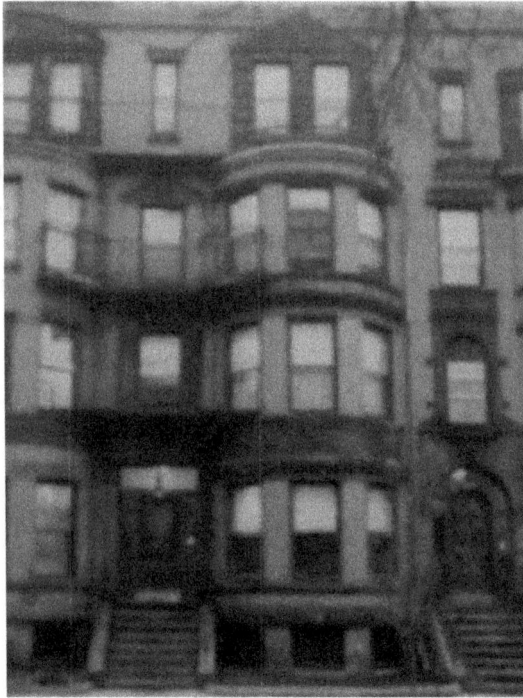

517 Beacon Street

Allen Lafayette Joslin's father-in-law, Loriston Shumway, was born in Oxford in 1806. He started as a farmer, but at home in the evenings also made shoes. The family, well known in Oxford, was part of the community in all its activities. At various times over the years Loriston Shumway was in business with other shoemakers in town, usually in partnership. He was able to introduce his son-in-law to the different processes involved in acquiring, then treating and preparing animal skins for the purpose of making various articles including shoes and boots. Shumway, being an accomplished cordwainer, may well have been the early influence which resulted in Allen Joslin's eventually branching out into manufacturing shoes.

After the death of Allen Joslin's wife, the large Shumway family – Loriston had eleven siblings and he himself had seven children– remained close to the young widower. The relationship continued even after his second marriage, because of the close-knit community of Oxford.

Although not directly related to the Shumways, Joslin was nevertheless deeply influenced by Ada, Allen Joslin's daughter from his first marriage. Letters between the two from his childhood through to his time at Yale attest to the love and affection which existed between them in spite of the age difference of 11 years. Ada moved with her mother to their city house at 517 Beacon Street in 1888 when Joslin was still at Yale in the class of 1890. However she was able to keep closely in touch with him during his years in medical school at Harvard University and beyond. During the early years of medical practice and then after his marriage when he was building his home/office, Ada remained close to her youngest brother. She never married, and only moved back to Oxford after her stepmother died in 1913.

The Proctor Influence

"The Proctors, they say, will have their way."

The Proctors were undoubtedly the most influential ancestors of Joslin. They make their appearance in the Joslin story some four years after the death of Allen Joslin's first wife, Lucretia, in 1863.

The Proctor family were joined with the Joslins through Allen Joslin's second marriage to Sarah Ann Emerson Proctor in 1867.

A typewritten account of Mrs. Sarah Proctor Joslin (12 January,1839 – 14 June,1913) can be found in the Joslin archives. The opening few sentences are informative.

"Miss Sarah A. E. Proctor was born in South Danvers, the name of which was changed to that of Peabody after she had married and removed from town. She was the daughter of Abel and Lydia (Emerson)) Proctor, and the seventh generation in the direct line of John Proctor, a victim of the Salem in witchcraft delusion.

From a child she showed the qualities which marked her mature years; energy and enthusiasm in her occupations, tenacity of purpose, independence of mind and executive ability to a degree rare in early life."

I have included this material for several reasons. Most importantly, it shows that many of the qualities for which Joslin was known were present in both his parents. To borrow a term from the veterinary lexicon, Joslin had a good pedigree. It is also noticeable that the writer of this piece on Sarah Proctor, possibly herself, had her own description for the trial of her seventh generation ancestor! More on this shortly.

Joslin was the only surviving son of this marriage. That the relationship between mother and son was undoubtedly profound is made clear repeatedly in Joslin's writings. However, there were other members of the Proctor family who were also an important part of the young man's life.

Clearly proud of his connection with this family, Joslin never shied away from its more colourful past as will be seen later in this narrative.

Abel Waters Proctor (1800-1879)

Two Proctor men in particular played significant roles in the Joslin story.

The first was Abel Waters Proctor, a wealthy leather merchant who owned some of the biggest tanneries in New England. He was Joslin's maternal grandfather.

The second was Joslin's uncle Thomas Emerson Proctor Senior.

Unlike the Joslins, the Proctors could trace their family history from the time of their arrival in New England from London in 1635. The first Proctor, John, was born in Yorkshire, England about 1595. He travelled with his wife Martha, aged 28, and two children, John aged 3 and Mary aged 1.

Also differing from the Joslin story, the Proctor saga becomes colourful almost straight away.

The Hanging

The early history of the Proctor family is dominated by one event, the hanging of John Proctor (1632–1692), the first son of the first John Proctor, during the Salem Witch Trials of 1692. Although the trials were discredited and discontinued with at least partial restitution of the assets to the relatives of those already put to death, the Proctors never forgot or forgave the injustice. Successive generations of the Proctors kept the memory alive. Even 250 years later Elliott Proctor Joslin referred to it in conversation, lectures and in his writings! Some might argue that he wasn't even a full Proctor. Or was the story told to a young Joslin as he sat on his mother's knee or on grandfather Abel's?

In addition to being hard-working and successful, the Proctors were known to be assertive and, if push came to shove, uncompromising.

The Rev. Nichols, one of the ministers of the church they attended, is credited with coining a phrase to describe the Proctor family or, perhaps more accurately, the Proctor men!

"The Proctors, they say,

Will have their way."

According to A Carlton Proctor who traced the Proctor genealogy from 1546 to 1982, from which I have this information, John Proctor appears to have been a colourful personality:

"John Proctor, son of the first John Proctor, was a man of large frame, with great native force and energy, was bold and fearless in language, impulsive in feeling, and sometimes rash and hasty in action. He was married three times and was the father of 17 children."

In spite of the universal view of the trials being an aberration limited to that period, the Proctors appear to have maintained the rage through several generations. Thus John Waters Proctor, during the centennial celebrations of the neighbouring town of Danvers in June 1852, more than 150 years after the event, devoted a large part of his welcoming address for the celebrations to the trial of his ancestor whom he defended vehemently, condemning his conviction by analysing,in forensic detail, not only the conduct of the court proceedings but also the character of the witnesses who had testified against the offending Proctor! As I said, 150 years after the event.

John Waters Proctor, a Harvard Law graduate, had practised as a lawyer in Danvers for many years. His connection to Joslin is through his younger brother Abel Waters Proctor, Joslin's maternal grandfather. That branch of the Proctor family had five children, three daughters bookended by two boys, John Waters, the eldest, and Abel Waters, the youngest of the five.

Abel Waters Proctor (1800–1879), had married Lydia Porter Emerson (1808–1883). They had six daughters and two sons. Their second daughter, Sarah Ann Emerson, was the second wife of Joslin's father.

Their son Thomas Emerson Proctor Senior (1834–1894) took over the leather business established by Abel Proctor at a young age. Abel Proctor suffered from ill health, as a consequence of which the education of his son Thomas was interrupted before college. Thomas Proctor went on to head one of the leading leather companies in New England. It is of interest to record some of his qualities because of the influence he had on Joslin during the latter's formative years.

Thomas Emerson Proctor Senior 1834–1894

At school Thomas Proctor was known for his scholarship, being particularly proficient in Latin and Greek as well as mathematics. He continued to study even after taking over the family business when he was no longer at school. In his early 20s, Thomas Proctor was elected president of the Leather Industry Cooperative in Peabody. Later he was elected to the leadership of the leather industries throughout New

England.

Thomas Proctor was a quiet achiever. He had a cool head in a crisis. One story about him records his reaction to the news that his leather factory was on fire. Instead of rushing out to the scene of the conflagration, Thomas Proctor instead went into the office to check that his fire insurance papers were in order!

He was offered the position of mayor of Boston on more than one occasion but preferred to restrict his activities and services to commerce.

Towards the end of his life he made what for that time was a significant donation of $100,000 (over $2 million in today's value) to the Massachusetts General Hospital (MGH) to be devoted to the care of the insane. At that time, Thomas Emerson's nephew Elliott Proctor Joslin was in the final years of his medical course at Harvard Medical School. He was to take up his internship at MGH few years later starting in the fall of 1897.

Thomas Emerson Proctor Sr. and his wife, Emma Esther (Howe), had lived at 327 Beacon Street, Boston, and it was no coincidence that Sarah Proctor Joslin had persuaded her husband to buy their city abode at 517 Beacon Street. This was in 1888 while Joslin was still at Yale. However, throughout his years at medical school from the fall (September) of 1891 to 1895, his mother encouraged frequent contact with his uncle who lived only a few doors away.

When awarded the Dalton Fellowship (for research while still an intern), Joslin in his letter of acceptance included the remark that the award will "have pleased [his] uncle, the late Thomas E. Proctor." The importance of contacts, integral to effective networking, was well and truly embedded in the young graduate's psyche from the very beginning of his career!

Ellen Osborne Proctor (1848-1902)

Another of his mother's sisters, Ellen Osborn Proctor (1848–1902), is seen to have been associated with Joslin in his early professional life.

Well travelled with several trips to Europe, particularly Germany, she was sufficiently proficient in German to translate some of the scientific papers from the European medical journals for her nephew.

She was unmarried and used her legacy for charitable purposes, including a research fund at Harvard Medical School for investigation of chronic disease. It is possible that Joslin was instrumental in persuading his aunt to do this. A grant from this fund was, in later years, awarded to Francis Madison Allen for his work on experimental diabetes in animals and prior to the publication of his opus magnum, *Diabetes and Glycosuria*. A further connection this aunt had with Joslin was that in later years she developed diabetes, said to be the cause of her death in 1902 at the age of 53 years. Some have suggested that this was the reason for Joslin specialising in the treatment of diabetes, but I could find no evidence for this in any of Joslin's writings or other sources in the archives.

Thus, at least two of the Proctor sisters had diabetes. It is known that Joslin's mother, who developed the condition in 1899, was obese. She lost 15 pounds using the diet initially suggested by Naunyn and supervised by her son. There are no details available on Ellen Proctor's diabetes. Their father Abel's condition was known to be in the category of what in today's terminology would be "morbid obesity." However he was not a diabetic.

Through another Proctor aunt, Mehitabel, Joslin had come to know James Phinney Baxter, Mehitabel's second husband.

In the last four editions of his manual for patients, starting with the seventh published in 1941, Joslin used an epigram which was the English translation by Baxter of a Persian poem.

"One who learns and learns,
Yet does not, what he knows
Is one who plows and plows,
Yet never sows."

I could not find any evidence of any contact between Joslin and Baxter other than the epigram. This may be because Baxter was an ardent supporter of the antivivisection movement whereas Joslin, aware of the benefits of animal experiments which had led to the discovery of insulin, was strongly in favour.

Clearly proud of his connection with this family, Joslin never shied away from its more colourful past and, like many other members of his mother's family, took a leaf out of the Proctor family handbook, to keep the memory of John Proctor, "of the 1692 notoriety" alive. (The label had been coined by John Waters Proctor and used in his Denver Centennial Celebrations address.)

Joslin recounted the story in several of his manuals and "dined out" on it in his lectures.

On one occasion, lecturing to an admiring audience in Britain, the tactful (or perhaps not so tactful!), Joslin thanked the English audience for sparing his ancestor!

He stopped short of mentioning that one of the presiding judges, Samuel Sewall, was English. Nor did he point out that the same Sewall was also part of the panel of judges who had convicted John Proctor and sent him to the gallows. Proctor's wife, the saved ancestor Joslin mentioned, only had her hanging postponed because of pregnancy but was later spared without any reason being given.

Neither did Joslin mention that Sewall had come to regret his decision to give credence to the accusations and had publicly confessed his regret, demonstrating his repentance by fasting and prayer one day each year to the end of his life. It is interesting that the yearly public "confession" by the judge was made in church during a Sunday service in the presence of the congregation. It was the same church where Joslin worshipped for most of his life – the South Church in Copley Square in the city of Boston.

Known for his mastery of the finer points of the polished delivery, the orator in Joslin was not going to weaken his message or his "punch line" by providing too much detail!! The valedictorian of the Harvard Class of 1895 never lost his touch.

Nor did he leave his polished delivery at the lectern, displaying equal facility when pontificating during informal discussions with visiting professional colleagues from around the English-speaking world, or at the family dinner table! (Except that at the dinner table, according to one of his grandchildren, they were not allowed to speak!).

History shows that his English cousins were captivated by the multitalented Bostonian. After all, the term Boston Brahmin was coined by none other than the popular Dr Oliver Wendell Holmes, a leading light in Boston medical circles when Joslin was a medical student at Harvard. And Joslin, according to Barnett, fitted that description to a T.

Thus, it is clear that the college student who was to become a doctor was influenced during his early years by several successful men, all of whom happened to be successful merchants: his father, two maternal uncles, as well as his maternal grandfather. Also, almost without exception, these men were leaders, respected by colleagues and the community.

As will be seen in this account, Joslin repeatedly demonstrated habits and practices of a merchant. Also socially adroit, he was comfortable in the company of industrialists, bankers and holders of high office in the commercial world, just as he was at ease in the medical establishment of clinicians, academics, medical researchers and–conspicuously ahead of his time–allied health professionals. His friendship with the Governor of Massachusetts facilitated many dealings he had with the bureaucracy of the city and state.

The Joslins in the Oxford Community

Much can be learned about the citizens of Oxford and their interest in the parts of its history they considered worthy of preservation and commemoration. The programs published in 1913 and 1963 for the 200 and 250th anniversary celebrations provided me with a wealth of material from this point of view. They carried photographs of buildings named after its distinguished citizens, monuments marking historic events, institutions valued for their contribution to the everyday life of Oxford's citizens, as well as a succinct exposition of its history and development.

The programs also contained details of the roles played by the Joslin family especially for the bicentennial event.

The Joslins were prominent in Oxford during the 200–year anniversary celebrations when three generations of the family took part. Joslin's mother, "Mrs A.L. Joslin", was in the reception committee, while his older brother, Homer, prominent as a senior merchant in the family shoe store "A. L. Joslin & Co.", was very active in community affairs. Homer's son Philip acted as an usher.

Ada Joslin wrote an impressive narrative poem for the town pageant. A verse from this poem was used as the epigram at the beginning of Joslin's memoir by Anna C Holt in 1969:

> "A green plain lying among the hills,
> Each one a watch tower high,
> Broad meadows, brooks and forests old,
> Where gentle streams flow by. "

Ada Joslin also wrote an essay on the vegetation of Oxford and its surroundings. Joslin himself did not attend the celebrations, which is not surprising given that he had, as usual, several irons in the fire, including his collaboration with Francis Gano Benedict in research projects on his diabetic patients. He frequently worked seven days a week and, except for attending church, did not let anything come between him and his medical commitments.

That Oxford holds Joslin in high regard is seen on the signage of several public buildings declaring, "Oxford, the home of Dr Elliot Joslin." He is remembered for his pioneering treatment of diabetes.

Equally highly regarded is Clara Barton, founder of the American Red Cross. She is also part of the Joslin history, as the first camp for diabetic girls was established on a property owned by her family. The Clara Barton Camp for diabetic girls runs every summer. It was Joslin's idea to establish a summer camp for diabetic girls, and he personally undertook to supervise their diabetic management which required adjustment of the dietary requirements as well as insulin dosage, depending on the girls' outdoor activities.

The summer camp for the young people also had another important reason, which was to allow the parents, especially the mothers of diabetic children, a break from their busy daily routine of looking after their children.

Later, Joslin handed over the job of the Director of the camp to Priscilla White. Following Joslin's example was always a challenge for all of his associates. White confided to some of her colleagues of being exhausted with the addition of the duties of the camp to her usual task of looking after the office practice in Boston. She said that she often sang to herself on the way back from Oxford so she would not fall asleep at the wheel of her car!. The camp is still run by the medical staff of the Joslin Diabetes Centre.

(I had the pleasure of being the physician of the camp in the summer of 1970. Apart from the joy of being associated with a wonderful group of girls, my wife and our two daughters were relieved to be away from the crowded inner city area of Boston for six weeks. An added bonus was the close association I had with Dr Priscilla White. Sitting with her and learning the finer points of treating diabetes in girls whose ages ranged from 10 to 16 was an invaluable experience. Dr White never forgot even the most minor details (which I often did,) of each patient, including blood sugar levels of any patient from weeks earlier!)

An interesting aspect of earlier commercial/industrial developments in Oxford in the mid-1800s, was the prominence of family-owned enterprises. Frequently, several members of one family would be involved. One such business started and controlled by the head of the family lasted for 40 to 50 years, even longer if continued by the eldest son as was the custom in the Puritan families. The program for Oxford's 250 year celebrations mentioned several such businesses.

The A. L. Joslin Shoe Store was started by Joslin's father in 1870. Allen Joslin's elder brother Orrin was associated with him from the beginning. Both remained active merchants to the end of their lives even though in later years Joslin's older brother, Homer, had joined and then taken over the leadership. The eldest son in a family joining his father's business was common practice in the New England Puritan families at that time. This Joslin enterprise ran successfully for over 40 years.

Allen Lafayette Joslin: a Quiet Achiever

Even though he was only 15 years old when he first arrived in Oxford from Thomson, Allen Lafayette Joslin quickly became fully involved in nearly every aspect of community life in Oxford; he was active in church affairs as well as projects in town, especially those related to the leather industry. No one was surprised, therefore, when in 1860 one of the leading shoe manufacturers of that period, LB Corbin, invited him to join the firm. His progress was rapid and within a few years he was made a partner in the firm of L B Corbin and Co. During this period he learned the finer points of shoe manufacturing on a larger scale as opposed to shoe making which he had learned from Shumway.

Although lacking the pedigree of the Proctors, Allen Joslin, still in his early 30s, was a rising star in the commercial sphere of Oxford and surrounding towns, most of which during this period had flourishing leather industries.

In 1870, together with his older brother Orrin, he decided to establish his own business. He selected a site adjoining the railroad just across from the passenger station. A building of three storeys together with the basement bearing the name A.L. Joslin Company was built within 12 months. Its location was ideal for receiving materials brought by the railway as well as dispatching the finished goods.

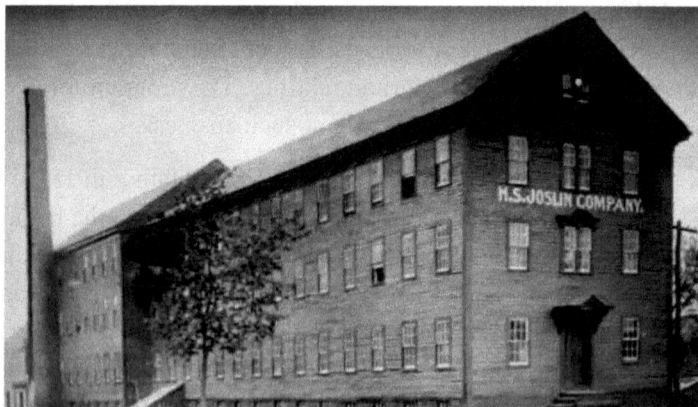

The Shoe Factory

Through the kindness of Mr Richard Croall (of Sydney, Australia) who, following in his father's footsteps, has spent a lifetime in the leather industry, particularly in shoe manufacture, I have learnt that the Joslin factory was typical of the buildings constructed for that purpose during that period. The basement was for receiving raw materials (animal hides), the first and second floors were devoted to the preparation of the large pieces of leather. This required heavy machinery for cutting the large pieces into specific sizes for the different sized shoes, slippers and boots.

There were different leather- cutting knives for different shoe sizes. The presses for knives required hydraulic power. It was very heavy work which could only be done by strong men. Thus the basement and the lower floors were largely occupied by male workers.

The finer work of finishing the process, like stitching and "clicking", provided employment for women and, at times, children as well. Thus the leather industry, in many of the towns during this period, involved entire families, a situation which may be difficult for today's citizens of Oxford (or, for that matter, any town,) to envisage.

A Family Tragedy

Unfortunately, just as it seemed that there was no stopping him, Allen Lafayette Joslin's stars were halted in their upward trajectory by an entirely unforeseen family tragedy.

On the morning of 8January 1863, the young merchant awoke to find the lifeless body of his young wife beside him. She had had a fever for the previous two days but had seemed better when retiring the night before. She had complained of a sore throat for a few days but had been too modest to mention the dark red rash on her chest and abdomen. Her face was flushed but clear.

She had scarlet fever.

Now known to be caused by a common bacterial agent called *streptococcus* which, in most cases, is eliminated with one course of antibiotics, scarlet fever has virtually disappeared from most developed countries. In the 1800s however, it was frequently fatal as it turned out to be in this instance.

Lucretia Miller Shumway Joslin was laid to rest in North Cemetery, Oxford. She was 26 years old.

The distraught father was left with a five-year-old daughter and a two-month-old baby boy.

The close-knit community rallied around the young man – the Shumways were one of the oldest families of Oxford. Allen Joslin employed a housemaid to look after the two young children and returned to work. The improvement in economic conditions in general and his business in particular meant that, unlike in previous times, remarrying for the sake of providing a carer for the children was no longer an issue for men in his position.

Allen Joslin's contribution to the Oxford community lay in the leadership he provided in virtually every aspect of the town's life.

In 1871 he was chairman of the Building Committee for the first Congregational parsonage built by an incorporated association. Members of the committee assisting him included George Daniels, the writer of the book on the history of Oxford.

In 1881, he became president of the Oxford National Bank which was originally incorporated as Oxford Bank in 1823.

From 1882 to 1883 he was a state senator and member of the Governor's Council.

From 1882 to 1890 Allen Joslin held the position of Town Treasurer of Oxford.

In 1885 he was elected Representative in Congress.

In 1889 he was elected president of the Agricultural Society responsible for organising the Oxford Fair.

In 1881 Allen Joslin's elder son, Homer, then aged 19, joined his business as a junior partner. He had grown up with the business and was "eminently well fitted to be a voice in the affairs of management". Homer went on to be the Assistant Treasurer and Clerk (to his uncle Orrin) and became a director when Orrin Joslin died in 1908.

After the death of Allen Joslin in July 1911 Homer took his father's place immediately, although he had practically exclusive control of all departments for some time prior to his father's death.

Allen Joslin's business acumen can be seen in the description of the Joslin enterprise by another leather merchant in 1913, as follows:

"When Allen Joslin began in a small way as a manufacturer he specialised in the production of pegged shoes for women, misses and children. He continued in this line for 23 years, building a reputation and establishing a standard of quality that has never been lowered.

With changing times and styles, the company developed, and the early 80s saw its original line increased by the addition of shoes with standard fastenings and the McKay sewed shoes, both new types being made in both women's and men's sizes.

In 1908 the Corporation commenced to give attention to the manufacture of Goodyear welt shoes for men. How well this standard type of 20th century footwear was received with the Joslin stamp of quality upon it is evident today – the corporation is practically specialising in this work, manufacturing under its own trademark and, for dealers in various parts of this country, lines of shoes for men retailing from $3.50 to $5, and special shoes at higher prices, that have an enviable reputation in the shoe trade."

Father and Son

Joslin's father remains very much in the background in his son's story. Yet casual comments by Joslin himself and Holt's account both show him to have been a significant influence in his younger son's life. He impressed on Joslin, even as a child, the importance of hard work and thrift. There is an oft-repeated story of the boy at the age of seven or eight years being taken to his father's shoe factory and being given the task of lacing 60 pairs of shoes and being paid only a few cents, which had to be deposited in a savings account at the local bank! Holt records that Joslin kept this account at the Webster's Bank in Oxford to the end of his life. So the lessons taught by his father were not forgotten. On the other hand, Allen Joslin was generous with his son, who on one occasion asked what he was to do with "the surplus".

The father remained a part of his son's life even in his senior years. Although frail, Allen Joslin came to Buffalo Hill to help with land clearing shortly before his death in 1911. It was he who suggested hiring a landscape architect when the young couple had found the job of clearing the newly acquired plot to be beyond their capabilities.

What Allen Lafayette Joslin demonstrated through his efforts in his own area of commercial expertise was the value of hard work and clean living, principles preached and practised by the puritanical New Englanders. Joslin's life showed that his father's example, teaching, and expectations were followed by his son to the letter throughout his life.

Part 2.
Youngest in the Family

An Adventurous Child

At the time of Joslin's birth, on June 6, 1869, the Joslin household consisted of his parents, an older sister Ada Luella 11, and a brother, Homer Shumway, 7. Ada and Homer were children of Joslin's father's first marriage. Joslin was the first son of Sarah Proctor Joslin, Allen Lafayette Joslin's second wife and, as it would turn out, Sarah Joslin's only child. There was a younger brother Abel, born in 1872, who died the following year. There is no mention of him other than in his mother's handwritten account of the family history, recording his birth on 7 October 1875, in Oxford, his death on 15 August 1876, and burial on 17 August of that year, and also a note which records that "Abel Proctor Joslin was baptised by Rev. Thomas E. Ball in the church at Oxford July 16, 1876".

The family had lived in the house built on Main Street by Allen Joslin in 1866. The household chores were done by a Swedish woman called Annette. Just how much hands-on mothering was done by Sarah is unclear. However, she was conscientious when it came to the children's attendance at Sunday School and church as well as school. The new addition to the family was a particular favourite of his older sister Ada who called him Small Fry, a name which persisted even when he was at college. That Joslin was a lively little boy is shown in an incident described by Holt. On the occasion of a birthday dinner some 50 years later Annette recounted the story of the redcurrant jelly, one of young Elliot's favourites. Wanting to surprise him, she called out telling him of the treat. What she had not realised was that he was two floors up. The excited little boy came hurtling down the stairs and stumbled just before he got to the jelly sitting on a low bench in the kitchen, and fell headfirst into the bowl. She got him cleaned up and cheered him up with a small cup of jelly even though he was not supposed to have dessert till after his main course.

Another incident, recalled and recounted at the same birthday dinner, was when the adventurous little boy went exploring in the woods in winter and fell into an icy pond. On this occasion Major, a big black dog who was a constant and devoted companion, sensed danger and jumped into the pond to drag his young master ashore. Again, it was Annette who, terrified on discovering the frightened little boy shivering and blue-lipped, hustled him into a warm bath. "I didn't tell Mrs Joslin everything," she said, with a twinkle in her eye.

There were frequent visits to the sprawling Proctor family mansion in Peabody. Sunday dinners with the extended family were a ritual. After dinner, Abel Proctor the grandfather, and Joslin's father Allen Lafayette Joslin, would retire to the drawing room and discuss business and community affairs.

Abel Proctor, then in his late 60s, was less active in business, having handed the reins to his son Thomas Emerson Proctor Senior some years earlier on account of his failing health. His son-in-law, on the other hand, had been a partner in the firm of Lament B Corbin for nearly 10 years. It is also entirely possible that the two men discussed the opportunities for Allen Joslin to start his own business. It is a matter of record that this in fact did happe, with the formation of the shoe manufacturing firm of A.L. Joslin and Company in 1870-71.

Participation and involvement in community affairs was part of life for all able-bodied men in those times. Building construction was with timber, and fire was a constant hazard. Maintaining a firefighting unit was essential, and every town had its team of volunteers. In addition, there were committees for improvement in farming conditions, and those with leadership qualities (already evident in Allen Joslin) were part of such groups.

Lydia Porter Emerson Proctor, Abel's wife, was proud of her son-in-law's reputation as a dynamic businessman in Oxford. She was a doting grandmother to all his children, but especially baby Elliott, her daughter Sarah's only offspring. He was, after all, the first Proctor born into the Joslin lineage. If both, the mother and her daughter, harboured secret hopes that the young man would carry the name Proctor together with the family name with distinction, they never said so openly. History shows that Joslin fulfilled this hope in ways neither his mother nor his grandmother could possibly have imagined.

Joslin was baptised in the church at Peabody by the Reverend Anthony at the age of six months. Religious instruction and practices were part of his upbringing from a young age. His Sunday School teacher, a young woman called Miss Ella Paine was an early influence. Amongst Joslin's memorabilia, Holt came across a carefully preserved birthday card with a picture of a spray of pink roses and red flowers. The young woman had written birthday greetings in red ink. A boyish scrawl records the gift: "Given me by my Sunday School teacher Miss Ella Paine, June 6, 1879," a treasured 10th birthday present which Joslin preserved for 80 years, showing it to Holt on his 90th birthday. Ella Paine was the daughter of the local doctor, Samuel Paine, a much admired figure by the entire community including, perhaps especially, the children, as recorded by Joslin in a school exercise when he was 14. He wrote:

"I live in a quiet little country town in New England where everybody knows everybody else and where the life of the majority of the people remains unchanged from year to year. As is usual in such a place the community is divided into many religious beliefs and consequently none of them flourish to any great extent but on one matter they all agree and that is this – love and reverence for the village doctor."

Joslin further described the doctor in a composition written during his time in Leicester Academy.

"He is an old man past 80 but still shows only in slight degree the traces of his active profession. It has been an active one for in a country town the people live so far apart it consumes much of his time in reaching them and when he is by himself he must improve every minute. He came to Oxford when a young man fresh from Yale medical school to study with an older doctor whose place he gradually filled. He has lived in the same house and driven the same chaise for so long that his house is a landmark from which all other houses get their position and his chase is known for miles around. One morning three weeks ago as I was walking to my boat I saw the familiar old horse coming towards me with its customary slow trot and with him, packed in every part of the carriage, four or five school children. All were laughing and the old man was the merriest of the party. Every day in the week you may see him doing something of this nature which shows another side of his character, namely, his love for all."

The essay is impressive not only for his composition but also for his maturity and powers of observation verging on the precocious. Not many 14-year-olds would have opinions on the different denominations of the Protestant faith, nor offer comments on the importance of keeping up with medical advances or the details of starting in medical practice. (Perhaps the essayist may be forgiven for overestimating the doctor's age. The elderly often encounter that failing in people younger than themselves! Paine was 76 at that time).

Holt speculates that Paine's immaculate appearance may have been a reason for Joslin's lifelong habit of paying careful attention to being well-dressed. According to Holt, Joslin," whether in his office or on the farm, had the happy faculty of never getting himself mussed up. He was one of those fortunate people to whom dirt did not adhere!" One doubts, however, that the village doctor's neatness of attire would have, at least in later years, matched that of Joslin who is said to have worn signature Brooks Brothers tweed suits with a vest, a watchcase and a chain, and high button shoes which required special laces. Barnett described him as being endowed with the manners and dress of a "Boston Brahmin".

As a child Joslin spent a good deal of time with his uncle Orrin. Although the eldest in his family–he was two years older than Allen– Orrin was less outgoing than his younger brother who devoted virtually the entire working day to business and community affairs. Orrin was good with figures and helped Allen with company accounts even though the latter had added the title of Treasurer to Head of the Company, A.L.Joslin & Co., with Orrin as the junior partner when it was incorporated in 1903. Orrin Joslin remained an integral part of the company until his death in 1908. He had also helped Allen's older son Homer when he had joined the firm in 1881 as a junior partner at the age of 19. Homer had gone to Philip Academy, and had been active in community and business activities in Oxford for many years prior to joining the family business.

The area around the town of Oxford was dotted with creeks and ponds. Webster Pond was a particularly popular haunt as it was known for its abundant variety of fish, perch and striped bass being the local favourites. Orrin frequently took young Elliott there. He would hire a boat and row into the small inlets he knew well. Watched by his enthusiastic nephew,

Orrin would build a fire, clean the fish and cook them "Indian style" on sticks. Whether the fishermen felt less confident of their success or Annette refused to believe tall tales, they always set off on their fishing expeditions with a lunch packed in the Joslin kitchen! Claiming the combination of the packed lunch with their fresh fish, the ever enthusiastic boy would recount to Ada how they had "feasted blissfully". On one he declared, "we brought home, bass and 49 other fish and felt very tired when we reached home." The age at which this accomplishment was claimed is not recorded! Was this an early indicator of the young man's narrative capabilities…?!"

Uncle Orrin also introduced young Elliot to sailing. He presented the 10-year-old with a small boat which the new owner proudly christened *Sea Foam*. Then, contrary to the suggestion by his uncle that he would benefit from some lessons first, he launched the vessel immediately! Furthermore, unable to control his exuberance, he also ignored the advice to be shown the basics of sailing. Instead, he had his new acquisition transported to a nearby pond called Mary De Witts to be launched immediately. Much can be learned from the logbook kept by the young owner.

"Logbook of the Sea Foam, schooner yacht.

Sea Foam Built 1879. Owned by Elliott P. Joslin.

Sea Foam was launched on a pond named Mary De Witts pond on a cold morning when a little ice was on the pond. She sailed very poorly but that was because the owner didn't know how to sail her. It was a very strong breeze.

Second Voyage. She was tried again but sailed no better. The owner was disgusted with her.

Third Voyage. She was tried again but did no better than the first two times but there was a boy who owned the yacht "Skylark" which sailed very fast. He told me to let down the fore and main sails and he said that he would hitch his little sloop on so that it could drag the Sea Foam ashore (as) it wouldn't sail. So we pushed off and what was my delight to see the Sea Foam pull around the little sloop and drag it through the water by its hind end [surely an original term to use for a boat part] at a very fast speed. Well after that the *Sea Foam* grew in my favour... "

Joining four other boys who also had boats, Joslin sailed Sea Foam with them in the deeper ponds-the shallower ones usually dried out in the summer. They decided to form a club and organise races. The annual membership fee was one cent per member. The accumulated funds, providing there was a surplus, were to be put towards the prize for the winner. The first race winner was not rewarded as the Exchequer was empty. Much to his delight, Joslin and *Sea Foam* won the next race even though according to the skipper he had to contend with "very rough weather". The prize awarded to him was a fish line.

Showing remarkable aptitude for recordkeeping by a 10-year old, Joslin had kept this piece of his early history and sporting triumph, neatly written in pencil and, according to Holt, without ever being corrected by an older person.

Orrin Joslin's main influence on his young nephew, however, was through his life-long devotion to his Protestant faith. He attended church regularly and was an active member of its Building and Maintenance Committee. Known and respected for his meticulous record keeping and scrupulous supervision of all monies spent, Orrin Joslin, for much of his life, also served as the treasurer of the Oxford Congregational Church. The current Congregational Church records his donations towards the cost of its pipe organ in 1905, in memory of his wife. The organ is still in service.

As a child Joslin was often allowed to sit with Uncle Orrin during Sunday services, frequently having been outdoors with him the previous day.

Two Doctors and an Attack of Measles

Joslin mentions two doctors during his early years, both of whom left a lasting impression on him for entirely different reasons.

At the age of seven Joslin contracted measles. A feared malady, the community remembered the devastation of life caused by the 1713

59

measles epidemic in Boston. Passive immunisation to prevent the condition had not been developed even though protection afforded to the afflicted after exposure was recognised, and attempts to achieve some protection by exposure was well publicised by many including Cotton Mather, the renowned and respected cleric and scholar (although he was also remembered as an instigator of the prosecution of the witches in Salem in 1692.)

The only practical method of limiting the spread of the disease was isolation of the sufferer.

It was during his period of isolation in an upstairs room of the Joslin household that he recalled his first impressions of seeing a doctor. Described as a young moustachioed man with neatly parted brown hair and a steady gaze under a wide brow, a picture which suggested a vigorous, strong personality, Dr Adams of Webster was making his first visit to examine the son of one of the town's more prominent merchants. As was common practice, the doctor used a horse-drawn carriage to visit his patients.

The shiny, immaculately kept carriage carrying the impeccably dressed doctor was drawn by a "spanking pair of high stepping horses." Keenly observed by the watcher in the upstairs room, the young medical practitioner stepped nimbly from his impressive mode of transport.

He was courteously greeted at the door by the maid and escorted to the room where he examined the patient in the presence of his concerned and doting mother. The doctor looked inside the boy's ears, a common and troublesome area for the rash. "All clear in there," he said. The boy was intrigued when he saw the doctor looking inside his bag and even more fascinated to see a hollow wooden cylinder in his hand. Joslin was too young to know that he was undergoing an examination (*auscultation*) of his chest with a wooden stethoscope.

There were no tell-tale signs of pneumonia, another feared complication of the disease. The doctor asked the mother if she had noticed the child averting his gaze from lamplight at bedtime, or sunlight during the day. Photophobia was a clue to inflammation of the brain (*encephalitis*), another feared complication which is usually fatal, even today.

The seven-year-old, obedient, compliant and remarkably composed for one so young, spoke only when spoken to, his mother answering most of the doctor's questions.

Free of all these complaints, Joslin received a clean bill of health from Dr Adams and returned to school shortly afterwards.

Many years later Joslin said that his main interest in the doctor's visit had been to look at the horses arriving and leaving. He wrote that it was from the time of this illness that he decided to pursue medical studies, crediting the doctor's horses, rather than the physician, for his choice of career!

A memento treasured by him to the end of his days was a photograph of the doctor with a handwritten note by Joslin at the back of the photograph, "Dr. Adams of Webster took care of me when I had the measles about 1876, and at that time I definitely decided to study medicine. Possibly influenced by the horses he drove."

Holt recalled that "in later years, Dr Joslin enjoyed telling, always with a chuckle, about this wholly unscientific manner of choosing his dearly loved life's work."

(Whether or not the photograph had been found amongst Joslin's papers by Holt is not recorded but may be an explanation for her comment explaining the note by Joslin at the back of the photograph as being written "many years later".)

Joslin was not to know that his practice in the City of Boston at the beginning of the next century would only lend itself to visiting patients in horse-drawn carriages for the first few years before being replaced by more modern modes of transport.

A more lasting and stronger impression likely to have influenced Joslin came from his observations on the village doctor, Dr Samuel C Paine, as recorded earlier.

Dr Samuel C Paine (1807-1888)

"...highly esteemed by all classes."

GF Daniels

George F Daniels' *History of the town of Oxford Massachusetts* records that Samuel C Paine was born on 1 February 1807.He had graduated from Yale (Class of 1828) and apprenticed with a senior physician until 1831 when he came to Oxford. For 50 years he was the principal physician in Oxford. Active in community affairs, Paine was, at different times, President of the Oxford National Bank, a representative and a Selectman as well as a Superior Presiding Officer and Moderator in many town meetings. He was active in church affairs and known for his benevolence towards the disadvantaged.

Daniels' book also reveals two other activities which reveal the seriousness with which the young doctor regarded his association with the town and its people.

Since the leather industry was the leading employer of Oxford's working population, Paine went into partnership with Samuel Richards and A G Underwood in a shoe manufacturing business in 1849. The business was conducted in a building called the Arcade. Richards had previously been an agent, but little is known about Underwood and his background in the industry. However, the venture was ill-fated as in 1850, barely a year after its commencement, a fire completely destroyed the Arcade. Paine did not continue the commercial association.

More dramatic was Paine's role, albeit a minor one, in Oxford's contribution to the American Civil War. On 12 April 1861 Fort Sumpter, an island fortification in Charleston Harbour in South Carolina was attacked by the Confederate Army. This incident is generally regarded as the beginning of the Civil War, which was to see bitter fighting for the next five years.

Three days later, on 15 April, the newly inaugurated President, Abraham Lincoln, issued a call for 75 troops for three months. Four days later a public meeting of the citizens of Oxford was held in town, presided over by the Honourable Alexander De Witt. After spirited addresses, five prominent citizens were elected to form a committee "to effect immediately the organisation of a volunteer military company."

Headed by De Witt, the committee chose as its first member the much respected Dr Samuel Paine. Within 2 to 3 days 45 volunteers had been enrolled "to respond to the call of the country for men to defend her against rebellion..."

Daniels' description also includes comments which indicate that the doctor was highly regarded. He says that Paine was known for "a superior mental ability, very decided moral convictions, early an antislavery voter, very social in manner and influential in the community, highly esteemed by all classes".

Paine died following a stroke on 1 April 1888. His eldest daughter Elizabeth had married Charles E Daniels, related to the writer of the book on Oxford. Charles E Daniels had been in the shoe business, as was the historian George F Daniels. The former had a business association with Loriston Shumway (Allen Joslin's first employer and the father of his first wife). The sparse details of Paine's life in Oxford as recounted by Daniels, while providing biographical details and a list of his contributions to the civic life of the village, give little insight into what this man gave of himself to the day–to–day life of the men, women and children of Oxford.

Paine had known Joslin's father from the time of the latter's arrival in Oxford in 1848 at the age of 15. Paine, the only doctor, and a prominent member of the community for many years, knew most, if not all, the families in the district. He had known the family of Lauriston Shumway even before Allen Joslin's arrival. He had delivered the shoe merchant's older two children, Ada and Homer. He had attended to their mother Lucretia, Shumway's daughter. He had been at her bedside during her short final, fatal illness, distraught that he wasn't able to help.

Paine had attended Allen Joslin's second marriage. And he had delivered Elliott, Sarah Proctor's first child. Paine was well known to the Proctors, Peabody being a neighbouring town. He had also attended the birth of her second child, Abel. And he had had the burden of comforting both the parents when the child had succumbed to a short febrile illness in his first year.

Holt had a photograph of the popular Village Doctor. She describes him as "a fine looking man with a shock of white hair and a full beard. The face that looks out openly on the world gives the impression of a kindly, intelligent man, carefully groomed, capable and one to be trusted." Unfortunately it was not included in her book on Joslin.

Joslin had treasured Paine's photograph and on the back had written: "Dr. Samuel C. Paine, who took care of me when I was born in 1869".

So the village doctor, with an association going back over the years, had done much for the Joslins of Oxford – and the Proctors of Peabody. Neither family ever forgot that. The prominent shoe merchant of Oxford and the wealthy tanner of Peabody always paid their debts.

Both men engaged in acts of philanthropy throughout their lives as did their descendants including Joslin. A home for disadvantaged women established in Peabody by the Proctors remains in service to this day.

Joslin's Early Education

The Puritans, well known for their work ethic and religious practices, also emphasised the importance of education. As early as 1800 the American colonies, especially in Massachusetts, had passed a law that any town with more than 100 children had to establish a grammar school. These were usually a one-room school with a single teacher instructing students in grammar, reading and writing, and cipher (arithmetic). Joslin went to the local grammar school in Oxford, and in later years was fond of pointing out the building which was still standing when his memoir was written by Holt in 1969. However, the Joslin School featured in many photographs of Oxford in the early 1900s was not the school he attended. This Joslin School was a donation by Joslin to the town in memory of his father Allen Lafayette Joslin who had died in 1911. The school eventually fell into disrepair and was demolished in the mid-1900s.

There are few details of his early years of schooling but clearly he was able to grasp the basics of primary school education in order to proceed to the next step which was to be admitted to an academy.

Academies were the next rung of the academic ladder after primary school. Now, more often than not, such institutions are referred to as high schools, though some still prefer the older, more traditional term, even if the practice is considered by some as an affectation of elitism.

Phillips Academy, which Joslin's older brother Homer attended, would certainly fall into this category. Situated in Andover, Massachusetts, it still heads the list of the best private schools in the country. It was founded during the American Revolution in 1778 and is the oldest incorporated school in the United States. Highly selective with an acceptance rate (currently) of only 13%, its alumnus directory includes luminaries from the elite of American society including at least two Presidents of the United States, prominent politicians and Nobel laureates. Phillips Academy also had secret societies, the membership of which was only by invitation. Long regarded as another tradition of the elite educational establishments, the practice was, in the case of Phillips Academy, officially disbanded in 1949. However, it is believed that at least one such society still exists within its student body.

As recently as late 2018, the death of arguably its most distinguished alumnus, President George H. Bush (Class of 1942), was featured on the school's website when he died in early December 2018.

Usually, attendance at academies like Philips is regarded as a feeder for college education. However, this did not occur in the case of Homer Shumway Joslin, who after his time there joined his father's business, as was the custom for the first son of New England families at that time.

There is little information on a college education being discussed for young Joslin, regardless of the thoughts he may have harboured after seeing Dr Adams' impressive horses during his bout of measles!

And why not Phillips Academy for him too?

Perhaps it was the mission statement of the Leicester Academy which may have swayed Joslin's parents. It would certainly have found favour with the pious, church-going Sarah Proctor Joslin.

The Academy stated that "the purpose of Leicester Academy is to promote piety and virtue; and, for the education of youth in English, Latin and Greek and French languages, together with writing, arithmetic and the art of speaking." In addition, it also had impressive teachers, possibly another reason that students not only from the neighbouring areas of Massachusetts, but more distant states, sought to enrol there.

The town of Leicester also has an interesting history.

The Early History of Leicester

Incorporated in 1730, Leicester was named after Robert Dudley, the first Earl of Leicester.

Though the Academy at Leicester could not boast of a status matching Phillips Academy, the town is proud of its history. It played a significant role at the start of the American Revolution.

The term "minutemen," a term for militia members who fought the early battles in Lexington and Concord, derives from Leicester's Colonel William Henshaw insisting that "we must have companies of men ready to march upon a minute's notice."

An early settler in town was Dr Samuel Green. Since medical training at that time was largely through an apprenticeship with an older experienced practitioner, Green trained many doctors in this manner in the early 1700s. This formed the first "medical school" in Massachusetts.

Green's house at 2 Charlton Street in Greenville, now a part of Rochdale village in Leicester, was also chosen as one of the houses to hide ammunition and equipment from the British troops who were advancing towards Lexington and Concord to engage in the early battles of the American Revolution. Another colourful citizen was Peter Salem, a freed slave who ensured his place in local folklore after killing a British Major, John Pitcairn of the British Marines. The Leicester town fathers memorialised Salem in his adopted town's street name of Peter Salem Road.

Letters From Leicester Academy (1883 to 1886): Lessons For Life.

Details of Joslin's time at Leicester Academy, where he started in the fall of 1883 at the age of 14, are contained in the memoir by Holt. It is clear that at least some of the material to which she had access has either been lost or not given to the Joslin Diabetes Centre archives, as I was unable to find copies of several of the letters written to the young man by members of the family as well as his letters home. For this reason, and because of the concise and lucid commentary by Holt herself, some of the material found here is quoted from her book.

Leicester was 12 miles from Oxford. There being no direct transport between the villages of Oxford and Leicester, the 14-year-old boy had to ride his beloved pony Flossie from home to school on Monday mornings. The pony boarded at the house of the local minister and was fed and cared for by the youngster through the week before the journey home on Friday afternoon. Punctuality was emphasised in schools (from primary through to college) which meant that Joslin had to leave home no later than 5 am on Mondays to get to school which started at 9 am sharp. In some ways this responsibility may have been as useful as, if not more useful than the lessons in the classroom, for it brought home to him what he never forgot–that self-reliance and discipline are essential elements of a productive life. The 3 to 4 hours' horseback riding twice a week as well as caring for his pony was the beginning of his love of horses and riding which remained throughout his life.

The Academy curriculum included Latin (Virgil), French and Roman history. Academically, Joslin's strength was his ability to write essays, a good example of which can be seen in a letter he wrote at the end of his first term of 15 weeks.

Calling it "My Christmas Vacation", he wrote:

"School closed on Friday, December 14, for the holidays after a term of 15 weeks. During the first week of my vacation I went to the foreign exhibition in Boston. The exhibition is on Huntington Avenue about a mile from the city. One country whose exhibit interested me very much was Sweden. In the basement it had a number of figures representing peasant life. In one of these groups was a sleighing party drawn by reindeer. In another a young man was laying his heart and future happiness before the mother of a pretty young lady who stands by, an interested spectator. Upstairs this country had a fine collection of furs.

On Christmas Eve there was a gathering at the church, and ice cream and cake were given to the company. I enjoyed it exceedingly as I officiated at the ice cream cans with a gentleman friend."

Then he goes on to describe an incident which, even by today's standards, would appear precocious for a 14-year-old. It appears that he served "a very slender lady who came for her glass of ice cream. We filled her glass heaping full and thought we had disposed of her for the evening. But she came again and again and yet once again at the request of a friend ("just to keep company") and we made the last glass the largest of all. It is curious how much refreshment small and delicate people can bear."

Whether this comment on the amount of food being consumed by a given individual was the result of his observations or experience at the Academy or, more likely, the puritanical influence of moderation in all things as was emphasised–and practised–at home, remains speculative. That he was conscious of quantities was further emphasised when in the same composition he commented on "A young woman, when she received a visit from her young man, took only five beans on her plate, cut these in two, and said she was making more of a meal than usual. But after dinner, as the young man was walking around the yard, on passing the pantry window he discovered his lady love helping herself to beans with a relish and with a very big iron spoon."

Having covered his visit to Boston and the function at church, the composition finishes with details of a visit from a friend to the Joslin home at Christmas.

"We were expecting a friend to come and spend Christmas with us and had looked for him all the day before, on all the trains and had given him up. At six o'clock of Christmas night he made his appearance, saying that he had missed trains coming through, and had spent the day waiting in different depots. Some family friends were spending the day with us and after he had refreshed himself he entertained us all by singing Negro melodies which he had learned in his Southern home. The rest of the vacation passed swiftly and pleasantly and 2nd of January came all too soon".

Letters to the young man from home, especially from his sister Ada, were less formal and serious. And more concise!

Signing the note "Aunt Jane," which was Joslin's pet name for Ada, she wrote:

"Home, Wednesday noon.

Dear Small Fry:

The house is very still because the racket is all gone to Leicester. Hope the old town won't crumble at the sounds. How do lessons go after two weeks' vacation?"

Then follow small bits of family news of interest to a boy away at school. The note ends with this broad hint.

"Supposing you send us a postal.

With love from the family,

Aunt Jane."

An interesting and possibly significant weakness in Joslin's academic capabilities was discovered during his early months in Leicester. He was asked to draw a steam engine. Here, for the first time, Holt mentions "a boy without mechanical interest or particular manual ability."

Once again the kindly Anna Holt claims that "through a dogged determination and stern self-discipline a creditable result was achieved." However, the drawing which still exists, suggests that Joslin may not have been the sole artist. The now yellowed paper has been carefully preserved. Done in pencil on a small sheet with signs of Joslin's struggle to produce the drawing is a revealing note by Joslin himself. "I had to draw a steam engine and had a terrible time doing it. I believe this is the final one. Davis – my classmate helped me. E.P.J." (Holt used his initials instead of his name throughout her memoir).

Over the years Joslin was heard on more than one occasion to say "I have always used my hands badly." This admission by Joslin may be a clue to more than one puzzling, and at times unexplained, incident in later years.

At or away from home Joslin was always aware of the code of conduct expected of him by his parents. According to Holt "the young man was sociable and appears to have been popular at the Academy". When invited for a night out by one of his classmates he had written home to ask his parents' permission.

Here is a letter written by his mother in response to a request by the young man during his early years at Leicester Academy.

"Dear Elliott,

Your letter came tonight and your father and I have considered the matter. You know our opinion regarding such parties when guests must go by carriage, and although you suggest a double sleigh yet that necessitates selecting a particular lady and I'd rather you would not, especially as you have once before this term. If the party were to be given in town our objection would be taken away.

I never allowed Homer and Ada and do not think it best for you. You can excuse yourself to Miss Bartlett stating the reason your parents have not been accustomed to their children attending parties in that way, when at school and in term time, the late hours being an additional objection. Under other circumstances we should be happy to have you pass the evening at Mr Bartlett's. I want her, Miss Josie, to understand that if we ever broke over our rule, we should most certainly do so in the case of friends we esteem as highly as Mr Bartlett's people.

My missionary meeting was a success. Mrs Wellington has asked me to read Saturday night.

You loving mother,
Sarah P Joslin."

(Here, Anna Holt inserted her own comment noting that the final two

sentences would have been of little interest–or comfort–to the young man after the denial of his request!).

Joslin, dutifully, did not go to the party.

It would appear, however, that in spite of all the reasons given by Joslin's mother, the real sticking point was that he was going to be taking a girl. Thus, when another invitation came from a Mrs George W Olney, from Cherry Valley, dated 29 January, 1883 and addressed to Master Elliott Joslin, Leicester, Mass. inviting him to spend the night at Cherry Valley accompanying her two sons Robert and Richard on the homeward journey after school on a Tuesday afternoon together with John Coolidge, another boy from the Academy and a friend of Joslin's, no parental permission was sought!

Once again (and not for the first time) Holt playing the role of an editor, suggested that parental permission was not sought by Joslin because "time, in this instance (was) of the essence, and the telephone was beyond the reach of a teenager of the day." One sees Joslin merrily skipping off to spend the night away from the Academy, with the approval of the memoirist (!), "we can only hope that Master Elliott went with the other boys and had a joyous visit." However Holt does concede that the invited group was "a strictly male party and well chaperoned."

.

The 16-year-old Joslin

By his third year at Leicester Joslin had matured considerably. He was taller, and his riding had made him fitter and stronger. Perhaps this was the reason for his retiring Flossie, his faithful and much loved companion for the journey to and from Leicester each week for the previous two years. Gypsy was a sturdier steed.

His final year in Leicester Academy was to see several significant changes in the life of the 16-year-old Joslin.

Most of these changes were described by him in the spring of 1885 when he wrote a long letter, eight pages in length, to Ada. Ada was on her way to England by ship, a journey which took around two weeks.

In part, the letter from the 16-year-old said, "I will try and tell you in this letter all the news of importance that has transpired at my end of the line.

I will first take up school matters. Thursday we finished our review of *Anabasis,* the rest of the class now read the fourth book in advance while I take up Greek composition for the rest of the term. I'm going to take it for one of my examinations at Yale"...

(*Anabasis,* a narration by Xenophon, referring to a military incursion by Cyrus the Younger into Asia in 401 BCE was clearly a class exercise in Greek recitation).

He then continues, "now I must go up and put on my giddy clothes, go down to Mr Kimball's and get a book on Nineveh. So good by [sic] for the present."

Soon the letter resumes with the statement: "I have come back you perceive and will not be interrupted until I harness up to take Mr. and Mrs. Frost and Mr. Kimball over to the prayer meeting at the School House..... Mr and Mrs Coolidge arrived from Saratoga last night, at least they were expected."

Then, abruptly he says what he may have been keeping as a surprise.

"I have engaged my room at Yale. $4 per day (real cheap isn't it.)"

Yale expected its students to organise their own accommodation on the premises of the college. Rooms were sparsely furnished and any extra furniture had to be purchased and transported by the student.

This letter records the first time that Joslin mentions Yale, although clearly plans to go there had been made some time earlier.

Interestingly however, the bulk of the letter, at least as quoted, complete with comments by Holt, was devoted to a visit to Wellesley College for the Junior Promenade. Just how Joslin and his college friend John Coolidge had managed to get themselves invited is not revealed. At the end of his letter, he mentions his birthday. Perhaps it was a present from Ada who was a Wellesley alumnus. It seems that the earlier parental discouragement of socialising with young women had slackened by this time.

At the end of the day, in Joslin's words, they "came into the scene of action." Clearly this is what he had been looking forward to more than anything else. It was a reception where they were introduced to various prominent visitors as well as at least one faculty member called Miss Freeman. As she spoke to the two young men for around 10 minutes, Joslin enquired if she remembered the girl who had her (the faculty member) as a student in her history class, whereupon Miss Freeman exclaimed, "What! Do you mean Ada Joslin?" When he told her that that was the young lady he was referring to, "she smiled on me now more than ever. I was very much taken with her indeed."

After supper he met another young woman who was Miss Sarah's roommate. And if you, dear reader, had reservations about my previous comment on his interest in young women, note Joslin's remarks following meeting the roommate.

"She's very pretty and I liked her very much. As she was then alone she wanted us to go to supper again, this time with her. So up we went John and I. The waitress recognised us as having been there shortly before that evening and looked a little bit shocked but we did not mind it and went on eating."

The New England reserve and propriety, very much in evidence throughout Holt's memoir, perhaps account for no mention being made of Joslin's interest in, perhaps even a weakness for, the opposite sex. Not even a passing comment! Clearly, just a smile from Miss Freeman had left the teenager weak-kneed.

It is interesting therefore to read in Harvey Cushing's biography by Michael Bliss (p.70) of a social get-together organised by Joslin and mentioned by Cushing in a letter to his father in 1893, saying "I have done more social mingling today than for a very long time. Joslin invited three or four medical embryos to dinner at his house where there were three or four unmarried women of the genus spinster which as you know abounds in this New England region. They were very pleasant however, and I actually found myself talking ….."

It would appear that the Yale College student from Oxford was no shrinking violet.

Towards the end of their visit Joslin described the beautiful gardens situated near Wellesley.

"The grounds looked beautiful. The azalianss [sic] and rhodadindrons [sic] are all out. I must have made a mistake in spelling but please overlook it."

Returning to Leicester a few hours later he continued, "At 3.45 started over the road with Gypsey, picked up the Oxford Minister and brought him along. As soon as I arrived home, after being received affectionately, I changed my clothes and went to work.

So ended my birthday. The family gave me a shaving set, very fine in every respect."

Joslin finished the lengthy letter with "had a good report of you while you were at Wellesley. I'm afraid it would make you high-minded if I should tell you." Clearly Miss Freeman had said more about Ada to her younger brother than is included in the letter.

The long letter closed with "excuse all mistakes, penmanship et cetera. We expect you will be in England tomorrow or next day. Good by [sic]. Elliott P Joslin."

It would appear from this letter that, in addition to difficulties with drawing, Joslin had shortcomings in spelling as well!

However, these drawbacks had not dampened his enthusiasm for writing. His aptitude in this area was recognised early in his time at Leicester, when in his junior year he had begun contributing articles to and editing the school paper *The Academy Echo*.He continued as the editor in his senior year. Articles were solicited from faculty members as well as students and a copy was produced every six weeks. The subscription price was $.25 and single copies could be purchased for six cents.

In his senior year Joslin was editor-in-chief, which required him to write editorials as well as articles. He even persuaded his sister for a contribution and, much to his surprise and delight, received a piece called 'A Story of Venice' which Ada wrote in the first person singular – in masculine gender! Whether or not the editor disclosed this to his readership is not known. Neither, for that matter, is there any information on whether *The Echo* invited letters to the editor!

The close attention paid to his progress by his mother is reflected in her recording his marks in different subjects during the winter and spring term of 1886, his last year at the Academy. For Virgil (Latin), French and Roman history Joslin scored 93 1/2, 94 and 93 respectively. He was noted to be punctual, but was marked down on deportment scoring 96. At the back of the card in handwriting recognised by Holt as his mother's was the comment, "Elliott's last report at Leicester and the highest he has ever had there." Interestingly, Holt also commented on the loss of the four marks for his deportment. She noted that the reason was not explained and "one wonders what caused the loss of those four missing points!"

Looking at various photographs of Joslin over the years one notices that when writing, his shoulders were hunched. He carried himself well, especially in public, as is seen in photographs of him addressing a lecture audience. In a photograph taken on the occasion of the 25th anniversary of the discovery of insulin, when Joslin attended the sixth annual meeting of the American Diabetes Association in Toronto in 1946, when he was 77 years old, he stood erect. Perhaps he had been helped in this regard by horse riding which remained his favourite pastime throughout his life.

The Graduation Exercises of the Class of 1886–Leicester Academy, Smith Hall, 2pm Thursday, 24 June 1886.

Joslin was selected to present a paper with the title "Lights and Shadows of American Life."

That he was highly regarded in the community is reflected in a letter from an older member of the congregation of the church he attended in Leicester who had been invited by Joslin to a celebration the day after his graduation.

(Even from an early age Joslin was conscientious in keeping records and documents. This letter was discovered some 70 years after it was written, with a handwritten note by Joslin at the back of the page. "What a nice letter from Mr Samuel May! He was one of the abolitionist school – a prominent May.")The letter reads,

"Dear Elliott Joslin:

We have a polite invitation for Friday evening next – which it would be very agreeable for us all, and doubtless will be in the power of some of us to accept. We think of your leaving our school and our town with no little regret – on our own account; but as it is to be unquestionably for your own advancement and benefit we cannot regret it on your account. We desire to assure you of our best wishes for your continued health and welfare in every way.

From the grosser temptations besetting the young everywhere, I do not presume to say a word of warning. Your excellent conduct, since you came to Leicester as a scholar, boy, perhaps young gentleman, certainly gives all your friends not only a present warm regard, but all confidence in your future. We wish to be counted of that number; and, with your parents and all your other friends anticipate for you, whether in College or elsewhere, a good and honourable record. Be sure our best wishes go with you where you go.

Very truly yours,
Samuel May.
Leicester, June 15, 1886."

Seventeen—year–old Joslin entered Yale College as a freshman with the Class of 1890 in September, 1886. His time at Leicester had seen him mature and develop self-reliance and a capacity for working with and managing people. The strict schedule he had had to follow in getting to school on time on Monday mornings bred in the young man the habit of rising early, which persisted throughout his life. His activities in Sunday School and church, which had included responsibilities as a teacher, had seen him develop people skills while still in his teens.

In the years ahead, Joslin's personal habits, self-discipline and a capacity for attracting loyalty would be noticed and commented on by colleagues, associates and patients as well as countless numbers of members of the public whose lives he was to touch.

His regular connection with horses, which began in earnest with caring for his pony, led to a lifelong love of horse riding. Even in later years he kept a stable of horses on his country estate, replete with farmhands and grooms. They all knew his favourite horses. In old age Joslin was often accompanied by a younger rider. The photograph of him on horseback shown later in the book was published in the *New England Journal of Medicine* in 1959, which had dedicated an entire issue as a tribute to the highly respected Bostonian on the occasion of his 90th birthday. He had sent it with his acknowledgement of the unusual gesture by the editor of the prestigious journal.

Joslin's Continuing Association with the Church.

Joslin's parents regularly worshipped at the Oxford Congregational Church situated on Main Street, and Joslin dutifully attended Sunday School every Sunday. The instructions and lessons remained with the boy into adulthood and inculcated in him a lifelong devotion to his faith. An early influence may have been his Sunday School teacher, Ellen Paine.

The Sunday school teacher was none other than the daughter of the Village Doctor Samuel Paine, the subject of Joslin's essay at Leicester Academy some years earlier.

The attendance at Sunday School continued even when Joslin was at Yale. He taught at the Congregational Church in Bethany, a small mill-town some 10 miles from New Haven where a new church had been built in 1832. At the end of his first year at Yale Joslin was made the assistant superintendent of the Sunday School.

It is also clear that he participated in the social activities associated with church and Sunday School more than at college where social activities were usually closely associated with sports. Although a keen spectator and one known to travel distances to watch college sports Joslin himself did not engage in any sporting activities. Whether or not this was lack of interest, or little if any sporting ability, or the frequent association of drinking with sports is unclear. It is interesting, however, that at the end of his first year at Yale, he wrote about his Sunday School activities, with information on College sports, almost as a postscript. The letter is dated 9 June, 1887.

"Last evening we had our final Bethany teachers meeting of the year at Dr Barnes. I took Miss Barnes, (you may have heard me speak of her). I was informed during the evening that the assistant superintendent had resigned and appointed me to fill his place. So I am Assistant Superintendent.

We danced the Virginia reel and had a fine time generally. You may see that Harvard Varsity has beaten our Varsity but just give us a show and I think we will get the championship yet. The next game with Harvard is the 25th. the Saturday after I come home and I think I should like to go there, rather than to the race. It would be cheaper for me, too. We '90's beat Harvard '90's, 10 to 2 yesterday. So Harvard does not get everything."

Good by, [sic] Elliott P. Joslin.

The role of the church in Joslin's life is shown repeatedly. Although he worshipped at the Old South Church in Copley Square in Boston for much of his adult life, the family connection with the First Congregational Church of Oxford was also maintained. Several items of interest attesting to their association can be found in the church to this day. In addition to the pipe organ donated by his uncle Orrin, an even more interesting Joslin family heirloom is housed in the same church.

This is the hollowed stone, mentioned earlier in this account, which was discovered by Joslin's father and his brothers during their childhood in Thompson. In 1947 Joslin commissioned his friend and well-known sculptress Amelia Peabody to design an angel pedestal to support the stone. The pedestal was cast by Italian stonemasons in South Boston. The impressive creation is now used as a baptismal font in the Congregational Church in Oxford. The font stands in front of the sanctuary. Given that the heirloom weighs some 800 pounds, one can understand the comment in the church's description of it on its website that "it is never moved"!

The baptismal font was a joint gift from Joslin and Mrs Clarence Dargneau (1910–1978) in memory of Ada Joslin (1858–1941), Joslin's older sister, and Louise Myall, related to Mrs Dargneau.

The tradition of church members supporting the maintenance of their places of worship, established from the time of the founding of the colony, is still followed, with families donating different items, usually in memory of their older relatives. Such items range from small pin cushions to electronic organs. In the Congregational Church a Baldwin organ donated in 1957 and an Allen organ in 1982 are further examples of the generosity of members of the congregation.

Part 3.
Yale

College Education

In September 1886 Joslin entered Yale with the Class of 1890. The college records show that he was the only student from Oxford. His college years in Yale became an integral part of his professional life. Therefore it is perhaps appropriate to look at the history and development of this prestigious institution.

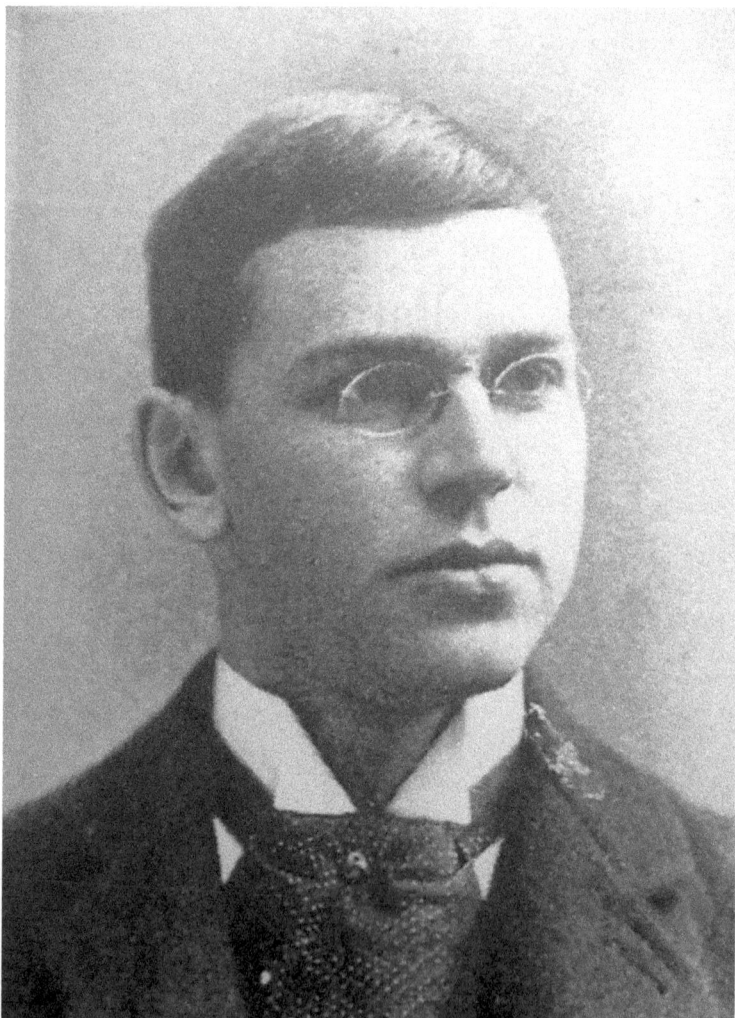

Yale Freshman - Joslin at age 17

Evolution of an early colonial educational institution–Cotton Mather, the Fund Raiser.

This august bastion of American education, situated in New Haven,Connecticut boasts among its alumni at least three Presidents of the United States of America as well as Nobel laureates and diplomats.

It is steeped in the folklore of the early English colonies on the eastern seaboard.

In 1638, a band of 500 Puritans fleeing from religious persecution in Anglican England established the New Haven Colony. Their religious leaders, especially John Davenport, were determined to pursue their dream of establishing "a theocracy and a college to educate its leaders". It wasn't till 1700, however, that a team of 10 ministers led by the Rev. James Pierpoint of New Haven met to fund a college. Each one donated a book towards the founding of "a college in this colony".

In 1701 the Governor and General Assembly of Connecticut passed "an act for liberty to erect a collegiate school... wherein the youth may be instructed in the arts and sciences and through the blessing of Almighty God may be fitted for Publick employment both in Church and Civil State."

Initially, the college operated in the home of the first rector who was the president of the school until his death in 1707, when it was moved to a small town called Saybrook situated at the mouth of the Connecticut River. The Collegiate School, as it was known then, was moved to New Haven in 1716.

By 1718 the increase in the number of students was straining the school's facilities beyond their capacity, and the need for providing more accommodation was recognised by its leaders.

Plans for expansion included the erection of a new building.

The project was placed in the hands of a committee. In charge of raising funds for the project was the redoubtable Cotton Mather, the brilliant but conflicted cleric well known for his oratory (in spite of a stutter which had led his father, the respected Rev. Increase Mather, to discourage the young man from pursuing his original ambition of becoming a doctor.)

This was the same Cotton Mather who in 1692 had given his support to the decision to hang those convicted of witchcraft in the notorious trials in Salem.

Mather, who had been associated with the institution from its beginnings, remembered a gift of 32 books made by a London merchant called Elihu Yale in the early years of the Collegiate School. Whether it was the man's unusual name, or the fact that his gift of books, mainly on religious subjects, had not attracted much interest, realising only a modest financial return when sold, is unclear. However, given that the gentleman had responded to the initial appeal, the optimistic fundraiser decided to approach him once again.

Yale's reply stunned not only Mather but the entire committee.

The London merchant's alacrity, matched by his generosity, was entirely unexpected by the conservative New Englanders. There were no books. Instead, a bulky, heavy consignment was delivered consisting of an unexpectedly large quantity of textiles. There were bales of muslins, poplins, silks, calico and other articles.

As was the custom of that period in the New England Puritan communities, most committees, though headed by the clergy, also included leading merchants. They were not slow to realise the substantial value of the merchandise. The bales of material were promptly sold in the markets of Boston for a return of 800 British pounds. This sum would remain as the largest single cash donation to the institution for at least the next 100 years.

To say that the committee, especially Cotton Mather, were buoyed by the success of his latest approach would be an understatement.

But Mather was not finished yet!

Deciding to ride his luck, he promptly despatched a letter of acknowledgement which, given Mather's command of the English language, accorded such fulsome praise that Yale needed no further encouragement to add to the largesse he had already bestowed.

As an added sweetener to extract a further contribution, Mather hinted at the possibility of Yale's name being given to the extension which had been financed by the merchant.

The strategy proved spectacularly successful.

This time, in addition to books, the shipment also contained what may be intriguing to some. It was a portrait of King George I. The explanation for this lies in the fact that Yale, himself a Protestant, had rejoiced in the overthrow of the reigning James through the Glorious Revolution of 1688, caused, at least in part, by the King's loyalty to the Church in Rome.

An opportunist by nature, Yale was not going to leave anything to chance. The scheming former slave trader – more on this later – still lurking within the latter-day philanthropist, gambled on the Protestants of New England favouring the Protestant King George over the current monarch.

The ploy worked!

So while the New Englanders rejoiced, the benefactor was no less pleased with the success of his strategy.

Thus for each party it seemed to be a win-win situation.

Truth be told, Yale could not believe his luck!

The prospect of securing a prestigious connection with the emerging school and, by association, he hoped, with the church, was beyond anything he had dreamed of at the outset of this exercise. Surely this would elevate him to the status of a man of generosity and unquestionable integrity!

Why else, he reasoned, would the Puritan pastors include his name in their school?

Surely this would make him the envy of the merchants in the commercial circles of London.

He may even have permitted himself the luxury of thinking that his scheming, cynical streak had succeeded in fooling the natives of another British colony as it had in the British territory in India.

From the point of view of the New Englanders, the association with the new benefactor was made in heaven.

With hindsight, one cannot help wondering why Cotton Mather, or for that matter, other members of the committee did not ask themselves why someone with no real connection to their school would be so conspicuously generous. A cynic may argue that the school's fathers had indeed been manipulated by the self-promoting diamond trader.

A rather comical incident occurred at the time of the Collegiate School adopting Yale's name.

So prompt was the dispatch of his final shipment, that to the consternation of the leaders of the Collegiate School, the gift arrived two days before Commencement. Neither the school fathers nor Mather had foreseen this. At that time articles dispatched from England to the New World were carried by steamship and usually took at least 2 to 3 weeks after leaving the English port, the time taken depending on the route followed, as well as the weather conditions. On this particular occasion poor weather conditions had caused the ship's captain to shorten the journey by avoiding some ports in Canada. Programs for the Commencement, carrying the name, Collegiate School, had already been printed.

The school authorities, including Mather, were caught entirely unawares. Anxious to keep the promise made to Yale, they hastily destroyed the printed programs bearing the name Collegiate School and replaced them with the cover page carrying, for the first time, the name Yale Hall.

Some years later, by the proclamation of 1718, it was declared that in acknowledgement of the benefactor's financial and educational support, the Collegiate School (has) changed its name to Yale College.

Then in 1787, to reflect its "elevated status", the name of Yale College was changed to Yale University.

Yale's alumni are referred to as "Yalies" or "Elies", the latter based on the founder's first name Elihu. The derivation of the name is Welsh.

So, while the benefactor and the beneficiaries were both satisfied with the exchange, forever tying the merchant to the institution, the association would come at a cost not anticipated by the founding fathers of the university. They could not have foreseen that this part of the history of Yale would, in the years ahead, become a source of continuing debate and controversy, even disquiet, at least in the eyes of some of its alumni.

Some detractors even question whether the 800 English pounds, one of the largest private donations, justified giving him "naming rights" to the New Haven institution.

So who was Elihu Yale? And what was in his history to arouse such controversy?

As it turns out, interested parties do not have to dig very deep to uncover details in the merchant's past which certainly raised eyebrows in the pious Neo–Puritan community.

Elihu Yale A Life in Two Parts

Wealth by Stealth

Elihu Yale was born in Boston on 5 April 1649. At the age of three he went to England with his parents. He never returned to America.

After a private school education in London he joined the East India Company in 1671 at the age of 22. The headquarters of this commercial enterprise were in the city of Madras now called Chennai. Starting as a company writer, a low-ranking employee with an annual salary of £10, he worked his way up to a senior position.

The peak of his career was reached when in 1687 he was appointed Governor of Fort St George, the company's major installation. Yale assiduously cultivated a patrician air with impeccable dress and a courteous manner. He garnished his grooming with lavish gift-giving, ("mostly at company expense", complained the London office), but managing cleverly to stay within the bounds set by the company.

Five years later he was dismissed from his position and charged with misappropriating company funds. He was found to have enriched himself at the company's expense by entering into secret agreements with local merchants and Indian princes. This was in direct contravention of the directives given by the company.

Yale was also found to have engaged in slave–trading. When in authority, he had started and maintained the practice of enslaving mostly young Indian men but also some women, and having them shipped to other colonies.

Yale's ill-treatment of the local people included ordering flogging and, on one occasion, death by hanging, of a youth for absconding with a Company horse.

Although demoted, Yale was not only permitted to remain in Madras till 1699, but, after paying a fine, was able to leave India with most of his ill-gotten gains which amounted to a considerable fortune. It was rumoured that by 1691 Yale had amassed a fortune equivalent to $5 million.

Thus, when he arrived in London, his wealth enabled him to join the diamond trade. Another example of the double standards Yale adopted in India was that he had acted as the vestryman and treasurer of St Mary's Church in Madras, a position which he hoped would deceive his employers, employees, and colleagues in the British company into believing that he was a paragon of piety, integrity and honesty.

Career Change?

In spite of the ignominious end to his employment in India, Yale, through the assistance of family connections and, perhaps surprisingly, some of the officials in the London office of the East India Company, managed to get into the diamond trade. He proved adept at this enterprise, which saw a rapid rise in his fortunes.

Next, he turned his mind to that which had haunted him since his dismissal from his position of Governor of Fort St George.

He harboured a desperate yearning for respectability.

With breathtaking hypocrisy Yale judiciously donated to various charities and courted popularity in business, social and church circles, with the sole aim of acquiring a reputation for concern for his fellow man. His sole aim and hope was that his cunning monetary donations might be interpreted as a generous trait in the character of a selfless individual. He wanted to be seen as a man of compassion and concern for the welfare of those less fortunate, while in reality he was driven by one motive and one motive alone, self–interest.

Leaving no stone unturned, and casting a net as wide as possible, he had sent a gift of books to the recently established Collegiate School in Connecticut, even though he had no memory of his time in America.

Whether Yale considered the proclamation of 1718, in a distant American colony, as his crowning achievement and for him, a public act of expiation of his sins, remains a matter of speculation and in some quarters, debate.

Yale died on 8 July 1721 in London. His tomb is inscribed with the lines:

> "Born in America, in Europe bred,
> In Africa travell'd and in Asia wed,
> Where long he live'd and thriv'd; in London dead.
> Much good, some ill, he did; so hope all's even,
> And that his soul thro' mercy's gone to Heaven..."

It would be mischievous to suggest that the words had flowed from the pen of Yale himself, the penultimate line bearing a fervent hope of redemption. Historians may or may not agree with the imbalance claimed between "much good" and "some ill".

The practice of buying favours through donations to the church practised in the Roman Catholic Church in those times may well have had an undeclared but hoped for fruition in the thinking of the comparatively new Protestant church and its adherents.

Several incidents over the years demonstrate that Yale continues to honour its side of the bargain in acknowledging the generosity of one of its founders.

In 1927 at Scollay Square, Boston, which is near the site of the donor's birth, the then Yale President Arthur Hadley wrote the inscription on a tablet erected in the square. It reads:

On Pemberton Hill, 255 feet North of this spot, was born on April 5, 1649 Elihu Yale, Governor of Madras, Whose Permanent Memorial in his Native Land is the College that Bears his Name."

On 6 October 1968, the 250th anniversary of the naming of Yale College was recognised by the presentation of a commemorative plaque to St Mary's Church in Madras, which had been founded by Elihu Yale, by the Yale Class of 1924, headed by Chester Bowles who at the time was American Ambassador to India.

As recently as April 1999, the University recognised the 350th anniversary of Yale's birth.

Yale University in American History

The early history of Yale records the part played not only by its students but also its staff, including its president. An interesting highlight is its active support of the American Revolutionary cause contained in the publication "A Brief History of Yale", by the prominent and popular archivist Judith Schiff who describes a citizen detecting the British fleet approaching New Haven harbour on 4 July 1779. The sighting was through a powerful telescope mounted in the steeple of the College Chapel. The college president and a substantial body of students joined the defence forces to defend New Haven the following day.

There is a slightly different version of events according to another account which claimed that in 1779 more than half the student body, led by President Naphthali Daggett, fought the British troops when New Haven was attacked. The story included the rather humorous incident of Daggett being easily overpowered by the British soldiers very soon after he had joined the fray. The invaders then forced the hapless leader to return to his quarters barefoot, the "dastardly British" having confiscated his boots with the sole purpose of humiliating him! Daggett, (Class of 1748), was President of Yale, 1766–77.

Another Yale alumnus, Edmund Fanning, (Class of 1757), a Loyalist and therefore serving with the British during their attack on New Haven, persuaded the invaders not to burn the city of New Haven, in the process saving his alma mater.

Yale alumni not only served as soldiers and officers during the American Revolutionary War, but some were also signatories of the Declaration of Independence on 4 July 1776. These included Lyman Hall Class of 1747, Philip Livingstone Class of 1737, Oliver Wolcott Class of 1747, Lewis Morris Class of 1746, and Roger Sherman who was Yale University Treasurer from 1765 to 1776.

Yale in the Time of Joslin

"From the date of the original charter in 1701, a course of instruction leading to the degree of Bachelor of Arts has been continuously offered at the College."

Catalogue of Yale University 1886–1887

Joslin travelled to New Haven on Thursday, 30 June 1886 to sit the examinations for admission to Yale which were only held in June and September. Persons applying for admission to any of the classes at the College first had to gain from the faculty permission to be examined, and then pay to the Treasurer a fee of $10. In addition, the person had to give to the Treasurer, on being admitted, a bond, executed by his parent or guardians, for $500 as security for the payment of charges arising under the laws of the College.

The Yale catalogue for the year 1886–1887, when Joslin started there, specified the "Terms of Admission."

The requirements of the College for knowledge of Latin and Greek, especially, would be intimidating by today's standards. In addition to grammar, the candidate was expected to be proficient in translating both languages into English and vice versa. The examination candidate had to be at least 15 years of age, and was required to present satisfactory testimonials of good character (preferably from the last principal institution). The College was inflexible in its application of these rules.

Joslin, clearly expecting to pass the entrance examinations, which he did, had arranged accommodation some time earlier. His rooms were in

Farnam Hall, a brick construction in the Old Campus at Yale which was named after Henry Farnam, a philanthropist and railways president.

During the freshman and sophomore years the emphasis was on Greek, Latin, mathematics and English, which occupied the teaching program for 12 to 13 hours per week. By contrast, only three hours of classroom work per week during freshman year and two hours per week during sophomore year were given to modern languages. There was a choice between French and German – Joslin had chosen German for no particular reason, though the choice turned out to be fortunate, permitting him in later years to read German scientific articles in medical journals.

In the freshman and sophomore years all the work was *prescribed.* The nature and the hours of study in the first two years were considered "essential for laying the foundation of a liberal education whatever the department or profession that may be pursued in after-life...." The college fathers felt that this form of study and instruction was "no more than is needed to give the student a proper basis of knowledge and discipline for the study of the elective courses which follow, and that knowledge of himself, and of the subject before him, which is needed for a judicious choice. The basis is necessarily a broad one."

The curriculum in Joslin's sophomore year also included rhetoric, which is a study of essays by English writers including Lamb, Macaulay and Addison. Joslin's aptitude in writing composition, in evidence since his early teens, came to the fore and, although the details of his core subjects in college are incomplete, it is clear that he was an outstanding student.

Chemistry and physiology were offered in 3rd year.

In the fourth (senior) year there was a course with the title of "physiological chemistry". One exercise described as part of this particular course is found in Harvey Cushing's biography by Michael Bliss. Cushing, who was a year behind Joslin, was asked "to go to the slaughterhouse and get a calf brain to show the class." Doubtless Joslin was also given a similar exercise and it is perhaps not surprising that given his difficulties with assignments requiring manual dexterity, details of such challenges are scant, if not absent, in his academic history.

(The practice of getting animal specimens from local markets has persisted in the medical course of many universities including Sydney University where as a "pre-med" student in the late 1950s I had to go to the fish markets in the inner city Haymarket area. Paddy's Markets, which are still in service, had a stall for dogfish which I purchased in order to carry out the prescribed dissection as part of our zoology course. The fish, which were preserved in formalin, gave off an overpowering, pungent odour which was immediately felt by the passengers in the compartment of the tram on which I travelled from the city to the university. The fumes were potent enough to make one's eyes water. The exercise was to cut through the bone of the spinal column as well as the skull in order to demonstrate the brain and spinal cord. The main challenge for the student was managing the very sharp scalpel without slicing his fingers, as well as coping with the profuse watering of the eyes from the formalin fumes which pervaded the entire dissecting room as scores of dogfish were unwrapped!).

The College routine was strict. The day began with Chapel at 8.10 am and attendance was obligatory. The first recitation was at 8.30, the second at 12 noon and the third at 5 pm. Joslin's program included geometry, Latin (Livy and Cicero's letters), Greek (Homer's *Iliad*), algebra and German. Any spare time between recitations was spent preparing for the next lecture.

Between 8 am and 5 pm there was little time for relaxation. Unlike some students who attended gym or played baseball or rowed, Joslin did not participate in any sports. However, he was a keen spectator and supported the Yale teams enthusiastically. The rivalry was keenest with Harvard, and Joslin was not averse to travelling to contests between the two schools, especially in baseball. Clearly he felt that this was enough as far as participation in non-academic subjects was concerned. He referred to this aspect of College life as "the day of the bulldog and the big pipe and all that sort of thing. I did them all." Clearly he had no inclination for engaging in any sporting endeavour himself.

The Joslin papers do not provide much information on his thoughts or opinions on his course or on the subjects he studied. In letters to family he restricted himself to results of class exercises and examinations. An exception was his letter to the family at the end of his first year in June 1887, when a few days after his 18th birthday (6 June 1870), he wrote:

"Dear Family:

I was very glad to get all of your birthday letters. The eventful time passed off very quietly and I did not tell anyone of it until evening. My last recitation has finished and now I am preparing for the examinations. The other day I was very fortunate in an examination with Prof Richards. I received "4" the highest mark attainable. In my other studies, in French I am either first, second, or third. In Latin, I was told I did very well and the same in Alcestes. Of the remaining two, in Cicero's letters I think I have done well but in Greek composition not quite so well. During his term I did not cut a single recitation. I think I shall be satisfied this summer. I would not write this to anyone save the family, but thought you might be interested, and please do not mention it and I mean it.

(Years later, EPJ had this laconic remark typed on the letter: "I think it might be safely mentioned now. November, 1936.)"

Attendance at Sunday School continued even when Joslin was at Yale. He taught at the Congregational Church in Bethany, a small mill town some 10 miles from New Haven, where a new church had been built in 1832.

It is also clear that he participated in the social activities associated with church and Sunday School more than at college where social activities were usually closely associated with sports. Although a keen spectator and one known to travel distances to watch college sports, Joslin himself did not engage in any sporting activities. Whether or not this was lack of interest, or little if any sporting ability, or the frequent association of drinking with sports is unclear. It is interesting, however, that at the end of his first year at Yale, he wrote about his Sunday School activities, with information on college sports, almost as a postscript. The letter is dated 9 June 1887.

"Last evening we had our final Bethany teachers meeting of the year at Dr Barnes. I took Miss Barnes, (you may have heard me speak of her). I was informed during the evening that the assistant superintendent had resigned and appointed me to fill his place. So I am Assistant Superintendent.

We danced the Virginia reel and had a fine time generally. You may see that Harvard Varsity has beaten our Varsity but just give us a show and I think we will get the championship yet. The next game with Harvard is the 25th, the Saturday after I come home and I think I should like to go there, rather than to the race. It would be cheaper for me, too. We '90's beat Harvard '90's, 10 to 2 yesterday. So Harvard does not get everything."

Good by, [sic] Elliott P. Joslin.

Affectation or Advantage: Yale's Social Activities

"... To be adored by cheering blue-jacketed Yale men, violets in the buttonhole and their blue-frocked ladies, violets at the bosom, on sunny spring days when no one had a worry in the world...."

The core of social activities in college was tied to sports and all that went with it, including the post-match celebrations where drinking, rowdy behaviour and partying was the norm for the fans and perhaps some of the college men as well. Social experiments with drinking – the use of illicit drugs was not part of the scene at that time–and "easy women," by fans and occasionally college students, though frowned upon by the authorities, were as difficult to police then as they are now.

Yale College's continuing interest in, and association with, its alumni is well known. A Class Secretary gets annual reports of progress in the professional and personal aspects of every individual. From the institution's archives I was able to obtain Joslin's yearly reports submitted in a form designed (by the College) for easy completion. Joslin always mentioned his family as well as details of his practice. In later years he would mention his writing and progress of his children. His first son, Allen Proctor Joslin, much to his father's pleasure and possibly at his insistence, had gone to medical school as Joslin noted in his yearly report to the College. When Dr Allen Joslin went on war service, this was also included. Still later, he wrote of the service of his son-in-law,

Major Otto, the husband of his daughter Mary.

In a rare admission of just how busy he was in the latter part of the 1920s, probably as a consequence of the discovery of insulin for treating diabetes, Joslin apologised for not coming to a function organised by the College, exclaiming, "Heavens, what with lecturing, writing, seeing patients and attending several committee meetings, I just haven't the time."

Social activities during school hours were limited consisting largely of gossip and banter when the students gathered around "The Fence." Most colleges of that period were surrounded by a perimeter fence of timber or brick construction. The students either sat on or leaned against the structure. Pranks were hatched, becoming the stuff of gossip.

In those days Yale College was situated in the centre of town, and on market days the local farmers often tied their teams to the fence. A popular prank for the youngsters in the College was to free the tethered animals. There is no record of Joslin's being party to any such activity, let alone being a ringleader. It is clear that his social activities were almost completely centred upon Sunday School and church.

Yale's Secret Societies

Yale's secret societies were based on English fraternal societies whose early history is obscure. They are said to have started in the Middle Ages when trading had increased and the grouping of people of several trades as a guild became part of the urban culture. For example, those belonging to an odd assortment of trades were grouped together under the name Odd Fellows, giving rise to one of the earliest fraternal societies. Perhaps the best-known fraternal order indigenous to America is the Elks, which was initially, but no longer, an all–white organisation. What has remained common to all such societies is the perception of exclusivity.

In Yale, the oldest secret society, Skull and Bones, started in 1832, and remains active to this day. However, it is no longer secret, its membership being published each year. The story of how the society took its name is often repeated for reasons which should become clear soon enough. It is said that the skull and bones were from the remains of Geronimo, the Apache warrior who died in 1909. Some members of the society were stationed at an army outpost near the warrior's tomb. The grave-robbing posse, which included Prescott Bush, the father of the late President George H.W. Bush and grandfather of President George W Bush, is said to have spirited away the remains to New Haven, storing it in the society's clubhouse aptly dubbed The Tomb. Needless to say, the authenticity of this account remains unconfirmed!!

Generally regarded as groups supporting the College, the secret societies also provide help and support for its younger members, especially in opening doors to opportunities for professional development and advancement. Thus, for many of its alumni, Yale was a stepping stone to a professional career.

To some, including Harvey Cushing, Joslin's contemporary, election to one of these societies, preferably the elite Skull and Bones or Scroll and Key, was of utmost importance.

"I don't know whether you or anyone, except a Yale graduate, knows what it is to get an election to Skull and Bones or Scroll and Key," Cushing told his father. "It is the greatest honour a man can receive in College and is one thing more than any other sought after by everyone from the time of entering college to senior year." Later in his career, when he was at Johns Hopkins, Cushing met William Welch, who told him that of all his professional associations and accomplishments, his membership of the Skull and Bones fraternity was, without doubt, the highlight of his professional life!

However, unlike William Welch*, and many others including Cushing, (whose flame of ambition in professional as well as social spheres remained undimmed throughout his life), Joslin showed no interest in social position or status, at least at this stage of his life.

*(*William Henry Welch, 1850–1934, was a larger than life character who bestrode the American medical scene in the late 19th and early 20th century. A brilliant pathologist, Welch, together with William Stuart Halsted, surgeon, William Osler, internist, and Howard Kelly, gynaecologist, was one of the "Big Four" founding fathers of Johns*

Hopkins Hospital and Medical School. Welch was also known for his large appetite, including "five dessert dinners!")

The Yale Club in Boston, of which Joslin was a member and which he used for meeting friends and contemporaries, was no more than a social facility for him. Today's Harvard Club, which is open to Harvard graduates and their guests, would have been an obvious choice for him, but I could not discover any reference to his use of the club's facilities. In recent years, staff of the Joslin are known to belong to the Harvard Club. In Joslin's time however, those who visited him were, more often than not, guests at his home in Boston or his country retreat, Buffalo Hill in Oxford.

(During my fellowship we used the squash courts at the Harvard Club where Bing Brinegar and I enjoyed many games. I also got to know George Cahill, who was a keen competitor and very generous with advice on why I should remain in the United States! Even though I did not follow that particular suggestion, we remained friends. He was the Director of the Research Laboratory and one of the most brilliant men I ever met.)

The most prominent social event of Joslin's college years was his European trip in June 1888 his sophomore year. It was his first overseas trip.

The journey, which in those days was by steamship, took several weeks. A prominent steamship company, the Cunard line, was named after its founder and proprietor Samuel Cunard, later Sir Samuel Cunard. Cunard was a prominent businessman from Halifax, Canada. Today the Cunard Company owns vessels including the "Queen" ships (Queen Mary, Queen Victoria and Queen Elizabeth), which travel from Southampton in England to their original destinations in America as well as to many other parts of the world.

On Joslin's first trip, instead of today's diesel-powered vessels, coal was burnt to provide steam. In order to conserve this resource, which was expensive, most vessels used wind power on the ocean, saving the steam for guiding the vessel when steaming into port. Even with such measures the quantity of coal needed filled the bunkers, and extra supplies had to be carried on the decks.

Joslin crossed the Atlantic Ocean to Europe 16 more times over the next 73 years, the last in 1961 at the age of 92. That records have been kept of the number of times Joslin travelled abroad is perhaps indicative of such travel reflecting the social and financial status of those able to afford to do so. Although the first trip was a holiday with hikes in the snowfields in the Swiss Alps and shopping – he had been accompanied by his mother and sister Ada – the later trips to Europe were largely devoted to observation of medical teaching and practice in various centres on the Continent, especially in Austria, Germany and France, as well as participating in scientific conferences.

This first trip was one which Joslin remembered to the end of his life, even down to the details of what they had bought while shopping–a large oil painting of a "sea scene". He kept a photograph showing the three of them in Switzerland where they had met up with friends from England. Holt records this time as follows.

"At this time EPJ was 19 years old. The picture shows him standing erect, full of life and energy, at the head of the line of climbers with his Alpine "Stock" clasped firmly in his hand. His sister Ada likewise looks very businesslike and ready to start out with her stock well under control. Mrs A.L. Joslin is most properly (or perhaps improperly) arrayed for a walk in the mountains in a close–fitting silk basque, full, long skirt and small fashionable hat. She has a cane and wears kid gloves as do the other ladies of the party. One cannot help wondering just how much "Alpine climbing" these ladies so attired really were able to enjoy. There are eleven people in this jolly group and on the bottom of the photograph EPJ wrote: "1888, with the Sharlands in Switzerland."

"In the Fall, [as noted by Holt], refreshed by his European travels the young student returned to New Haven for his Junior (third) year at Yale, prepared to work and study harder than ever."

Details of Joslin's studies in his junior and senior years at Yale are scant. Details of his curriculum are important as possible clues to his choice of the course he would study at university. Many, if not most, students chose subjects in their third and fourth years to prepare them for the course they planned to follow upon entering university.

Details of the courses offered to the Yale Class of 1890 during their junior and senior years are found in the college "Prospectus of Elective Courses 1887-1888," a copy of which I obtained from the Yale archives.

This is where the controversy, or at least discussion, on just when Joslin decided to pursue medical studies becomes interesting, even a little confusing.

For juniors, the College offered four hours of instruction on zoology in the first term. The syllabus indicated that in addition to lectures on classification of animals, there would also be lectures and recitations on physiology. Huxley's, and Martin's *Elementary Biology* and Huxley's *Elementary Physiology* were recommended texts.

There is no mention of Joslin's taking any of these courses. One possible explanation may lie in the first line in the relevant section of the prospectus: *"Dissection of a small number of typical animals."*

It is difficult to escape the conclusion that the 19-year-old Joslin, even though he was a son of a leather merchant and familiar with the processes of preparation of hides following the slaughtering of animals, showed no interest in any such exercise, especially one likely to require manual dexterity. Whether he was also squeamish about dissecting animals, an activity which challenges most medical students, is not known.

A course in botany during the second term was limited to 20 students "who pass the best examination in Gray's *Lessons in Botany*".

In Joslin's defence, it may be argued, as it often is amongst medical students during the early part of their course, that such subjects have little relevance to medical studies–"I'm not going to be treating animals!"–But regardless of the pros and cons, the subjects are part of the preclinical years of the medical course in many if not most universities in English-speaking countries.

Physics was offered to seniors for two hours–two exercises each week, mainly practical work in the Sloane Physical Laboratory with measurements especially in heat, light and electricity, each occupying two hours.

"Recitations and discussions on the theory and methods of physical measurements, the use of instruments, and other special topics."

The prospectus stated that preference for allocating this course was given to students who attained high standing in physics and mathematics.

In spite of the high mark scored for mathematics as mentioned by Joslin in his first year, there is very little information on, or evidence of, proficiency or interest in any of these subjects, as one would expect of a student planning to go to medical school.

In third year, the syllabus included a chemistry course which incorporated laboratory work. Chemistry was offered to seniors for four hours in the second term when "a special laboratory fee [was] charged ..."

Physiology at that time included recitation which may be intriguing to today's medical student. Advances in scientific knowledge over the intervening years have made it a well–developed science, the mechanisms of various processes within the human body having been elucidated sufficiently for them to be understood rather than having to be learned through recitation. An example perhaps of knowledge by acquaintance being replaced by knowledge by explanation.

In the senior year there was also an optional introductory course in physiological chemistry especially designed by the head of the department. It was at this point where, in my opinion, Joslin's time at Yale may have been significant in his decision to become a doctor.

On 25 June 1890 Joslin graduated with a Bachelor of Arts (AB). He had just turned 21. In 1914 Yale conferred an honorary Master's degree on Joslin, the first in the Class of 1890 to be so honoured.

Career Choice

"Do not go where the path may lead, go instead where there is no path and leave a trace."

Ralph Waldo Emerson

Just when Joslin decided to become a doctor is unclear. Was it his own decision – "a light bulb moment"? Unlikely, given that there is nothing in the history of his time at school or in his involvement in Sunday School or church affairs to indicate an impulsive streak in his personality. Neither is there any evidence of his father's expressing an opinion on a particular career for his second son, let alone suggesting one which was so decidedly different from the range of occupations followed by the family. I could not discover any information on the occupations followed by any of the Joslins in the generations before his father's.

The Proctors were prominent leather merchants and their public profile was certainly higher than the Joslin family's. Thomas Emerson Proctor Senior was an admired and respected leader of the industry, not only in the local district of Peabody but also in the state of Massachusetts and beyond. Like many prominent businessmen, he was also a philanthropist. His donation of $100,000 to the Massachusetts General Hospital enabled the institution to establish a facility to care for the insane.

Although there is no evidence that Sarah Proctor Joslin doted on her only son – just as there is no evidence that she did not lavish unstinting affection and care on the two older children of her husband's first marriage – she did pay close attention to young Elliott's progress, including his school work, right down to the marks obtained for different subjects. Doubtless she would have spoken to her children about her older brother Thomas and his prominence in the community as an example of a man who was admired and respected, just as Joslin's father was in the Oxford community. She may well have told them that her brother's ambitions of going to college had been thwarted by her father's failing health. Abel Proctor had stopped work prematurely, with the eldest son having to take the reins of the family business, thus never making it to college. There is no evidence in any writings or in the Joslin papers that anyone in his family suggested medicine as a career for Joslin.

I believe that a possible clue to Joslin's decision to become a doctor may lie in the history of the development, within the precincts of Yale, of a particular branch of the emerging science of physiology as well as, and perhaps, more importantly, the influence of one particular individual. His name was Russell Henry Chittenden who was described as "Yale's most distinguished scientist."

There is some support for this in Holt's memoir of Joslin.

Holt wrote: "During his Senior year E.P.J. met and talked with the Professor and evidently discussed with him at some length his plan for a medical career. Thus it was that he came to realise how valuable the advanced course [meaning the course devised by Chittenden] would be to his future work, especially when the teaching was conducted by the man himself."

As one who had devoted the bulk of her working life as an assistant and then the head librarian of Harvard Medical Library, Holt's observation on Chittenden's influence on students deserves to be quoted. "Professor Chittenden ," she said, "held a great influence over the minds of the students."

Even though Holt ascribes the primary role in this important decision to Joslin, it is just as likely to have been the influence and persuasive powers of the impressive professor. Joslin had shown no particular interest in a scientific career of any sort during his college years. There had never been any mention whatsoever in his letters home of pursuing medical studies. That he was not only popular but admired by the student body for his marks, usually being at or near the top of the class, was revealed in a note from a fellow student. There had been an impromptu quiz for Joslin's class at which Joslin had excelled. Writing home to his mother in Ohio, the student, Harvey Cushing, a year behind Joslin at Yale, said, "Joslin and a man named Mix will lead the class in the examination...."

Chittenden's reputation of scholastic accomplishments and scientific achievement was well known, not only within Yale but also in the wider academic circles throughout America. The students were receptive to the advice and ideas of the much admired teacher.

Chittenden's habit of recognising academic capability and conscientiousness had brought Joslin to his notice. Already recognised as one of the most brilliant students in the Class of 1890, Joslin was receptive to Chittenden's opinion on the value of devoting a whole year doing laboratory work as a useful adjunct to, and preparation for, medical studies. The acute intellect of the college senior quickly recognised the opportunity to be ahead of the pack from the very beginning of his medical course. The acceptance of the suggestion transformed Joslin, the college graduate, into an aspiring medical student, or possibly already, an aspiring doctor. Either way, the die was cast.

So, was it Chittenden who saw the makings of a physician in the young man known for his work ethic and a natural talent conspicuously better than most? Did he see in Joslin, "a young man of outstanding ability" which he was known to do when looking for suitable students for his optional full year course in physiological chemistry? Whether or not the professor knew of the family background of the student is unclear. A look at the admission list for his class would have shown that Joslin was the only one from Oxford in the Class of 1890. There is no record of anyone from the Joslin family having gone to medical school or even college for that matter. Oxford was known for its agriculture and the emerging prominence of the leather industry. It would not have been difficult for Chittenden to find out that Joslin had come from a wealthy home and was the son of a successful merchant.

Apart from his father the most prominent influences on the young Joslin were his uncle Orrin, and in all probability, his maternal uncle Thomas Emerson Proctor Senior. As far as his maternal uncle was concerned, following Joslin's father's buying a home in Beacon Street in 1888, the contact with him would have been more frequent, as Thomas Proctor was also living in Beacon Street. Thus all three exemplars–his father, grandfather Abel Proctor and uncle Thomas Emerson Proctor senior– were men prominent in the leather industry.

It is tempting to speculate that Chittenden, who had also harboured ambitions of becoming a doctor but had fallen in love with studying and teaching physiology, saw in Joslin the twin talents of a superior intellect and unshakeable piety – both attributes, at least in those times, considered essential requirements in a doctor. Did he see in Joslin the very antithesis of some of his own character traits described in an essay he had written?

"... Not greatly inclined to mingle with other children, but preferred the quiet of my own with a tendency to play alone; altogether too serious, with a fondness for books and stories, with a rather vivid imagination for a child and *an ambition to be a minister or a doctor.*"

Joslin's affability and popularity. as well as an enviable ease with people younger (remember he was a Sunday School teacher, even assistant superintendent!) as well as men older than himself, as described in the letter by Samuel May when Joslin left Leicester Academy, would have been noticed by Chittenden.

I can find no other reason for Joslin's sudden interest in a scientific subject, certainly not an interest so intense as to make him decide to spend a whole year in a laboratory. I could find no letters or notes in the archives relating to this decision either at the end of his years of college or even during the year with Chittenden.

If there were other influences and factors causing Joslin to take this fateful step I was unable to find them, and so they must remain in the realms of more conjecture and speculation than I have allowed myself. Suffice it to say that the 21-year-old Joslin returned to Yale in the fall of 1890 for a full year of work in the laboratory. Little did he know how pivotal this year would prove to be in his professional development. Neither could he have realised that it would also be a burden he would carry in his later years. A burden which, in the opinion of some, would prove to be almost a millstone around his neck.

So who was this persuasive scientist and teacher whose counsel had such a profound effect on Joslin?

Yale's Most Distinguished Scientist

Dr. Russell Henry Chittenden had studied Physiology, a branch of science of which he could justifiably be called the leading American authority at that time. The course he introduced in 1874 for the senior year was Physiological Chemistry. The lecturer, as well as the Chief Supervisor of Laboratory Techniques and Studies, was Chittenden himself, referred to by Bliss in his biography of Cushing as "Yale's most distinguished scientist."

Appointed Professor of Physiological Chemistry in 1882 when only 26 years old, Chittenden had studied in Heidelberg from 1878 to 1879. This year in Heidelberg had a profound influence on the then 22-year-old scientist. He had spent this time in the laboratory of Wilhelm Kuhne.

Kuhne (1837-1900), with a faultless academic pedigree, having studied under Claude Bernard in Paris and worked in the laboratory of Rudolph Virchow, "the father of modern pathology", had delved deeply into the chemistry of digestion. He had discovered the digestive enzyme trypsin and coined the term "enzyme". The charismatic German was deeply impressed by the young American. Their association and friendship endured for the next 22 years, ending only when Kuhne died in 1900. Returning to Yale, Chittenden was awarded a Doctorate in Physiological Chemistry in 1880. In 1890 he was appointed Professor of Physiology. His book *The Nutrition of Man*, published in 1907, was hailed as a classic.

Chittenden received many citations and awards as well as prestigious positions in scientific circles, but at the centre of his being was a lifelong dedication and devotion to teaching physiological chemistry, and it remained his primary interest to the end of his life.

Convinced that this branch of science, especially when combined with laboratory and classwork, as in the course he provided, would be of great value to students pursuing studies in medicine, he sought, even pursued, young men of outstanding ability to spend one whole year on this one subject before embarking on the course provided in medical schools at that time.

In a comprehensive essay on Chittenden published by the National Academy of Science, it is recorded that "Chittenden is credited with influencing a generation of distinguished scholars at Yale and other institutions to do laboratory research work as part of their medical training. Chittenden persuaded unusually gifted students to study for a Ph.D. and/or to do laboratory research work as part of their medical training." Many believe that this was an important factor in the development of physiology and physiological chemistry in America.

The influence of Chittenden on Joslin was clear to all who knew him, even without knowing the teacher. This included Holt, who concluded her comments in this chapter of Joslin's life and his association with the remarkable man with the observation that "all his life afterward Dr Joslin held Prof Chittenden in the highest regard and often quoted some of his wise sayings. Students literally flocked to this [Chittenden's] new laboratory."

Unlike the regimentation of the formal studies during his four years at Yale, the year in the laboratory was very different. There was close contact with Chittenden himself as well as others who were working in the laboratory on their own projects.

Joslin, who had a natural ability to impress people, even at first meeting, thrived in the atmosphere of comparative informality in the laboratory. Conversations over coffee or during meetings after hours brought him into contact with other gifted students.

Two of these went on to distinguished careers of their own. Graham Lusk, developed a worldwide reputation as a physiologist, and Lafayette B Mendel, the peerless successor to Chittenden himself, remained lifelong associates and friends. Lusk gave Joslin great assistance during the latter's foray into laboratory research carried out in the New England Deaconess Hospital in the early years of his medical practice.

Joslin also met students who chose the elective term offered in fourth year, even though their work was quite different from those doing a full year. It was at this time that Joslin became acquainted with a student who was to become an associate and a friend for the rest of his life. His name was Harvey Cushing.

Joslin's first scientific paper based on laboratory experiments was written as a result of studies carried out during his year with Chittenden. It is the first entry in the publication *A History of Joslin's first 100 years through its Publications.*

In 1891, the scientific journal, Transactions of the Connecticut Academy 8:38–65, (1891), published the paper with the following title:

Chittenden R.H, Joslin E.P, Meara F.S. On the ferments contained in the juice of the pineapple (ananassa sativa), together with some observations on the composition and proteolytic action of the juice.

As is common, the paper was largely written by Chittenden himself, with Joslin's name included to reflect some of the work done in the laboratory.

Although the vast majority of Joslin's contributions to medical journals were based on clinical findings and not laboratory data, this paper is important because it introduced the recent college graduate to the laboratory. Even more important to him was to be associated with the distinguished first author. He had had his first taste of seeing his name in print, a joy known perhaps only to those who have experienced it.

In Joslin's case, his first experience of seeing his contribution published may be seen by some as the kindling of a flame which burned brightly to the end of his life and led to his greatest contributions to medical literature and, arguably even more importantly, to the wider diabetic community throughout the English-speaking world.

Part 4.

Harvard

Departure from Family Tradition

There is not a single mention of the reaction of Joslin's family to his decision to become a doctor. Certainly the first Joslin to go to medical school, his writings never commented on this difference between him, his older half-brother Homer, or indeed his father, his uncle Orrin, or any in the generations before them. Similarly, although not the first in the Proctor line to go to college (at least one Proctor had gone to Harvard and had practised as a lawyer in Danvers), Joslin was the first one with Proctor genes to become a doctor. It is surprising that Sarah Proctor Joslin, demonstrably interested in and ambitious for her son – her only son – is not mentioned in this connection by either the memoirist Holt or the biographer Barnett. I choose to believe that they had as much difficulty as I did in prising personal details out of the archives and papers of the very reserved New Englanders!!

Harvard Medical School had been established in 1782, but in the early years the doctors went through a very different program. This consisted of formal lectures for 1 to 2 semesters and then an apprenticeship with a practising physician. There was no academic preparation and no compulsory medical examination. Neither were there tuition fees, the students being required to buy tickets to each lecture. There were no teaching hospitals.

After several locations in the city, in 1883 the school had relocated from being next door to the Bulfinch Building of Massachusetts General Hospital to Exeter Street near Boylston in Copley Square. It was here, in September 1891, that Joslin found himself in a group of students in the crowded premises which were to fit him for his life's work.

The building had been erected in 1883, and at that time was considered the acme of convenience and suitability. However, increasing student numbers as well as advances in medicine, especially laboratory work, had necessitated expansion of facilities so that even after the relatively short period of eight years from the time of its construction, the Exeter Street buildings were proving inadequate.

What would be even more interesting and perhaps intriguing to an observer today would be how mixed the group was. The explanation for this lay in the very flexible conditions of entry at that time. It was possible to get into medical school as long as the candidate could pass an entrance examination. Some were even less strict. For example, New York College, considered one of the best medical schools in America in the second half of the 18th century, – one of its most distinguished alumni being the previously mentioned William Henry Welch, a founding physician of the Johns Hopkins School of Medicine – only required the applicant to be able to read and write! For Harvard, the students had to pass a written entrance examination. A college degree from Yale, especially, as in Joslin's case, supplemented by the extra year with Chittenden, made him almost overqualified. However, to comply with the regulations, Joslin went through the motions of completing a simple written examination.

A singularly conspicuous feature of the Harvard student body in Joslin's time, which would be obvious to an observer today, would be the complete absence of women. Harvard Medical School did not admit women till 1945.

(Joslin's first female associate and the only woman in the "original seven," Priscilla White, was refused admission to Harvard and went to Tufts Medical School instead. She never forgot that. It was said that many years later, when she had gained worldwide fame for her work on childhood diabetes and the obstetric aspects of the condition, she was offered a professorship at Harvard.

When I worked with Dr White in 1969 and 1970, doing ward rounds of pregnant diabetics at the Boston Lying-In Hospital, the obstetricians in the team were from Harvard. They virtually worshipped the ground she walked on. I never saw anyone else accorded such profound respect and admiration. I never asked her about her opinion of Harvard Medical School!)

Medical teaching at that time was going through a period of transition. The traditional earlier didactic instruction was being replaced by increasing laboratory work and introducing the student to experimental methods and tools, thus encouraging him to develop lines of enquiry into possible causes of disease. This was copied directly from the European medical schools and universities where didactic teaching had been done away with years earlier. Indeed, visiting European centres, especially French, German, and Austrian, had become common practice for American medical graduates. Joslin himself had gone to Europe, although his reasons for going, at least on one or two occasions, were different and personal as will be seen later in this account.

Even though the curriculum had been extended, largely due to the efforts of the visionary Charles W Eliot, the 21st president of Harvard University, the great names of medical education were still household names in Boston. These men held major positions in the teaching faculties as well as in the hospital hierarchy. They also moved in the higher social circles of Boston.

The Boston Giants of American Medicine in Joslin's Time

In Joslin's time didactic teaching still held sway, primarily because of the reputation and authority of the leading medical men of Boston who, in addition to their private practice, conducted clinics in hospitals, taught medical students at the bedside and lectured in medical schools. Outpatient clinics were for patients who did not require admission to hospital. Hospitals were originally built for the poor who could not afford to have a doctor visit and treat them at home.

An advantage of this form of tuition was the influence of the leading medical men of the era on medical students. The calibre of the men who taught Joslin was such that the students could not help being influenced.

Surgery was taught by Dr John Collins Warren, grandson of John Collins Warren, who introduced ether anaesthetic to surgery. Another surgeon-teacher was Frederick Cheever Shattuck, as was John Homans. As previously noted, in the farming community of the New England Puritans it was a custom for the first son of the family to follow the father's profession. A similar practice was followed in the medical community. John Homans' son for example, also called John, described a sign useful for detecting thrombosis of the veins in the legs. Homans' sign is still used by doctors at bedside examinations.

Another of Joslin's teachers in medical school as well as in the outpatients department was a physician, Reginald Heber Fitz. The part played by Fitz in Joslin's postgraduate career was pivotal to the direction taken by the aspiring physician. More than simply an instructor, Fitz became a guide and a confidante who, a few years later, had to take Joslin under his wing. In my readings, the importance of Fitz's role in the Joslin story has not been recognised previously.

In first year, Dr Thomas Dwight (1843-1911), the rotund, popular exhibitionist with a winning smile, taught anatomy. Dwight had followed the brilliant Oliver Wendell Holmes as the Parkman Professor of Anatomy. The Countway Repository collections include medical images of Dwight at work. Possessed of not only abundant knowledge but also unlimited enthusiasm, Dwight, according to the recollection of one of his students, used models of bones and viscera as "graphic accessories to vivify and help the student visualise the spoken word...." These were predecessors of today's images delivered by video and audio devices via the Web as aids to students' learning.

Affectionately called Tommy (behind his back!), he was an expert at making plaster casts which he did in class, talking at the same time, to show the surface anatomy of different parts of the human body. He would be elbow-deep in the wet plaster, often his back to the class until, with wet plaster on hands, arms, dustcoat, even his face, having completed the exercise, he would triumphantly turn to face the youthful audience, beaming and pointing to his handiwork. The students, loud in their applause, would cheer and clap and Dwight, playing, even encouraging the theatrics, would take a bow with a flourish–often more than once!! So medical studies weren't (and aren't) as dull as some may imagine.

Experiences such as this become the stuff of reminiscences at medical reunions and sometimes also at medical conferences where more is learned at social activities by comparing different aspects of current medical practices with colleagues from other centres and countries than the latest advances in medical knowledge presented in formal lectures.

Histology and embryology were taught by Dr Charles S Minot. Years later, the teacher was to meet his student Joslin in a role reversal when Joslin was called upon to look after Minot's son, George, which is a story in itself to be explored later.

Medical pharmacology was taught by Dr Edward S Wood.

Physiology instruction was by Dr Henry Pickering Bowditch, who had studied with Claude Bernard in Paris and who is assured of a place in the medical history of America for establishing the first laboratory devoted to experimental physiology. Needless to say this particular course, taught for a term, was not nearly as comprehensive as that pursued by Joslin with Chittenden. However Bowditch, who had a long and distinguished career on the staff of Harvard Medical School, kept in touch with Joslin during and after his medical course to provide guidance and advice.

It is not difficult to understand that these men were regarded with awe and admiration by the students.

The extra year after college made the early semesters in medical school much easier for Joslin. Microscopy of cells and tissues required in first year was a repetition of work he had done more thoroughly and under closer supervision than required at Harvard. Joslin was clearly ahead of most of the class as Chittenden had predicted. Indeed, according to Cushing's biographer Michael Bliss, "keeping up with Joslin was to become one of Cushing's self-imposed goals."

However, it was not all plain sailing for the confident medical student. Never keen on manual exercises, working on human corpses (cadavers) proved a challenge. Even though he passed the required examinations, Joslin never enjoyed the hands on aspect of much of the surgical side of the course. His proven aptitude in communication, written as well as verbal, was quickly noticed by his teachers. Joslin, in turn, went out of his way to do extra work in this area, limiting attendance at surgical "demonstrations" or watching operations and occasionally assisting at operations to a minimum. The same went for the other duty of medical students, namely giving ether to render a patient unconscious for surgery to be carried out.

The use of ether as an anaesthetic had been pioneered in Massachusetts

General Hospital, and the hospital has never ceased to celebrate its role in the development with yearly celebrations of the seminal event of 16 October 1846, which are held in the Ether Dome designed by Boston's leading architect Charles Bulfinch in 1818. Indeed, the term *anaesthesia (without sensation)* was coined by one of the physicians of the hospital, the renowned Dr Oliver Wendell Holmes.

Prior to the use of ether, anaesthesia had been attempted with alcohol, and sometimes a simple blow to the jaw to render the patient unconscious!

(Ether, no longer in general use, was still employed for minor operations in the early to mid–1960s. I recall my personal experience acquired during clinical training after graduation from the medical school in Sydney University. I received instruction in dripping the ether solution from a bottle with a narrow metal tube attached to its screw-top, onto several layers of soft cloth held in place within a wire mask which was placed on the face of the patient (who always looked apprehensive to the point of sheer fright). Breathing in the fumes from the cloth held over his face, the patient would gradually lose consciousness, at which point the planned minor surgical procedure, usually circumcision, was carried out by my senior associate.)

Joslin Meets Miss Higgins and Dr Reginald Heber Fitz

One incident which requires special mention occurred in Joslin's second year. Medical instruction given in lecture form in medical school was supplemented by practical or clinical teaching. This meant instruction in the outpatient clinics in the hospital, in this case the Massachusetts General Hospital.

These clinics, where members of the public were treated by a senior surgeon or physician, small groups of medical students were expected to attend to watch their professors in action. Here the students were shown how to examine patients for different conditions. For example, they were shown the methods for detecting abnormal enlargement of abdominal organs like the liver. After first looking carefully, (inspection) the student was shown how to feel for any swelling, (palpation) before the act of tapping (percussion), then auscultation, the act of using the stethoscope to listen for sounds such as the heartbeat.

It was in these clinics that a student could discover, to his dismay, that book learning alone did not necessarily translate into becoming a good doctor. In order to combine the theoretical with the practical, he needed to acquire additional skills including careful observation together with various manual techniques. He was taught how to combine the theoretical with the practical, and the necessity for correlating all these pieces of information in order to reach the correct diagnosis. Many an academically accomplished student came up against hitherto unexpected difficulties. During these clinical years in my medical training, more than one accomplished student known for scoring high marks in written examinations during the early preclinical years of the course found himself at sea when confronted by a real, live person as a patient.

It was in this setting that Joslin had the experience which may well have at least been a factor in determining the professional path he followed some years later.

On 2 August 1893 Joslin, with six of his fellow students, headed for the outpatient (medical) clinics at the Massachusetts General Hospital.

It was a Wednesday, a typically hot and humid summer's day in Boston. The MGH premises were not air-conditioned. The group of seven young men had arrived early. They knew that their teacher had a reputation for punctuality.

Reginald Heber Fitz arrived at two o'clock sharp. Conservatively but immaculately dressed, his appearance was matched by his manner. He was quiet and kindly. And he was known for his acute perception in the diagnosis of disease. His fame persists to this day as the person who made the original observation on one of the commonest ailments to afflict mankind – appendicitis.

Fitz turned to the nurse in attendance. "May we see the first patient please."

A moment later the nurse came in from the waiting area with a young woman. That was an era when the medical profession was held in awe by members of the public. The patient's diffidence was matched, no, out-matched by her appearance.

Fitz remained silent: almost as if he wanted the appearance to be burned into the memory of the students.

The patient, a young woman in her 20s, wore a blank expression. Her skin was pale, but more remarkable was her general appearance because her body was just skin and bone. She turned to look at Fitz. She had sensed compassion and warmth in the manner of the senior man. Neither was it missed by the aspiring doctors. Fitz asked her to sit on the low wooden couch which was part of every cubicle and on which the patient could lie down to be examined. All this took place in less than 2 minutes but the impression created on the young men would be a lasting memory. This is an important part of medical training which can only be learned from experience, not from books.

Fitz turned to the students. "Gentlemen, Miss Mary Higgins is 26 years old. Her parents came from Ireland."

He did not have to draw attention to the woman's appearance, perhaps as much out of concern for her modesty as from the necessity to emphasise to the students the importance of careful observation. Even the uninitiated, aspiring doctors would not have failed to notice the listlessness, the sunken eyes, the languid movements from profound lethargy and tiredness, but most of all, how thin she was. Perhaps Fitz wanted the students to appreciate the plight of refugees or people who were not privileged like they were.

Fitz turned to the students and surveying the entire group asked,

"Do any conditions come to mind as you look at Miss Higgins?" Silence.

Fitz persisted."Would anyone like to ask Miss Higgins a question?"

One of Joslin's classmates was Francis Denny, a confident, moustachioed young man who came from one of the wealthy families of Boston. Denny asked if the patient had a cough.

"A reasonable thought," said Fitz. "You are thinking of..?"

"Koch's," said Denny, not wanting to use the word "consumption" or tuberculosis in front of the patient. (The germ causing tuberculosis was first described by a German physician called Koch. Hence the name Koch's for tuberculosis).

(Denny, whose family had bought him an expensive German microscope, was keen on bacteriology. He followed through on this early interest and eventually became a bacteriologist for the Massachusetts Public Health Department. Another Denny with no connection to medical education will illuminate these pages later, in case you're tiring of my medical stories!)

Fitz turned back to the patient, who now appeared far less nervous than she had been earlier, and with a twinkle in his eye asked, "Miss Higgins, have you lost interest in food?"

"No, can't get enough to eat."

Fitz turned to the students, not wanting to keep them in suspense any longer,

"Gentlemen, you have just seen your first patient with diabetes mellitus."

Once more there was silence. The entire group was speechless.

The effect on Joslin was profound.

Fitz made further comments to the nurse, but more to the patient, explaining that she would be taken to the office of the dietician for advice on meals.

But Joslin couldn't remember anything. In fact, he could not get the appearance of "this waif-like working girl of Irish ancestry" out of his mind.

He couldn't wait to get to his textbook of internal medicine. The one in use in medical schools throughout the English-speaking world at that time was written by William Osler from the Johns Hopkins School of Medicine in Baltimore.

Diabetes was not as clearly understood or as thoroughly studied in the late 1800s as it is now. Since then there has been a veritable explosion in studies and research into the condition. Today there are complete textbooks, some of 2 or 3 volumes, devoted entirely to diabetes.

Joslin, however, was not satisfied with Osler's description of the disease even though it was remarkably detailed for that period.

Seeking more information on the condition, he turned to Fitz who directed him to the medical library to search American and European scientific journals for articles on diabetes. In addition to providing information, these journals made Joslin aware of the centres where research on diabetes was being carried out.

Burning the midnight oil, Joslin – remember he was still only a second year medical student – studied diabetes in detail.

His earlier exposure to German helped in this regard. Joslin also had a much–travelled maternal aunt who was proficient in German and translated articles from scientific journals for her nephew's benefit. Younger than Joslin's mother, Ellen Osborne Proctor (1848-1902) later made a generous bequest to Harvard Medical School for medical research.

Searching the literature, the intrepid medical student was delighted to discover that his chief, Reginald Fitz, also had an interesting publication arising from a lecture he had given on diabetes in which he had drawn attention to the presence of glucose in the urine of a patient with epilepsy.

Joslin had already been elected to the Boylston Society of Harvard Medical School which had been endowed by and named after the well-known Boston merchant. Membership to this student organisation was by election, and a mark of admiration of the more accomplished. On 17 February 1893 Joslin read his paper on diabetes before the Society.

After his graduation, when he was on the teaching staff of the university, the Society elected Joslin as its president.

It is clear that he had spent a great deal of time on this particular project because, within four months of giving this lecture, it was published in the popular *Boston Medical and Surgical Journal* on 29 March and 5 April 1894 under the title *"Pathology of Diabetes Mellitus"*. Several aspects of this early single- author article invite comment.

119

The article describes much more than the pathology of diabetes. It is in fact a comprehensive dissertation on virtually all aspects of the condition known at that time. Written in lucid prose, the clinical and experimental information on diabetes of that period is presented in chronological order. Actual details of pathology are scant as the more significant advances in this area were to be made later. The references are up to date, several being journal articles written in the same year as Joslin's (1893).

Ever correct and courteous, Joslin referred to the authors of the referenced articles by their surname, but when it came to Fitz he referred to his supervising physician as "Dr Fitz"! The mark of respect would not have escaped the senior physician. (Had Fitz actually encouraged Joslin to do this project it would have been acknowledged in the article.) He was quick to record the assistance of Bowditch, the Professor of Physiology and at that time the Dean of Harvard Medical School, whom Joslin had approached for information on research done in the laboratory of Claude Bernard, with whom, possibly unbeknownst to the student, the American physiologist had worked in the earlier years of his career.

Two additional noteworthy points the article raised were firstly, whether Joslin had grasped the importance of the work of von Mering and Minkowski on pancreatic diabetes and secondly, whether the medical student, possibly overawed by the distinguished men who were his teachers in medical school, would be hesitant about approaching Herr Professors, should at some stage in the future he would have the opportunity to do so. The discussion in the paper would support the view that he had understood the significance of the removal of the pancreas. As to the second question, again his article showed that Joslin was not backward in coming forward!

In the course of preparing his paper, Joslin came across the work of a researcher in Paris called Lepine. He noticed in Lepine's report that the work had been carried out in the laboratory of Claude Bernard, the leading French scientist who at that time was working on pancreatic diabetes. At that time Bowditch also held the Chair of Physiology at Harvard Medical School. So was there any hesitation on Joslin's part to approach the Dean to ask about Lepine? Evidently not, for as often happened to Joslin, good fortune paved his way. Some might say he made his own luck.

As it turned out, not only did Bowditch know of Lepine, he had actually worked with him during his own tenure in Paris. Joslin's article made a point of mentioning this .Whether or not he revealed just how he had come upon the information is not stated. This was, after all, the ex- editor of the Leicester Academy's school newspaper, and like all good newspaper men he protected his sources!

So, no! The Harvard undergraduate was certainly not socially awkward- or backward.

I believe this project was made for Joslin. He was good at writing essays. As already mentioned he was active in this pursuit in high school at Leicester Academy. His letters home were essays in themselves.

Joslin's appetite for getting published had been whetted by his first paper co-authored with Chittenden after his extra year at Yale. However, this was the first time that he was the sole author. Doubtless he would have received accolades not only from his fellow students but also from the more senior members of the academic and clinical staff. He would not have been blind to the possibilities of more doors being opened because of this addition to his student record (CV or *curriculum vitae*).

Little did he know how important a role both Mary Higgins and Reginald Fitz would play in his professional life.

Joslin graduated from the Harvard Medical School in the fall of 1895. Although details of his results in the various courses and examinations are not recorded, Holt's memoir stated that he was "at or near the top of the class throughout his course."

He was the class valedictorian.

The Freiburg Incident or Joslin's "Damascus Moment"

One incident in his senior year affected Joslin deeply.

Failure, no matter how infrequent, affects the ambitious and idealistic individual much more than his successes. And it was such an incident described by Holt which haunted Joslin. Unfortunately, her account is sketchy to say the least, and unaccompanied by any documentation, references or sources. However, its authenticity may be deduced from the fact that Joslin felt unprepared to continue his course by serving an internship at the hospital, which is the usual practice. Instead, he took a year off so as to overcome the emotional trauma inflicted by the incident. I hope that my account may shed a little more light on the mystery, even with the risk inherent in all such speculations.

Holt's summary preceding the incident in Freiburg is as follows:

"For part of the training in obstetrics during the fourth year at medical school he served on the "District". This was in the poorest part of the South End of Boston. The program was supervised and directed by the Boston Lying-In Hospital. A medical student went to the home of a woman in labour to assist in the delivery of her baby at any time of the day or night whenever the call came. Conditions were usually squalid and on occasion, even dangerous to the young man when English was not spoken or understood by anyone else present in the home.

EPJ's time on the District proved to be a most unhappy experience. The man who was supposed to have headed the team of youngsters dropped at the last minute and E.P.J., who had led in excellence of performance thus far in his career was, on the strength of this fact, put into the top place. He was totally unprepared for this and, according to his own admission did poorly for the first time in his life. Being a perfectionist and highly conscientious, this failure to achieve his usual high standard of excellence distressed him almost to the limit of endurance. The worry over this persisted for months".

A more detailed description of the part of Boston city where the students had to do their practical training in obstetrics is provided in a letter written by Harvey Cushing to his fiancée Kate Crowell found in the biography of Cushing by Bliss. Clearly the Clevelander was sticking to his earlier decision to "keep up with Joslin."

"With Joslin I visited Italians, Portuguese and "Chews" in various tenements of all grades of squalor. One young one we tore from his parents arms midst wailings and gnashing of teeth and packed him off to the City Hospital else the other four children who slept in the same bed with him would in all probability have been down with diphtheria as well in a few days, if they will not be anyway. Not even the good District nurse, who is of necessity more of a linguist then we, could make them understand that our intentions were of the kindest. I should not like to go there after dark.

Then we saw ten or twelve more sick families, fathers, mothers, infants and what not with various ills, urgent and otherwise. The ones we did most for were least grateful and those for which we could do nothing or perhaps could not recognise the trouble would overwhelm us with "God blessings" as is usually the case even with more intelligent parties in different grades of society. In one room about half as large as mine here there were living a father largely boosy and nationality unknown, an Italian mother and six children the oldest being so many years of age and the most recent arrivals twins. In that room was combined kitchen, bedroom – one bed and one cradle and a box or two – sitting room and I guess that's all the variety they needed.

Thus we wandered up and down the dark stairways in and out of courts pretty extensively throughout "Little Italy" and the Portuguese quarters till 7:30(in the morning). Joslin and I then repaired to Young's and ate enough for all day and here I am, and that's more about charity medical work then I've told anyone for a long time."

The practical aspects of obstetrics such as the techniques needed for delivering a baby were taught in-house by distinguished obstetricians. This was mostly done in Boston Lying-In Hospital, the forerunner of what is now Brigham and Women's Hospital. The Boston Lying-In was the first hospital of its kind in New England. Founded in 1832, it had a rich history, not only in medical advances such as the use of anaesthetics during childbirth as well as sterilising solutions to prevent puerperal sepsis, but also of distinguished men who practised there. One of the best known was Oliver Wendell Holmes (1809–1894). Apart from professional competence, he was known for his wit, literary flair and a gift for rhyming. For example:

So the stout foetus, kicking and alive, leaps from the fundus for his final dive.

Tired of the prison where his legs were curled, he pants, like Rasselas, for a wider world.

No more to him their wanted joys afford, the fringed placenta and that knotted cord.

Given Joslin's interest in the classics, there is little doubt that he would have warmed to Oliver Wendell Holmes, and probably vice versa. Unfortunately, the extremely popular and witty poet and obstetrician, even though active after retirement from "The Lying-In"(Hospital) in 1882, had died the year before Joslin did his term of obstetrics.

The teaching of obstetrics, especially delivering a newborn, is always carried out in the presence of an experienced obstetrician. Emergencies, potentially fatal not only for the child but the mother, at times for both, can be sudden and entirely unforeseen even in today's technologically assisted environment. If, as appears to have happened in this incident, a senior medical student, no matter how competent, is the only one present for the delivery, the risks are substantial and would be totally unacceptable in medical teaching and practice today.

Although no actual details are provided by Holt, except that "he was totally unprepared for this and, according to his own admission did poorly for the first time in his life", regardless of how much of a perfectionist Joslin was, he was, after all, entirely inexperienced in this field.

Even with the scant details available, it is clear that compared to today's medical training, practical obstetrics in Joslin's time, was very much a sink or swim experience. The details of the particular medical mishap, perhaps understandably, have not been recorded.

The fact that Joslin went to Europe after completing his university course is not in itself unusual. European centres, particularly Germany, France and Austria, became increasingly popular destinations for American and English graduates after completing their university courses in the sciences including medicine. For Joslin, this could have been directly or indirectly the result of knowing that Chittenden had also gone to Europe after completing his studies in Yale. Chittenden may have told Joslin of the profound influence of the German physiologist Kuhne on him, and the benefits of their lifelong association.

However Joslin, it seems, was still troubled by the obstetric incident and carried it into his year in Europe. Again, like the incident in Boston, actual details are scant. Holt records it this way:

"By 1896, he went to Europe once again to visit some of the leading medical centres in Germany and especially Vienna, Austria. In Germany he went the rounds of several laboratories, particularly in Berlin, Strasbourg and Freiburg, listening to and observing all that the "Herr Doctors" had to say and show to their students. But in the back of his mind the hurt of the fiasco at the Lying-in Hospital in Boston still rankled. He wondered whether he should ever be able to live down, this to him, dreadful disgrace. It is amazing how some small episode, wholly unforeseen, can almost instantly change one's outlook on life. This happened to E.P.J. on a cold, gloomy day that matched his feelings.

One morning as he walked along a street in Freiburg, deep in his own thoughts, he became conscious of the sound of runaway horses galloping towards him. At once he became all attention. From long experience with horses he knew what should be done to stop their mad race. As the frightened animals came abreast of him the young man dashed out into the street and stopped them in mid-flight. When it was all over suddenly the thought came to him: "Perhaps I'm worth something after all." His whole outlook changed, he cheered up and went happily on to a long life of devoted service to others."

So the monkey's off his back and the demon/s exorcised,just like that!

There are no details on whether the horses had bolted with or without a carriage or even if there was a carriage. Also, whether it was carrying freight and/or passengers. In fact, the very next line in Holt's book, has him sending his family a "long, newsy letter, characteristically well-documented…"

If the bolting horses incident marked an upturn in his fortunes, Joslin either did not recognise it as such, or kept it to himself. There was certainly no mention of it in his letters home.

The reason I have described this episode is because of the profound effect the obstetric mishap appears to have had on Joslin. The death of a patient, mother and/or child, is extremely distressing, not only for the family but for the attending physician/s and nurses. If in fact this is what happened, its effect on Joslin would be devastating. Remember, he was a medical student and therefore unqualified practically and, probably, legally.

Why then the paucity of detail?

Given the enormity of the staff mismanagement leading to this tragedy, with the understandable effect on the medical student/s in attendance, surely there would have been consequences. If such a thing were to happen today, given the existing litigious mindset in certain sectors of the community, the resulting train of events would pose serious questions for all concerned, including the hospital.

The pioneering work of the late Dr Priscilla White in the management of diabetic pregnancies, which was respected throughout the world and which put the Joslin name in textbooks of obstetrics and paediatrics the world over, would certainly have given this incident in the formative years of the founder's training a cogent historical significance.

Yet there was not a single mention of it in any writings by Joslin or during my time in Boston his staff, or in later years. Admittedly, having only read of it since starting this project, I have not asked the two surviving members, Donna Younger or Don Barnett, about it. Since Barnett's book covers only the period from the time Joslin started his practice, the incident occurring during his student days falls outside the period covered. However, given that there is some coverage of his student years, one may be forgiven for expecting a reference to this incident.

"The long, newsy letter, characteristically well-documented" is only reproduced in part. Although not addressed to anyone in particular, the reference to the sewing class, a pet project of his mother, indicates that he was answering a letter from her. He wrote of meeting up with a Harvard professor who was holidaying in Freiburg. Clearly missing American cooking and home news, Joslin spoke enthusiastically of the evening, which included dinner, as being "very pleasant." The most pleasant parts were the food and American news.

The routine of visiting hospitals, which took 1 to 2 hours, was described by him as "good cases and they show them quite well." Clearly German medical graduates had a lighter workload, and Joslin noted that the cases were worked up much more carefully. He also noticed the importance and prominence of laboratory work in the German centres. At that time MGH was in the process of building a new laboratory.

Joslin also took advantage of his travels in Germany to brush up on his German. He had employed the services of a German teacher and mentions taking her and her mother to the Hollenthall Valley for an outing.

Clearly he was socially at ease even when in non-English speaking countries, especially Germany. In fact, one gets the impression that from the very beginning of medical school he was a young man full of confidence, whether in the company of fellow students, or teachers and professors. It was the same with older men and women in the community, not only in America but, as seen here, also when away from home.

In the footnote of this letter written a few days later, was a detail which was to have a profound influence in his life. The letter was dated Tuesday, August 18, (1896). The footnote on Thursday, August 20, 1896 said, "Have heard from Frank Denny and he goes to Vienna in about 10 days. I may join him shortly."

(Is withholding this gem of information just to keep you interested, dear reader? Perhaps I'm being influenced by one of Joslin's writing tricks...!)

Early European Influences on Joslin

"Give me a dog... "

Oskar Minkowski 1889

During this journey, Joslin visited centres in Berlin, Strasbourg,

Freiburg, and especially Vienna, Austria. There is little evidence that at this early stage of his career the trip was for any reason other than observing case presentations in different hospitals, visiting the hospital laboratories, and "sitting in" at outpatient clinics to see first-hand the famous professors treating patients. The cities mentioned in Germany were famous throughout the medical world, and this first professional European trip turned out to be the beginning of Joslin's lifelong association with Europe and its many medical luminaries.

By far the most important contact during this initial medical visit was with a man who was to become a guide, some would say a role model, for Joslin for his entire medical career.

Bernhard Naunyn (1839-1925), a German pathologist born in Berlin, had been working in Strasbourg since 1888. When Joslin visited him in 1896 the German professor, who had been appointed to the University Chair of Internal Medicine in 1888, was finishing what was to be one of his most famous contributions. It was a detailed dissertation on diabetes titled *Der Diabetes Melitus* [sic] which was published in 1898. How much direct contact Joslin had with Naunyn during this first visit is not clear.

What is clear however is that Joslin, in a detailed study of diabetes for an oral presentation to the Boylston Medical Society on 17 November 1893, was familiar with the ground-breaking studies on pancreatic diabetes which had been carried out in Naunyn's hospital laboratory. The importance of establishing an association with European medicine was clear to the young physician. Joslin's history would show how active and dynamic this relationship turned out to be.

Another acquaintance made during this visit was with one Oskar Minkowski. Academically accomplished, but by nature reserved, the Harvard medical graduate would undoubtedly have been left speechless with the brilliance of Oskar Minkowski. The irrepressible researcher would have needed little persuasion to recount the drama of the discovery of the connection between the pancreas and diabetes.

The story is beautifully related by Dr Viktor Joergens in an article on von Mering in the on-line diabetes textbook *Diapedia*, in the form of a first person account by Minkowski as follows:

"In April 1889, I went to the biochemical Institute to read some chemical publications, which were not available in our clinic, and I met von Mering in the library. He had recently recommended Lipantin, an oil preparation with 6% of free fatty acids as a replacement of cod-liver oil because he thought that the free fatty acids may be the most important substance acting in cod-liver oil.

Von Mering asked me, "Do you use the Lipantin frequently in your clinic?" "Oh no," I replied. "We give only good butter to our patients and not rancid oil."

"Don't laugh", he said. "Healthy people must metabolise lipids and if the pancreas doesn't work correctly, we have to give metabolised lipids to them."

"Did you prove this in an experiment?" I asked him.

(This conversation was followed by a discussion on how to do the experiment, and finally, Minkowski mentioned that this question should be studied in a dog following pancreatectomy.)

"This is not so easy," continued von Mering, "since the enzymes of the pancreas may still go into the intestines when you perform a ligation of the ductus pancreaticus."

"What I mean is, we should take out the whole pancreas!"

"This operation is impossible," von Mering replied.

Since I did not know about Claude Bernard's publication stating that no animal would survive total pancreatectomy, and due to my young age, overestimating my capacities as a laboratory surgeon, I exclaimed, "There are no impossible operations. Give me a dog and I will take out his pancreas today."

Von Mering replied, "Okay, I have a dog and you can try it." The same day, I performed pancreatectomy in Naunyn's laboratory with the assistance of von Mering. The animal survived and initially seemed to be doing well. The day after the operation, von Mering had to travel to Colmar because his father-in-law was suffering from severe pneumonia.

He had to stay for one week. In the meantime the dog, which had been clean before, started to urinate more and more frequently in the laboratory. I reprimanded the laboratory assistant for not walking the dog frequently enough, but he replied, "I do walk him frequently but this animal is funny. As soon as it returns, it urinates again even immediately after having done it outside." This observation led me to examine the urine of the dog."

Did one of the two contribute more to the discovery? Without the controversial discussion on lipid absorption – which had no relation to the final discovery – the experiments would not have been carried out. Von Mering provided the dogs and they performed surgery together in Naunyn's laboratory. By chance von Mering was not present when the laboratory assistant reported to Minkowski that the dogs were suffering from polyuria. Both collaborated to write the papers. The data collected in April were – shame on our medical journals today – already published by June 1889. The paper was brilliantly written, a masterpiece of a succinct publication – the title and the first sentence provide the full message. Both travelled together to the first World Congress of Physiology in Basel where, on 11 September 1889, Minkowski and von Mering presented one of the diabetic dogs – the highlight of the conference.

Neither of the two claimed to have more merit than the other in the discovery of pancreatic diabetes. They continued to collaborate, and von Mering invited Minkowski to write two chapters in his textbook (Textbook of Internal Medicine 1st Edition, 1901). Von Mering described the discovery of pancreatic diabetes in his chapter on diabetes: "we both found that dogs became diabetic following pancreatectomy" (p985).

They were very different characters – the quiet Minkowski with Jewish roots in Lithuania and an East Prussian education in Königsberg (the city of Immanuel Kant), and von Mering, the extrovert tall nobleman from Cologne, respected as a scientist and admired for his brilliant skills as a swordsman.

Both derived academic benefit from the discovery, but it took more time for Minkowski to be nominated for a senior appointment by a university. This eventually happened in 1906 in the tiny University of Greifswald. Before this he had worked as a Head of Department in a Catholic hospital in Cologne.

von Mering died young, but Minkowski continued to carry out research on diabetes. He was repeatedly nominated but never awarded the Nobel Prize. The esteem of the scientific community for Minkowski was reflected in the unanimous decision to nominate him as the inaugural chairman of the first German Insulin Committee.

This account illustrates what is a frequently debated topic in medical circles, namely the comparative merits ascribed to the different participants in a medical discovery–in this case the critical connection between the pancreas and diabetes. Jorgens was frank, even blunt:

"Whereas Minkowski is commemorated by academic societies (the European Association for the Study of Diabetes awards an annual Minkowski Prize), the memory of Freiherr Josef von Mering has been relatively neglected and he misses all the postmortem honours Minkowski received: no academic prize – no fellowship – no keynote lecture – no street – no monument – no postage stamp."

Bernhard Naunyn, the head of Minkowski's department, somehow managed to downgrade von Mering's contribution to the discovery of pancreatic diabetes in his autobiography by pointing out that Minkowski performed the surgery – his first pancreatectomy in a dog – and von Mering only assisted. But Naunyn's view may be biased, given that Minkowski was one of his preferred collaborators and that Naunyn – a leading figure in diabetology in Germany at the time – claimed some of the success for himself. He mentions in the first edition of his textbook, *Der Diabetes Melitus* [sic], that "the work following this great discovery was mainly carried out by Minkowski, and several others involved will have to be commemorated". Undoubtedly, he was talking about himself."

Viktor Jorgens, in my opinion, fittingly gives unstinting praise and credit to von Mering, calling him "an outstanding bench to bedside scientist with a broad interest in many fields and whose importance in medical history is "truly underestimated". He goes on to comment, "Since he could be called the "grandfather of SGLT inhibitors" for his work on Phlorozin his name may yet become better known in the future," albeit belatedly.

Although the importance of establishing an association with European medicine was clear to Joslin, history shows just how active and dynamic this relationship turned out to be. He visited Europe regularly throughout his career which spanned some sixty years. Between 1896 and 1961 Joslin made fifteen more visits to different European centres. These visits are another way of plotting the upward trajectory of Joslin's reputation and renown from a mere Boston physician to a world authority on diabetes, a pioneer in its management and, in later years, a revered elder statesman especially of the medical community, not only in America but in England and Europe as well.

From the Harvard Medical Library Archives housed in the Countway Library I was able, with the assistance of Dr Donna Younger of the Joslin Diabetes Centre and Mr Jack Eckert of Harvard Medical Library, to access their material on Joslin, and was delighted to discover two handwritten letters by Minkowski and Naunyn to Joslin. Joslin had an admirable capacity not only for establishing contact but, with regular correspondence and his sincere manner, to nurture the relationships which thrived for long periods, many to the end of his life.

Joslin Meets Elizabeth Denny

Vienna was at the top of the list of Joslin's destinations. Dubbed "the Mecca of medicine" by none other than Rudolph Virchow, it was, at least for young American physicians, the European Mecca in the 19th century. Brilliant men had worked there and made contributions and discoveries which altered medical thinking in several areas and remain influential even in today's practice of medicine.

Of particular significance, especially from an obstetric point of view, was the discovery by Ignaz Semmelweis (1818-1865) of the cause of puerperal fever, an infection which led to the deaths of hundreds of mothers of newborn babies until Semmelweis discovered that the infection was carried on the unwashed hands of medical students, doctors and nurses going from the autopsy room to the bedside of women in childbirth. Semmelweis was ridiculed for his claims by the medical authorities of that period and commtted to an asylum for the insane. He died from beatings inflicted on him by guards in the asylum. Today his statue in Vienna, and the Semmelweis University in Budapest named in his honour, bear testimony to his lifesaving scientific discovery. They are also a stark reminder of man's inhumanity to man.

Vienna was a favourite destination for medical men interested in other branches of medicine also. One interesting example was Sir Arthur Conan Doyle, author of the Sherlock Holmes novels, a literary favourite of Joslin (as was Nabokov–for *Lolita*!) Doyle, who was also a physician, studied ophthalmology in Vienna in 1890.

Frank Denny was a classmate from medical school. In Barnett's book there is a photograph of him in a group of students at MGH which also includes Joslin. Glad of the company of someone from home, the two men did the rounds of the hospitals and clinics together. Social activities will no doubt have been much more enjoyable, especially in the company of a fellow graduate–and one who spoke the same language.

Whether or not the two men remained together throughout September, October and November is unclear, although it must be remembered that Vienna at that time was famous not only for its medical and scientific attractions but also for its arts, theatres and restaurants. The Vienna Opera House remains a much sought-after destination to this day, provided one is fortunate enough to secure admission tickets! Certainly the night at the Vienna Opera was the highlight of the Triennial Congress of the International Diabetes Federation I attended in 1979.

In terms of the Joslin story, the significance of his time with Frank Denny lies in the fact that at Christmas 1896 Denny's three sisters had joined the two young men. There is no information to suggest that this was not the first time that Joslin had met any of the Denny sisters. Holt in her memoir of Joslin writes that the group consisting of their brother Francis

133

(Frank) and Joslin together with the three of them spent seven days together holidaying in the Swiss Alps. Continuing Holt's description: "The young people including EPJ made a merry but dignified party with an aura of 'Boston Properness' still surrounding them. A set of old photographs taken in 1896, shows them in the Semmering Pass in the Alps preparing to go for a sleigh ride. They are bundled up to the ears and beyond. The deep snow on the pine trees in the distant white-capped mountains may have been slightly reminiscent of their own White Mountains of New Hampshire when mid-winter really held them fast in its grip".

After the holidays the young men went back to work again and, as often happens with people away from home who have lived in very close family accord, EPJ, at times became homesick. A letter to his family dated Berlin, May 2, 1897, describes one such spell when he wrote:

"It was a great treat to have Frank Denny here and to be able to talk with him about medicine and America. I do not believe you know how very much I have been alone and unless you have tried this way of living for some time you can't know what it means to not freely discuss what you are most interested in."

The letter mentioned several other American students joining them for dinner one evening with Joslin noting that they sat and talked "..from 8:45 to 1:45 without looking at our watches or even realising the time....It is not very long – I'm thankful to say – until I get home.

Yours – Good night, Elliott."

Unexpected Bounty

What a journey!

Upon reflection, this Europe sojourn of 1896 may well be viewed as the most important ever taken by Joslin. It would not be an exaggeration to say that three life-changing events took place in a few short months of his stay there during the latter half of that year.

Firstly he had overcome the depression which had engulfed him following the obstetric incident. Then he had been given new insights in the management of diabetes during his visits to European teachers and researchers, especially Naunyn and Minkowski.

And last but not the least, he had met a young woman who had aroused in him thoughts and emotions which were to culminate in life-changing events for both.

Even though Joslin never spoke specifically of this European trip, it clearly turned out to be an eventful journey in more ways than the new medical graduate could possibly have imagined.

Part 5.
1897

Dr Elliott Proctor Joslin MD

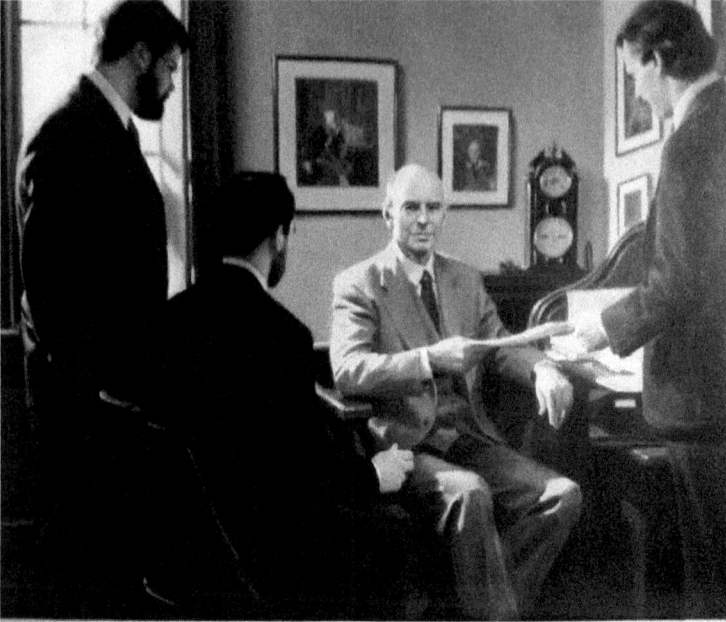

Joslin with a group of interns

Joslin's Internship

In the fall of 1897 the recently graduated Joslin began his internship at the Massachusetts General Hospital. The clinical chief at the time was Reginald Heber Fitz. Already well acquainted with him as a student and remembering the effect of Mary Higgins on Joslin, Fitz suggested a project in addition to his ward duties. He asked Joslin to look at the records of all diabetics admitted to the Massachusetts General Hospital between 1824 and 1898. Case-oriented approach to investigation of disease was a much used method of study by professor- physicians in the early decades of the 20th century. Osler, the author of the textbook of medicine in use at that time, emphasised the benefit of identifying the natural sequence of medical conditions, usually referred to as the natural history of the disease. Keeping track of the patient (follow up) would further clarify the development of new features (signs and symptoms) of the condition.

A ledger listing 10 to 12 characteristics of a condition at the time the patient was first seen and new signs detected as the disease progressed would help in understanding the condition. Medical records at the time of Joslin's internship were being scrutinised to find ways to improve them. The popular concept of doctors' handwriting being difficult, if not impossible, to decipher perhaps arose at that time and was, in many cases, justified. This was one of the improvements suggested by the senior men at the time of Joslin's internship, and the importance of this lesson was not lost on the young graduate. In later years Joslin was well known for his insistence on the need for accurate and legible entry of laboratory values of tests on patients in a flow sheet format.

The eager intern's search for diabetes in MGH patients over the 74 year period (1824 -1898) was not particularly successful. Only 172 cases were discovered and, in all probability, underestimated the frequency of the condition. There is little information on methods of classifying the diseases of patients admitted to the hospital at that time. It is possible that diabetes was not the main reason for their admission and therefore not recorded. It is well known that diabetes, especially in the adult, is frequently silent in that it does not cause any symptoms and therefore may not be recognised.

This exercise, however, produced interesting results many years later in Joslin's professional journey.

Joslin's First Presentation at a Scientific Meeting

"The doctor ordered me to taste my urine"!

Never one to vacillate, Joslin completed the study within six months. That he received much guidance and advice from Fitz is evident not only in the clear and orderly presentation of the information but also in the substance of the article. More importantly, as described below, prior to its publication Fitz had accompanied Joslin to an oral presentation of the paper at the 49th annual meeting of the American Medical Association held at Denver, Colorado 7–10 June 1898.

The journal article, six pages long, together with six tables, was published in *The Boston Medical and Surgical Journal* the following month on 23 July 1898. It contained a concise description of the main manifestations of diabetes and a dramatic illustration of the remarkable increase ("explosion" in some journalists' jargon) in the variety of ways it affected individuals. As in his Boylston Society paper, Joslin traced the history of the condition in detail. He also noted that until 1851 the diagnosis of diabetes was made only by tasting the urine. That was a duty usually delegated to the house physician (resident medical officer/intern) by the senior (attending) physician! One suspects that in private practice during house calls the patient may have been given that task! Joslin, ever the diplomat, did not dwell on this particular point.It is probable, however, that the patient was occasionally called upon to use this method, for in 1831 the statement appears "on tasting as directed to do so by the physician….. It was found to be sweet." If Joslin had hoped for audience reaction, even participation with enjoyment of a lighter moment, he had, for once, misread the mood of the staid audience of physicians. He finished his presentation by noting that treatment options were minimal and there were no drugs available at that time. "The only drug which has been persistently used in the treatment throughout this entire period [till 1898] is opium".

More interesting–and revealing–were attitudes prevailing at that time as recorded during the discussion which followed the conclusion of the presentation. The first two questions were both related to race, namely "the Negro race" and "the Jew" or "the Hebrew race."

One physician commented, "I notice the Doctor said that no cases occurred among the Negro race." The ever alert Joslin was quick to reply, "One case reported."

Even more thought-provoking was another "racial "(today it would be "racist") observation.

"I would suggest that the Hebrew race probably have this disease more than any other people on account of their love of high living. It is a well-known fact that they eat largely of such foods that are irritating more than any other class of people. They are given to parties, they congregate

140

together and have frequent and irregular meals. I believe it is from that fact that they have this disease more than any other people."

Clearly, that was an era of little racial diversity.

The conclusion of the discussion was as follows:

Dr Stockton of Buffalo," I rise to call attention to the historic value of the paper. I think this paper is a very useful illustration of the principle expounded this morning in the general address in medicine by Dr Musser.

Dr Joslin – "In reading my paper, much was necessarily omitted on account of lack of time. The printed article will contain answers to the preceding questions."

Joslin, probably instinctively from looking at such a large number of diabetics at this early stage of his career, suspected that there was much more to the condition than he had realised. He may well have been overwhelmed by the volume of clinical information he had collected and would have struggled to put it in any kind of perspective without the help of Fitz. Whether or not he was satisfied with his presentation to the American Medical Association is hard to say.

Joslin never forgot Fitz's influence on his career. I have a copy of a handwritten letter from him to Fitz's son, also called Reginald, signed as " a House Pupil of your Father R.H. Fitz at the M.G.H. 1894-1896."

His time at Strasbourg had repeatedly come to mind, especially after acquiring Naunyn's textbook which he had bought upon its release only a few months before he presented his paper in Colorado. Joslin had not forgotten the comprehensive study of the treatment of diabetes through dietary restriction described in an earlier book by the same writer. During Joslin's recent visit Naunyn had spoken about the forthcoming publication providing a fuller, up-to-date description of the subject.

The 1898 publication of *Der Diabetes Melitus* [sic] guaranteed Naunyn a place in the history of diabetes, even in the history of medicine. The tome of 551 pages published by Alfred Holder of Vienna–the copy I consulted online was printed in 1906–presented a comprehensive and succinct description of diabetes, including results of laboratory investigations pertinent to the way the thinking on the condition had developed in light of experimental findings up to that time. The investigation of the role of the pancreas which I described earlier and which had been carried out in Naunyn's laboratory by Minkowski and von Merrin was, deservedly, given prominent exposure.

Joslin was keen to show the material he had gathered to the German professor, especially as the new graduate's project "was begun for the purpose of seeking evidence with regard to the *pancreatic origin* of this disease.".

However, the possibility of visiting Strasbourg presented a problem because he was already committed to the next step in his medical apprenticeship.

At that time the pathway for medical training after completing the year of internship was to join the practice of a senior physician and learn the ropes of day-to-day management of patients with conditions which today would be called general medicine. In practice, even doctors known for their particular expertise in a given field still practised as today's primary care physicians or general practitioners.

Joslin had already secured such a position with the distinguished Dr James Jackson Putnam of Boston. Never one to leave a task unfinished, he persuaded Putnam to let him go to Strasbourg. Doubtless out of respect for the senior man he would have told him the reason. Putnam, being fully aware of the benefits of guidance from European experts as he himself had experienced, agreed to Joslin's deferring the start to his assistantship for a few weeks.

Neither Putnam nor Joslin was to know that this relatively short study leave would play a crucial role in a critical but tragic relationship between the two men 15 years later.

Within days of completing his internship in the fall of 1898, Joslin left for Strasbourg.

Unlike his previous meeting with the distinguished professor, the new graduate could now approach him armed with a body of information for which, at this stage of his career, he could justifiably plead lack of perspective and experience. And who better to guide him than the widely respected and eminent German?

According to Holt, the purpose of the visit was "to work and study under the best authority on the subject to be found anywhere". The clinical information gathered from his study of the MGH patients provided a platform for some intensive tutoring. Naunyn's opinions on diabetes inspired Joslin with insights into the condition none of his supervisors in Boston would have had the knowledge or experience to provide at that time. The knowledge of diabetes in America was not nearly as advanced as it was in Europe. Certainly there was no one with the experience of Naunyn. Neither had anyone in America published a book on the subject to match *der Diabetes Melitus*.

In fact, there was no English-speaking textbook on the subject in the English speaking world in 1898.

Just what, if anything, Naunyn said about Joslin's MGH study is not known. What is evident is the message Naunyn was able to impress upon his young visitor.

This was an attitude of optimism to replace the doom and gloom view so widely held at that time, especially in the management of diabetic children. Joslin was shown the results of the improvement possible in adults with diabetes, especially those who were overweight, which, though not as common then as it is now, was nevertheless present in a large number of patients. Simply by restricting the amount of food eaten, especially the starchy and sugary items, the sugar in the urine all but disappeared and the patients felt much better.

The effect was the same in children, but it was clear even then that the condition was different in the young ones compared to adults. Once again, *unlike many children today, children in those days were usually not overweight.*

The outlook for the young ones was pathetic, with death resulting from coma even after minor infections like a cold. Most children did not survive longer than two years. Even in these, Naunyn showed Joslin that restricting the diet reduced the loss of sugar in the urine, admittedly at the cost of further weight loss and the risk of semi-starvation. At that time there was little if any alternative to this, and the only defence for this strategy was that it bought time in the hope that a cure may be found. History shows that this, in fact, is what happened, but tragically not until 1921 as recounted later.

The critical effect of this time with Naunyn was that Joslin could see that there was a reason for hope. The deeply religious American had something to offer these patients. Joslin read the Bible every night. The importance of faith, hope and love (charity) did not need to be emphasised to him. The importance of providing hope to any person who is afflicted by a serious illness, especially one with the ever present possibility of death, can never be overstated.

Whether or not Joslin realised that this journey he had undertaken was to change his life is not clear. What is clear is that he was convinced that he could offer meaningful hope to patients with diabetes.

The article he wrote on his return made no mention of the MGH study. It was an eloquent piece of prose to present reasons for hope and optimism in the treatment of this hitherto hopeless condition.

Little wonder then that the German physician "for ever thereafter strongly influenced Dr Joslin all through his long medical career, and whose wisdom he so often quoted".

According to Joslin himself, Naunyn was "...the most noted specialist in diabetes at the beginning of the 20th century. Following my visit to his Clinic I attempted to use his methods and even now [1960] can think of no guiding principles superior to those which he then employed. Of course that was more than 20 years before the discovery of insulin...".

The influence of Naunyn on Joslin was evident from the beginning of the latter's entry into medical practice in 1898. It is seen in the very first of 17 papers he wrote in the eight–year period between 1898 and 1906, (*Boston Medical and Surgical Journal* 139:176–177, August 18, 1898.) Given that Joslin had only just returned from Germany a few weeks earlier, the paper may well have been suggested by Naunyn. For someone who had not seen many diabetics except for the medical records of the patients he had studied during the previous 12 months, the statements in this paper raise interesting questions and may even have raised some eyebrows in the conservative Boston medical establishment!! For someone with such limited experience in diabetes, the article could almost be interpreted as exhibiting unjustifiable zeal and confidence. Was he a self-appointed champion of the views of his new-found hero?

Barnett quoted excerpts from Joslin's article in his book as follows:

"..textbooks (state) so frequently that diabetes is incurable that the practitioner loses all his enthusiasm the moment a patient with the disease presents himself."

In contrast to this gloomy picture is the hopeful view of Naunyn in the following quotation, that cases apparently severe at the onset when subjected to a vigorous treatment, take a proportionally favourable course, while others running a severe course are, as a rule, those subjected late or not at all to careful treatment... in my opinion a broader, more definitive purpose should be put in the treatment, namely the strengthening of the deranged bodily function, at least the checking of further disintegration of the same. This change of view is our first step towards an improved treatment of diabetes. Barnett observes that this quotation reveals both Dr Joslin's admiration for the work of the Strasbourg professor and the need to bring optimism to the treatment of patients with this disorder.

Joslin Starts Medical Practice

To say that Joslin began his medical practice with a challenging schedule would be an understatement! He did not allow himself to "test the waters", so to speak, but dived headlong into a program which even experienced practitioners would have found daunting.

As was common practice, he started as an assistant.

James Jackson Putnam (1846–1918) had studied neurology in Europe and London. He was known for his reputation for sound scientific judgement and unimpeachable integrity. Becoming his assistant also opened more doors for Joslin. Like most physicians with a speciality, Putnam's practice also had many patients with the commoner maladies for which the afflicted seek the opinion and treatment of a doctor. Neurological disease is much less frequent than the commoner complaints of say, infections in the lung and the gastrointestinal system. Putnam himself tended to concentrate on the former leaving the simpler and non-neurologic problems to his assistant.

As assistant to Dr Putnam, Joslin had to visit patients at home and in hospitals. This involved travelling between the bigger hospitals, including Massachusetts General and New England Deaconess as well as smaller ones such as Corey Hill and Faulkner. If not during the day, certainly by the end of it, the assistant had to report to the senior man regarding his patients' progress.

In addition to all this Joslin was also treating his own patients in his home office at 517 Beacon Street. Putnam was incredulous when he saw the amount of work his assistant could get through in a 24-hour period.

"Be a Leper"

The strong work ethic inculcated in Neo-Puritan youths from an early age and which persisted throughout life certainly applied to Joslin as it did to many of his contemporaries. Holt recalled that "E.P.J. always enjoyed work for its own sake as well as for the results it brought. None of his accomplishments during his entire life was gained without long hours of thoughtful, hard work. He used to talk about the teacher of Economics at Yale, Professor Sumner, who, when discussing with his class the eight-hour-day labour law, remarked that he could not complete his work in eight hours but needed to keep at it for at least 10 hours. His young student (Joslin) made his own mental note of this statement, deciding that if it took a brilliant man like Billy Sumner 10 hours to do his work, he (Joslin) would have to take 12, anyway."

Joslin was not unique in his work habits. His contemporary Harvey Cushing, known in medical school for his meticulous note- taking and beautiful anatomical drawings achieved through painstaking and laborious effort, when asked by his fellow students the secret of his success, was characteristically blunt. "Be a leper," he said, "that is what I have decided to do." After that Cushing is said to have refused practically all social invitations "that would have wasted his evenings."

During his time as assistant to Putnam, Joslin, in 1900, wrote an article on the findings in one of Putnam's patients who had contracted meningitis. It was a report which in all probability stemmed from Joslin's acting more like a hospital medical officer under the supervision of the senior man. The only article written jointly with Putnam was published in his first year as Putnam's assistant. This paper in 1898, was based on a patient with an anatomical anomaly of the stomach associated with melancholia, an anachronistic term for depression. Putnam, a neurologist, would have had an interest in the associated psychiatric disorder as at that time psychiatry was not as distinctly separated from neurology as it is now.

It is interesting that in addition to all the new tasks he had to perform as an assistant medical practitioner throughout 1898 and 1899, Joslin continued to publish, mostly in the *Boston Medical and Surgical Journal*, articles on gastroenterology.

His appetite whetted by the diabetes studies he had carried out on MGH patients, he embarked on a similar study of gastric ulcers treated at the same institution from 1888 to 1898.

At a reunion after his death, one of Joslin's former assistants Dr Albert Horner observed that "before Dr Joslin specialised in diabetes, his contributions to gastrointestinal disorders was great." Indeed, at the beginning of his career as a physician, most of Joslin's publications were on gastrointestinal diseases.

Putnam, who had graduated from Harvard Medical School, had retained his connections with it, including commitment to teaching students. This was an advantage to Joslin and probably a reason for his seeking to join the older man, as he was able to maintain his own connections there.

Thus he continued to teach medical students at the bedside and in group tutorials. His association with his alma mater also continued through working on different committees. He also remained in touch with medical students through the Boylston Society and as a faculty adviser.

Joslin's interest in note-taking was emphasised in a paper he wrote for the *Boston Medical and Surgical Journal* in 1894, in which he included a list of 491 cases shown to the third class of the Harvard Medical School. His aptitude for record-keeping of large numbers of patients found its zenith in the remarkable Joslin "Register" (also called Ledger) of patients seen in his practice. In later years the register provided information not only for his voluminous writings, but also proved useful for several other purposes, including the life insurance industry.

Academic Appointments

Joslin's first appointment at Harvard Medical School was immediately after his internship in 1898, when he became Assistant in the Department of Physiological Chemistry. He could not have foreseen but doubtlessly remembered the advice and encouragement of Chittenden which was proving not only accurate but almost prophetic. This appointment brought him into contact with William Pickering Bowditch, the Professor and Head of the Department and Dean of the faculty. The nature of medical politics is such that Joslin's earlier contact with Bowditch in the course of preparing his Boylston Society presentation back in 1893 would have been remembered by the older man and would certainly have helped Joslin onto the first rung of the academic ladder.

Two years later, in 1900, he became Assistant in the Theory and Practice of Physic. (Physic is an old term for medicine. Although largely considered archaic, it is still used at Harvard. The Chief of Medicine and Chairman of the Department is still called the Professor of Theory and Practice of Physic.)

(During my time in Boston I was delighted to meet, and, on several occasions, see patients with Professor George Thorne who occupied this position. It was a special association for me because he was also the editor- in- chief of Harrison, the textbook of medicine which was the recommended text in the Faculty of Medicine at Sydney University.)

Joslin remained on the staff of Harvard University and progressed through the academic ranks to Clinical Professor of Medicine in 1925. When he reached the age of 68, he followed the usual precedent of becoming an Emeritus Professor, a position he held for life.

It is clear that from an early stage in his career Joslin had harboured private ambitions which did not include senior academic positions. This is supported by Donald Barnett's account in his biography of Joslin, in which he said that the position of the Dean of Harvard Medical School had been offered to Joslin in the early 1900s but Joslin had declined. His forceful personality as well as a remarkable capacity for time management, people management and administration were evident even at this stage of his life.

Popular as a leader and effective as a committee member, Joslin was co-opted into a committee for raising funds for extensions to student accommodation. He was elected as the spokesman to launch an appeal for funds from the public, and on more than one occasion broadcast the appeal on Boston radio. Even allowing for the quality of the taped recording at that time it is interesting to hear his voice on the radio. Although there is no record of his having any actual training for this, his voice was well modulated, clear and forceful in his conviction in the worthiness of the cause being promoted. Even at this early stage all who came across him, including the senior men at Harvard, could see a bright future for this multitalented and dynamic young physician.

In the Harvard archives I discovered correspondence from Harvey Cushing seeking Joslin's advice when, upon arriving in Boston from Johns Hopkins, he had difficulties with the bureaucrats at Harvard Medical School and the associated teaching hospital, Peter Bent Brigham, in his efforts to establish the hitherto unrecognised specialty of neurosurgery.

Joslin's enthusiasm for the role of the library in medical teaching established a lifelong connection with the Harvard Medical Library. In later years one of his closest younger associates, Anna Holt, became first the assistant and later the chief librarian of the Harvard Medical Library. Thus Joslin's association with that library continued from the beginning to the end of his medical career.

Many patients in the late 1800s and early 1900 were treated in one of the many smaller hospitals in Boston. Joslin was quick to establish contacts in several of these, including Corey Hill and the Faulkner Hospital, both of which were in the Jamaica Plain area, close to the Longwood Avenue Harvard medical establishments. Emily Denny, an older sister of Joslin's wife Elizabeth, was a secretary to the Board of Governors of Faulkner Hospital.

Joslin was associated with the New England Deaconess Hospital (usually referred to as the Deaconess) from its very beginnings before the turn of the 19th century. He was also its Chief Physician, a position he retained to the end of his life.

Boston has always been known as a Mecca for excellent medical meetings, and this was so even in Joslin's time. Local meetings were usually scheduled weekly. There were also national meetings which were held annually in different American cities. He tried to attend them all.

He maintained his contacts in Europe and, once he had finished working with Putnam, visited European centres particularly Paris, Vienna and Germany regularly.

The archives of the Massachusetts General Hospital hold several old copies of publications from Harvard University of notices of public lectures on wide-ranging subjects, varying from precautions for avoiding pneumonia to treatment of diarrhoea. Joslin was a frequent lecturer.

One other aspect of Joslin's association with Putnam is of interest. It is clear that he was much liked not only by the senior man but also by his wife. His wife was a Cabot and the Cabots were prominent in Boston social circles. They were part of a very select group of Boston's citizens known as *First Citizens.* Indeed, such was the esteem in which they were held, that they were the subject of a well-known jingle:

"And here's to good old Boston,
The land of the bean and the cod,
Where Lowells talk only to Cabots,
And Cabots talk only to God."

Needless to say, Putnam's new assistant, already known in medical circles in Boston but now in the public eye, would have been noticed as much for his impeccable bearing and courteous manner as for his conscientiousness in the care of his patients.

It is equally clear that the young man was very welcome in the home of the Putnams. Joslin had become very fond of Frances, the youngest daughter of the couple, born on 20 October 1897. In her memoir Putnam's wife wrote "Dr. Joslin was struck by Frances' quiet good nature as an infant. He gave her a silver lucky piece on a blue ribbon along with a note that was signed "Your would-be admirer, Elliott P Joslin."

Not that there ever had been any doubt about Joslin's being a success not only in his career but in life, but once he started medical practice it became increasingly clear that, with each stage of his progress professionally, he impressed all those around him with his work ethic and his capacity for relating to others. In short, he was quickly recognised as an ideal "go-to person." This would also account for his involvement in the number of activities and commitments which would be beyond most people at this stage of their lives and professional responsibilities.

Little wonder then that there seemed little time for anything else.But, as in the past, the highly organised and self-disciplined young man made time. His commitment to the religious side of his life was steadfast and regular. Since moving from Oxford to Beacon Street in Boston, Joslin had become a regular member of the congregation of the Old South Church in Copley Square in the city. He was a deacon of the church and discharged the duties of the office faithfully to the end of his life.

And there was more!

Part 6.
Elizabeth

Elizabeth Elliot Denny Marries Joslin

The New England reserve of Joslin's memoirist Anna Holt and his younger associate Barnett may be held to account for their reticence in the matter of one Elizabeth Denny.

If Joslin was smitten after the meeting mentioned earlier in this account he didn't say so – would the New England properness frown on such forwardness? However, it was after the visit of the young women that Joslin spoke of his loneliness. It is the only time this is mentioned in any publication.

I found no record of any further contact with Elizabeth, the youngest of the three sisters or for that matter any interaction with any of the Dennys. However, given Joslin's history of socialising with young men and women in his different social circles, it is more than likely that he did keep in touch with the Dennys. My enquiries and search for details of any overtures of friendship by Joslin – dare I say courtship – met with an impenetrable wall of silence. There was a total lack of any notes, letters or photographs in any publication. I never saw any letters from Joslin to Elizabeth, or vice versa.

Yet clearly there was much interaction between their first meeting and the four years which followed because towards the end of my search I discovered a copy of one of the "Joslin Moments" titled, *Elliott P Joslin, MD, marries Elizabeth Denny.*

The wedding took place on 16 September 1902.

According to the "Moments", Joslin had met Elizabeth Denny while hiking in the Swiss Alps. According to Holt however, the couple had met earlier when Joslin had gone from Freiburg to Vienna to join up with his Massachusetts General Hospital fellow intern Francis Denny in August 1898.

Joslin had made a second trip around Christmas that year when the three Denny sisters had come to Europe to join their brother for Christmas at around which time they had all gone for a hike in the Swiss Alps. Holt's description is as follows, "the young people, including EPJ, made a merry but dignified party with an aura of Boston "properness" still surrounding them. A set of old photographs taken in 1896, shows them at the Semmering Pass in the Alps preparing to go for a sleigh ride. They are bundled up to the ears and beyond. The deep snow on the pine trees in the distant White Mountains may have been slightly reminiscent of their own White Mountains of New Hampshire when midwinter really held them fast in its grip. After the holidays the young men went back to work again....."

No mention of any romance there! However, there was a footnote: "The youngest sister in 1902 became EPJ's wife and the treasured and beloved 'Aunt Elizabeth' of several generations of the Joslin and Denny families."

In all likelihood the Dennys would have first heard of Joslin from his classmate Francis Denny. Holt speaks of the Dennys being somewhat taken aback by Joslin's insistence that the marriage take place sooner rather than later, which was in keeping with his personal motto of "do it now." Clearly a compromise was reached, and the usual 12 month period for preparations was reduced to 6.

"The Joslin Moments" is valuable for a photograph of the couple, not a formal wedding photograph but one clearly taken the same year. Joslin is in a three-piece suit, a high neck shirt and tie with a watch chain visible on his waistcoat. Elizabeth Joslin is in a full length dress held in at the waist, neck and wrists. Her attire, in vogue in the early 1900s, was in keeping with the Victorian style of dress for women, being simpler and less fussy than the elaborate frilly garments of the Edwardian era. Also reflecting the fashion of the times, her hair was tightly styled with a centre part. In spite of the formal attire Joslin looks relaxed, and the faded photograph shows a hint of a smile, a decidedly infrequent feature of his photographs until very late in life. Very much a well-dressed, prosperous Boston couple!

Next to this photograph taken during the year of their wedding is a group photo taken in the late 1950s showing the Joslins with friends and several of their grandchildren. This was taken at Buffalo Hill Farm, the Joslin country estate in Oxford.

Following his marriage, Joslin moved from his parents' city house at 517

Beacon Street (where he had started his medical practice in 1898) to an apartment at 421 Marlborough Street. He continued to practise in the Beacon Street house (which had been considerably modified to accommodate the needs of his practice) until 1905, when he moved his office and residence to the newly built premises at 81 Bay State Road.

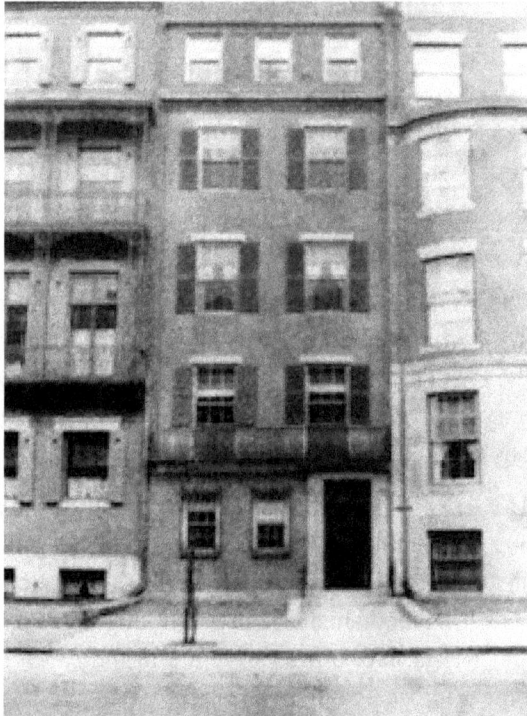

81 Bay State Road

The Dennys were a well-known and moneyed Boston family who could trace their origins through several generations over more than 200 years back to England. The family lived in fashionable Brookline which provides homes for the wealthy even to this day. A house in the most sought-after area in Brookline, called Pill Hill because of the large number of doctors residing there, is still listed in their historic homes as being built for Emily Denny, one of Elizabeth's older sisters. Incidentally, the architect of the house was a descendant of Ralph Waldo Emerson, who was related to Joslin through his mother, Sarah Ann

Emerson Proctor. In the Joslin archives I discovered several letters written (in longhand) by Joslin to Emily, clearly a popular aunt in the Joslin household. A further connection between Joslin and Emily Denny was that the latter was a senior secretary at the Faulkner Hospital, one of the many smaller hospitals Joslin used for his private patients.

(The adjacent suburb of Allston does not have the same reputation for wealth. Accordingly rents for apartments in Allston are considerably lower. My wife and I had rented an apartment in Allston, separated from Brookline by one cross street and a 30% reduction in the monthly rent! The difference in wealth and status in different parts of the neighbouring suburbs was still very much in evidence 70 years after the time of Elliott and Elizabeth Joslin).

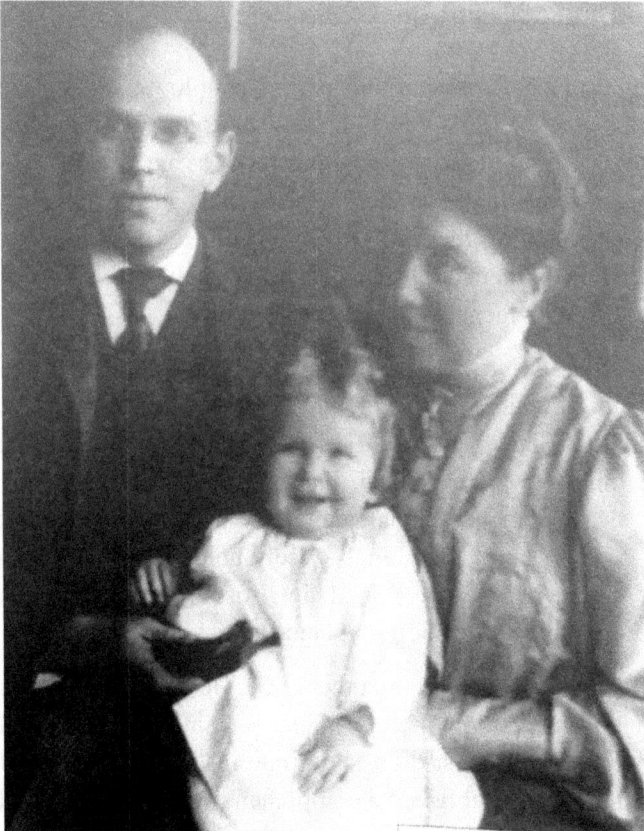

Joslin with wife Elizabeth and daughter Mary

Their first child, Mary, was born on 3 March 1904 then in 1906 a son Allen and in 1908 their youngest, Elliott.

By 1904, Joslin had been an assistant to Putnam for six years. He had been married for two years and with the birth of his second child, as well as the pressures of starting the construction of his home/office, not to mention his own ever expanding and increasingly demanding private practice, he realised that the time had come for him to pursue his own goals.

In 1904 Joslin ended his tenure as assistant to James Putnam. However he maintained a close association with the Putnams throughout his life.

Birth of The Joslin Clinic 1906

Joslin, like other doctors of the period, employed an assistant upon starting his practice. He involved his assistants in most, if not all, aspects of his work. In addition to assigning tasks as needed to care for his patients, especially in the smaller hospitals, he made them feel part of his team by encouraging them to work with him on his clinical research projects. Many of them published scientific articles as his co-authors. He kept in touch with them even after they left him.

Joslin's first assistant was a young medical graduate, Harry W Goodall. Goodall stayed with Joslin from 1904 to 1908. The second assistant was Dr Frederick A Stanwood, 1908–1912, then Dr F Gorham Brigham, 1912 – 1915, followed by the fourth, Dr Albert A Horner, 1915–1920. In addition there were occasional temporary assistants as mentioned by Barnett, who spoke of a Dr Hugh Greely helping out with a particular patient. Albert Horner remained in Boston, eventually becoming Physician-in-Chief at the New England Baptist Hospital.

One of the ex-Joslin staff members, Dr George P Kozak, a senior physician during my time there, who has remained a close friend, is still in practice at "The Baptist" as a senior internist and diabetologist. While at the Joslin, Kozak published a comprehensive textbook on diabetes as well as one on the management of diabetic foot problems. (*Clinical Diabetes Mellitus*, W.B. Saunders & Co. 1982 and *Management of*

Diabetic Foot Problems, W.B. Saunders & Co. 1984).

In 1920 Joslin employed Dr Howard F Root as an assistant, and later as an associate. Root remained with Joslin for the rest of his life as the second member of his team. Over the next 30 years Joslin appointed five more physicians. These six physicians together with the founder became known as "The Original Seven".

When I took up my fellowship at The Joslin in 1969, five of "The Original Seven"– Joslin and Root had died – were still in active practice. I consider that time and my association with each one of those remarkable physicians as one of the greatest privileges of my professional life.

The Marlborough Street apartment to which Joslin and his bride had moved after their marriage was convenient, being just around the corner from his office and close to the Harvard Medical School and the nearby hospitals. But the couple wanted a larger home. Even though there is no evidence at any time in Joslin's life that there was any shortage of money, the funds for the new home were partly provided from his wife's legacy. The block bought on Bay State Road overlooked the Charles River. At that time this was just a tidal stream which at low tide, especially during hot, humid summer months for which Boston is notorious, brought into the area a most unpleasant, sulphurous, rotten- egg odour.

81 Bay State Road was chosen as the site where, between 1904 and 1906, the couple built a five-level townhouse incorporating Joslin's office for conducting his practice as well as accommodation for his young and growing family.

During the late 19th century new homes in the Bay State Road area became known for the Revival style of which there are five main types: Classical, Renaissance, Georgian, Federal and Tudor.

According to a current website which had a section on the history of Bay State Road, "81 Bay State Road was the home of Dr Joslin who lived in this 'Classical Revival' house." Barnett, who had visited the house, referred to the area as "classically beautiful 19th-century Back Bay Boston." At the time Joslin first moved to 81 Bay State Road it was part of a Harley Street of London type address for many doctors. It also had some of the most magnificent mansions in the area especially those facing Charles River". Barnett recalled that the house was a "deceptively large residence."

For 50 years Joslin would live and practise at this address, where his life's work would reach heights few could have imagined.

The Joslin Clinic, as 81 Bay State Road came to be known, became the destination of literally thousands of patients from Boston and beyond for the next 50 years. It was also the destination for scores of physicians from different parts of the world, including Europe, Britain, South America, and Canada, as well as American physicians from Massachusetts and other states.

These doctors stayed a few days to a week to observe the methods used by Joslin and his associates to treat diabetes. Later, through fellowships awarded to younger physicians, The Joslin became a temporary home for these graduates, most commonly for one year but occasionally (as in my case,) for longer.

Today 81 Bay State Road is part of the inner campus of Boston University with residences and fraternity houses. Joslin is remembered with his former home/office being called Joslin Hall, which is used as a dormitory for graduates.

The five-level brick construction with a basement was completed in 1906 shortly after the Joslins had had their second child, a son whom they called Allen Proctor Joslin, following the custom of giving the eldest son, the first name of his paternal grandfather.

Outwardly, 81 Bay State Road was architecturally similar to the adjoining houses. However, the internal structure was custom designed to serve as a fully equipped office for Joslin's practice as well as a residence befitting a popular and successful Boston physician.

At ground level, just inside the front entrance, there was a small laboratory and an office for several secretaries. Joslin had learnt the value of laboratory analysis and tests, initially from his time with Chittenden, but even more so from his visits to Europe, especially Germany.

The second floor afforded space for his office which included an examining room and a toilet. The waiting area for patients was in a spacious hall outside Joslin's office. On the same level was located the dining room which had French doors opening to the view across the Charles River to Cambridge situated beyond. The dining room was wood-panelled in light oak. There was a long dining table and a fireplace in the far wall. Holt recalls that Mrs. Joslin always sat with her back to the fire with "the Doctor" at the opposite end and the children and guests along the sides. Past the office, still on the second floor, was a wide, curved staircase to the third floor, where directly above the dining room was a living room, also with a large fireplace. The master bedroom, on the third level, overlooking Bay State Road, was directly above the doctor's office. It is said that Mrs Joslin would tap gently on the floor with the heel of her slipper when she felt that EPJ had burned enough midnight oil and needed to be reminded that he really should stop work and come to bed. The fourth and fifth floors were devoted to the nursery, maids' quarters and guest rooms.

Joslin himself never spoke of his ambitions as such. Rather, he pursued with unrelenting vigour his plans in every area of his life, not only as a physician but also as a religious and responsible member of the community. Even at this early stage of his career Joslin was a physician, a tutor of medical students, a lecturer (to the public) on common health issues, as well as an active member of his church and a committed family man. As will be seen, he was not only going to build premises for his practice and his home but was going to build much more on both fronts– and with minimal delay! The destiny of the son of a shoe-manufacturing merchant from Oxford was clearly going to be different from his father's, as it would be from that of his mother's family, the Proctors. Despite this, Joslin never forgot his roots. As noted by Barnett, the use of agrarian metaphors, especially in his manuals for patients with diabetes, had its origins in his childhood in Oxford.

A Private Ambition: Buffalo Hill

"Those who lose dreaming are lost."

(Australian aboriginal proverb.)

Almost immediately after completing the construction of his home/office in Boston, Joslin and his wife started planning a country retreat. It would appear that Joslin was determined to go back to Oxford, for there is no mention of any other location being sought for this purpose. This, more than anything else, indicates the strong ties between Joslin and the village of his early years, even though he had left home for boarding school at Leicester Academy in 1883, when only 14 years old. Undoubtedly the beauty of the village, which it retains to this day, would have been a reason, but even more so it was Joslin's happy childhood which drew him back to the historic town.

The idea of establishing a country estate was clearly a departure from the mindset and practices of his father, who had stopped building projects once his business premises and the family home on Main Street had been completed. The family home in Oxford continued to be used by his father, and later by his older brother Homer for many years after the death of Joslin's father.

As his plans evolved it became clear that Joslin had an entirely different vision for his personal and professional life. He had dreams. He was going to be more than just a successful Boston physician. Much more!

"The actual location for their country house was found after a diligent search by the couple. The young doctor and his wife went prospecting by horse and carriage all about the countryside carefully considering various locations. They even inspected old farmhouses which could be renovated to serve as their future country retreat.

At long last the spot was found on a rocky hilltop overlooking the town of Oxford. The land was bought..." (Holt).

One aspect of Joslin's marriage which has become increasingly clear, not only through my reading but looking at the way he charted his professional and personal (domestic) progress, is the unfailing and patient cooperation of his wife Elizabeth. Indeed, apart from the naming of the country estate, one sees only Joslin's hand in virtually every aspect of construction and development.

Elizabeth, though present, is silent. Her silence was one of the more challenging aspects of my research and a reason for nearly giving up on it.

Just as the selected site was described as "rocky", so, as it turned out, were the early experiences of the young couple in taming the inhospitable plot–rocky!

The area had been a long-neglected pasture. It was overgrown and home to wildlife, not the animals the city-bred mother of three imagined. Somewhat apprehensive of living in a house which, compared to her city dwelling, seemed like living in the wilderness, she feared that there may be wild animals to contend with and asked her husband about the "beasties." When Joslin asked what animals she feared, Elizabeth answered, "wild buffalo." Although, at the time, keeping a straight face, he hastily reassured his bride on that score, the incident was recalled with much hilarity in the years ahead, which she accepted in good humour. However she may or may not have favoured the name Buffalo Hill for the recounting of the reason for it over the years!

Buffalo Hill remained in the family for several generations and, although in the intervening years parts of its land holdings have been sold, the house, still in good repair, is used by Joslin's grandchildren and great-grandchildren. It is preserved by the Historical Commission of Oxford as a homage to its founder, regarded by the town as one of her finest sons.

At first the land was cleared by hand by members of the family working during weekends. Even Joslin's father Allen now in his late 70s and somewhat frail joined in. Too weak to wield a metal crowbar, he used a sturdy wooden pole to dig out the smaller rocks and stones. The pole, now labelled, became a treasured family relic in the Joslin household. Joslin used it as a prop in his oft-repeated story, especially to the grandchildren, about the building of Buffalo Hill.

Details of the actual construction of the farmhouse are scant except that it was "a traditional New England farmhouse" built between 1908 and 1911.

The Oxford Reconnaissance Report of 2007 describes the farm house design as "vernacular". Vernacular architecture refers to designing buildings using local materials and designs so as to achieve a construction compatible with the surroundings as well as suitable for the purpose for which it was built.

The long barn had an apartment at one end, built for a caretaker to live there during the summer and oversee haying operations. Later a second house was built (around 1920) for year-round accommodation of caretakers.

The report also contains an intriguing detail. It records "a cottage on the property, located at the corner of Brown Road and Dana Road was built for Dr. Priscilla White, one of the original founders of the Joslin Clinic. Dr. White was a pioneer in helping pregnant diabetic women have healthy babies."

I did not find any mention of this cottage for Dr White in any publication, nor in conversations with Dr Donna Younger, who had worked with White from 1961 and succeeded her on retirement. Nor did Dr. White herself ever mention it to me at any time during her weekly visits to the Clara Barton Camp for diabetic girls when I worked there in the summer of 1970.

Actual details of the interior design of Buffalo Hill are not available, but clearly the house was spacious enough "to welcome family, friends and guests. No matter how many people were already staying in the house, Mrs Joslin, the quiet and perfect hostess, always quickly and efficiently made another place at the table for the unexpected new arrival, and found a spare bed somewhere for the guest who had been persuaded to spend the night even though wholly unequipped. Toothbrushes, nightclothes and slippers were almost magically produced. This delightful custom of hospitality still endures." (Holt 1969).

The Landscaping of Buffalo Hill. A Yalie to the rescue!

Landscaping of the property is a fascinating story and reveals hitherto unseen facets of Joslin's character. In some ways the landscaping became just as challenging as building the house, perhaps even more so.

It had quickly become clear that the task of clearing the land around the newly built farmhouse was beyond the best efforts of the family. Not only was the work arduous, but even reaching the site each weekend was difficult. Transport was restricted to trains, trolley cars and horses. The final part of the journey to the house was usually on foot. Despite the best efforts of the family, all they had to show for their backbreaking labour was a rough landscape pockmarked with tree stumps, holes, hollows and boulders, leaving the inexperienced prospective owners frustrated and perplexed. Neither of the couple had anticipated the task being so difficult.

Reluctantly, Joslin had to face the reality that the DIY exercise was impractical. He followed the advice from his father to hire a landscape architect. His father had supervised construction of various public buildings – including improvements to the first Congregational church in town – in the early years of Oxford, not to mention the erection of his own shoe manufacturing premises and the family home on Main Street. He had remained in the background as Joslin, in his exuberance, had charged into the project without consulting anyone! Clearly, the father had wanted his younger son to learn from experience!

It is interesting that while acknowledging the difficulties posed for the couple, Holt does not see the problem as proving particularly difficult for Joslin, and records it as follows:

"Soon after the house was completed attention centred next on the ground surrounding it. The rough pasture with all the humps and hollows left by the land clearing operations still remained. To a perfectionist such a condition was most distressing and must be remedied forthwith. EPJ dearly loved a challenge and here was a big one already at hand. As neither the Doctor nor Mrs. Joslin ever before had encountered just such a problem as this – literally to bring order out of this vast chaos – the answer to their perplexity must be to hire a good landscape architect for the undertaking. As usual with EPJ, no sooner said than done, and while they were about it, why not include plans to beautify the centre of Oxford as well? Dr Joslin always delighted in doing this sort of thing for the pleasure of others and cheerfully footed the bill when the time came to do so."

This version of events was typical of Holt's tendency to sanitise Joslin's mistakes. Her account does not accord with the facts as recorded in other documents such as the Oxford Historical Commission and Reconnaissance records and the Olmsted papers. It is clear that important practical aspects of the project had escaped (by a considerable margin) the physician's and his wife's assessments–assuming she was consulted!

Accepting his father's advice, Joslin turned to the best-known landscape architect in Boston. In 1911 he commissioned the firm of Olmsted Brothers. And included his plans for beautifying Oxford! The plans and specifications for the latter are recorded in the annual report of the town of Oxford, 1913–1914. They include suggestions which, even in the very conservative and ordered ways of society at the time, appeared somewhat prescriptive. For example, the recommendation included "all houses be offset in specified styles of architecture, painted in various specified colours away from white, be set a uniform distance away from the street, fences be built along the front of each lot, kerbstones set with prescribed widths left for driving entrances." Finally, advice was provided on suitable shrubs and trees, adapted to the climate, to be planted in various strategic locations along Main Street.

John Charles Olmsted (1852 - 1920).

Olmsted was the senior partner of Olmsted Bros Landscape Architects, a firm he had established in Brookline in early 1898. He was a graduate of Yale and Sheffield School of Engineering.

Olmsted had had a tragic and traumatic childhood. His father, a doctor, had died of tuberculosis in Geneva where John had been born five years earlier. His uncle, Frederick Law Olmsted, had married his brother's widow and adopted John. The youngster's tumultuous life became more settled when he came to stay in his new home in America – a house in the middle of Central Park then under construction under the guidance of his stepfather, the legendary Frederick Law Olmsted! The traumatic early years had resulted in a shy, almost withdrawn, personality.

The Olmsted brothers, (actually cousins), although less well known than their father, had quickly established a reputation mainly through the projects completed by John Charles Olmsted, the older and the senior partner who was the one Joslin had commissioned. The choice could not have been better.

In 1903 John Olmsted had been commissioned to beautify a part of Seattle. The results were amazing and had made him an admired figure in that part of the country. The writer Valerie Easton, describing the project in detail, had heaped unstinting praise on the architect in an essay published in the *Seattle Times* as recently as 2003. Easton had spoken of the architect's acute sensitivity to the "extraordinary landscape advantages…., views of wooded hills and distant mountains…"

John Olmsted himself assumed charge of landscaping Buffalo Hill. Perhaps he was excited by the substantial acreage to work with. Or had he been charmed by the outgoing and popular physician and his wife?

Olmsted, some 20 years older than Joslin, would undoubtedly have heard of the latter as he had been practising in the Brookline area over the previous decade, especially as the offices of the Olmsted Bros' architect firm were also situated in Brookline.

The architect listened carefully to the plans, ideas and hopes of his client.

Just what he thought of Joslin's ideas for beautifying Oxford town is anyone's guess. Perhaps he knew that the town fathers were unlikely to tolerate the suggested plans, but did not want to be the one to deliver the bad news. Or perhaps he did agree and could see the obvious commercial advantages of the possibility of securing another lucrative commission and the chance to beautify another town. That was not to be. Regardless of whose idea it was, the independent- minded town fathers gave it short shrift and vetoed the lot except for the suggestions of trees and shrubs! Clearly the high regard for his father, who had remained prominent in the town affairs in Oxford, was not sufficient to sway the town elders when it came to the son who, after all, had never really taken any active role in the affairs of Oxford, unlike his older brother Homer who had continued the family tradition of active participation in virtually all aspects of life in Oxford since taking over the family shoe manufacturing business.

Olmsted, however, was impressed by Joslin's choice of the design for the farmhouse, which was clearly sympathetic to the surroundings and faithful to the purposes of the building. He quickly saw the natural beauty in the rugged surroundings.

Apart from around 45 acres of suitable land and the cleared area to accommodate the buildings and the gardens around them, the remainder of the property was wooded. There were wetlands along the edge of the property where Dana Road was built later. There was a large marshy area created by water draining from several valleys. This area drained south towards what was later called Brown Road (and later still, Joslin Road). A large pond, several acres in size, was thought to have possibly been created by beavers.

The ponds, the wild woodlands and marshes were the very stuff of the extraordinary landscape advantages for which Olmsted's practised eye was noted. His love of trees had been a feature of the beautification of Seattle and they were not going to be sacrificed on the Joslin farm. Neither would the marshes be cleared nor the ponds interfered with in any way which might diminish their role as a habitat for wildlife. Riding trails would give right of way to the natural lie of the land and the vegetation. Trees were to be cherished and protected, not felled.

If Joslin realised the architect's sensitivity to and concern for the environment, neither he nor Holt ever said so in any of their writings.

Correspondence in the Joslin family papers indicate that design consultations were held over a period of three years. The architect could see what Joslin had envisioned. He could see that the approach to the house was important, and sensed that Joslin wanted the construction of the approach to be such that the house would come into view after a curve at the end of a long driveway. Olmsted was sympathetic to his client's desire for a dramatic effect which he thought would be achieved by the driveway being constructed on an impressive scale, lined by beautiful trees.

On 4 May 1911 Olmsted's correspondence arrived containing plant lists. The plans for the construction of the driveway were supplemented with details of plantings as well. The original plans, which included a boundaries survey, a topographical plan and a planting plan, according to the Oxford Reconnaissance Report of 2007, unfortunately, were destroyed.

However, an 18-page letter from Olmsted dated 19 October 1910 "illustrates the considerable thought that was put into the design of the entry drive and the character of the plantings around the house." More than once the architect had to apply gentle restraint and persuasion, while reminding Joslin that he was designing what was meant to be a *working* farm. Fully aware of his client's desire (or was it a fantasy?) for a winding driveway, Olmsted wrote:

"Considering that it is your conception to treat the place primarily as a farm, the landscape gardening treatment that could require expense for maintenance may be irksome to a farmer at a minimum, it seems best that the approach drive should be on a straight line so as to be obviously convenient and farm like..."

Then relenting a little, perhaps to lessen what was a fairly forthright reminder to the new owner of the priorities in the project, namely: first that while the house was a summer home for his family, the land was to be used for a working farm, and secondly, what a new owner at times appeared to forget, that the cost of maintaining the property could become, as Olmsted tactfully put it, "irksome".

Here the architect was heeding a principle clearly enunciated by the revered Frederick Law Olmsted as one of the "Ten Design Principles" namely, *so long as considerations of utility are neglected or overridden by considerations of ornament there will not be true art.*

He then proposed a compromise.

"It will perhaps seem utilitarian to have the drive without any shade trees so the hayfield would need to be sacrificed slightly in that regard."

Trees on its border were going to make driving the large farm vehicles difficult. Olmsted advised Joslin to buy a 10-acre tract of land which would give him a much better approach both topographically and in terms of views of the house, as well as ease of access for horse-drawn vehicles and later, tractors and (even later), motor vehicles.

The architect's thoughtfulness in giving careful consideration to reconciling domesticity with the wildness around the house, as well as the utilitarian functions of various areas near the buildings, did not escape the notice of Joslin's wife. Whether or not Elizabeth brought this to her husband's attention is not known, but what is clear is that the experience of working with this brilliant professional was an eye-opener for Joslin.

He quickly realised that he had markedly underestimated the scale of the task.

The planting plan was detailed and precise. It provided actual quantities of the proposed species of trees with numbers keyed to the accompanying plant list. Views of the hills to the west and a proposed seating area south of the house were clearly marked. The plan managed vegetation so as not to lose this scenic vista to the south-west. Also included in the plans were an icehouse and a poultry house with a chicken run. These additions to the landscaping contract were a result of Joslin's asking Olmsted's advice on where to place different parts of the farm. Olmsted also advised on where to locate the arable and pasture lands and their proximity to the barn.

Joslin, now convinced that Olmsted was going to more than fulfil his dreams as far as Buffalo Hill was concerned, followed his advice to the letter. The additional acreage suggested by the architect for the driveway was bought promptly.

Joslin accepted all advice given for Buffalo Hill and the location of the driveways and planting of scores of trees, ornamental shrubs and vines which were, on maturity, to provide an impressive vista dominated by oaks and lindens lining the entry to the property. The plantings around the house included extensive lawns and a croquet court off the northern end of the greenery.

There was a grass tennis court to complete provisions of facilities for exercise. Joslin often said that exercise chased away obesity. He himself exercised mostly by riding horses on his property during weekends. During the week, at work, he preferred to walk whenever possible. In his office, between floors, Holt recalls that he took the stairs, often two at a time.

More than one writer, and several staff members I spoke to when I was in Boston, said that Joslin never put on weight. An erect 5'10" in height, which at that time was considered tall, his weight throughout his adult life was unchanged at 140 pounds. In his 80s going into his 90s he dropped to 125 pounds. Abstinence from alcohol and abhorrence of cigarette smoking were second only to his lifelong habit of abstemiousness.

The Gentleman Farmer

The records do not show the size of the initial purchase but Joslin had clearly planned to acquire a substantial holding, and gradually added small parcels until he had a property of some 300 acres which he considered an appropriate size for the country estate of a gentleman farmer.

Joslin took the farming aspect of his new acquisition seriously. At different times of the year the farm was a hive of activity. Fields were prepared for hay and the rotation of crops was observed strictly. A farmer from Maine was employed to supervise the preparation of the fields for hay and location of crops. Potatoes were planted in order to break up the soil. The substantial harvest was sold and, in the winter months, given away free to the needy.

Holt recounts a story of Joslin's personally delivering a large bag of potatoes to a Cambridge matron who, during World War I, was finding food rationing an unbearable hardship as she was entertaining some hungry young men from the US Navy for Thanksgiving dinner. Joslin never spoke of such acts of kindness and generosity, and only those closely associated with him, as Holt was, knew of them.

The poultry farm also flourished. "Joslin is our leading farmer," declared an Oxford resident in the 1930s, mentioning a constant supply of farm fresh eggs to several businesses in town.

The stables were manned by hired hands. Joslin, who had ridden horses since childhood, had a lifelong love for these animals. The weekly 12 mile journey every Monday and Friday from Oxford to Leicester

171

Academy and back had forged an attachment to horses which lasted a lifetime. His desire to have the facilities to keep horses and ride regularly on his own property had been a strong incentive for buying Buffalo Hill.

That he was able to combine the need (and desire) for a summer retreat with a large parcel of land for farming and a stable of horses showed a side of his character and personality distinct from his academic ambitions in the field of medical practice and research and his aspirations of being a writer.

Hard work was a way of life not only in his medical practice but also at home. The grounds of Buffalo Hill needed constant care, and Joslin would do many of these jobs himself. He also expected other members of the family, including the young ones, to do their share. Work was rewarded with some form of recreation such as a horse ride. Ponies were available for the young. The older members, including his mother and older visitors, would sit on the wide veranda enjoying the sunset behind Dudley Hills.

The farm was well equipped and staffed. In the early days there were the usual farm animals, but by the mid-1900s only a flock of sheep remained. A tractor replaced draft horses but the riding horses were kept throughout Joslin's long life.

Buffalo Hill remained an important part – Holt called it a talisman – for Joslin's descendants for more than 100 years. Many a family picnic was held in its grounds. Girls and boys from the diabetic camps were also regular visitors during the summer. The grooms had been thoroughly instructed in the practical aspects of diabetes by Joslin. The girls' camp was held on the property named after Clara Barton, an Oxford resident remembered as the founder of the American Red Cross. The boys' camp was named after Joslin.

Buffalo Hill also accommodated houseguests, including many medical friends visiting from America, Canada, Britain and Europe. Charles Best, the co-discoverer of insulin, had spent part of his honeymoon there. Elizabeth was a capable and quietly efficient hostess. Guests, including unexpected ones, not only found a comfortable bed but also toothbrushes, night clothes and slippers!

Given Joslin's penchant for garnering financial contributions for his various medical projects, one cannot help but wonder if the lavish facilities of Buffalo Hill were at least partly designed to make it suitable for this purpose.

Did Joslin override Elizabeth's influence at Buffalo Hill, or was she the one with the final word on domestic matters? The Puritan households were known for the husband being in charge of outside matters including business (and farming,) but it was the wife who held sway in household matters like children's education, supervision of servants, entertainment of guests and other social activities. But did her authority extend to matters such as fundraising by her husband's negotiations in the parlour?

Did any notable donors receive an invitation to the country retreat? What about George Baker, to whom Joslin dedicated the third edition of his textbook? Or did the New York banker's well-known reserved manner discourage social engagements? Joslin's method of soliciting funds from patients was well known and employed by physicians on his staff. This was almost formulaic in letters to patients following a visit to the clinic– "report (results of laboratory tests), affirm, solicit." But it is hard to imagine Joslin using this approach when dealing with men like Baker and Vanderbilt.

Whether or not the country estate was seen by Joslin as simply a pastoral entity in his overall plans for family life is unclear. In actual fact however, Buffalo Hill turned out to be the most enduring legacy for the descendants of Elliott and Elizabeth Joslin.

More than a century after its completion the Joslin descendants retain possession (held in trust) of the country property, albeit slightly reduced in acreage. The architect- designed homestead and its beautiful approach lined by the trees planted 100 years earlier endure to the present day. That Joslin's dream was realised can be seen in the description contained in the Oxford Reconnaissance Report of 2007:

"The house and barn area are approached by a long entry drive flanked by a double row of oaks and lindens, which are the original trees from the 1911 planting design by the Olmsted Brothers. Cropland can be seen through the trees to either side. The design of the drive heightens the visitors' experience of arrival, ending in a circular drop-off area by the house, then continuing on to the barn and beyond." There is a cornfield across the drive from the house. The report notes that "the interior of the house is very much as it was during Dr Joslin's tenure, including original furniture. The property is under chapters 61 and 61A, and is held in trust by members of the Joslin family."

In his senior years Joslin liked to look beyond Buffalo Hill to the distant hills, perhaps recalling, as was his habit, a favourite biblical saying, "I will lift up mine eyes unto the hills from whence cometh my strength."

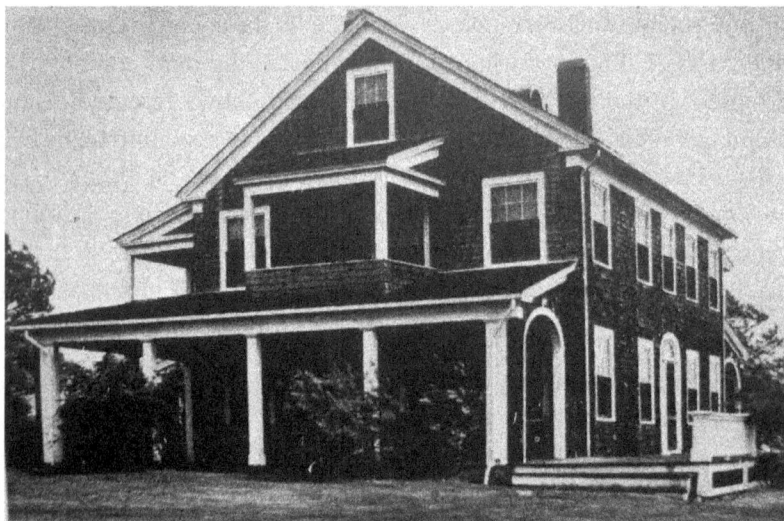

Buffalo Hill

Part 7.
Shadows Fall

The Death of Allen Lafayette Joslin

Two significant family events overshadowed the Buffalo Hill project.

On 19 July 1911, a hot and humid Wednesday when the north-eastern part of the country was in the grip of a heatwave, Vermont recorded a temperature of 105°F and the humidity sapped the energy from adults and children alike, Allen Lafayette Joslin, then aged 78 years, who had been frail for some years, was too weak to get out of bed.

Joslin's mother knew that the busy young physician's routine started earlier than 7am. But she also knew that he was aware of his father's deteriorating condition. Joslin cancelled his commitments, and leaving his assistant Dr Frederick Stanwood to attend to his other duties, travelled to Oxford to join Ada, Homer and his mother. He was at his father's bedside when Allen Lafayette Joslin died.

Following the death of his younger brother Orrin three years earlier, Allen had realised that it was time to allow his older son, Homer Shumway, to take full responsibility for the family business in Oxford.

Joslin, known for his New England reserve, seldom spoke of his parents, and the only direct reference to his father is in Holt's memoirs. He remembered his father's generosity, and in his letters when in college had spoken of the generous allowances and on one occasion had asked what he was expected to do with the surplus. Referring indirectly to the father's prominence in the affairs of Oxford, Joslin said, "His success was due to the fact [that] the worse things were, the better he was. He always came to the fore in a crisis."

Allen Lafayette Joslin was laid to rest in the North Oxford Cemetery.

A photograph of Joslin's father in the *Worcester Magazine* of 1913 shows a man with deep-set eyes and a steady gaze looking into the distance. There was frontal baldness (which Joslin inherited) and a luxurious moustache. The article accompanying the photograph was written by Ada Joslin for Oxford's bicentennial celebrations in 1913.

In his memory, Allen Joslin's wife and children gave to the town of Oxford a gift of land on which the Joslin School was erected. The school, now referred to as Old Joslin School, was demolished in 2007 and replaced by the present Allen Joslin School located on Maple Road, a stone's throw from its junction with Main Street where the house of Joslin's childhood, built by his father in 1866, still stands.

Memories of Childhood

Just after the completion of the farm house, Joslin's uncle Orrin Franklin died in his sleep. Joslin had been particularly close to his uncle, who had been his frequent childhood companion. He remembered his walks in the woods, going fishing and the boats that he had been given by Uncle Orrin. He also remembered sitting next to him in church.

Not quite as prominent as his older brother Allen Lafayette, Orrin had been entrusted with the finances not only of the Joslin shoe store but several community organisations and churches. His donation of pipes for the church organ in the current Congregational Church in Oxford honours his memory.

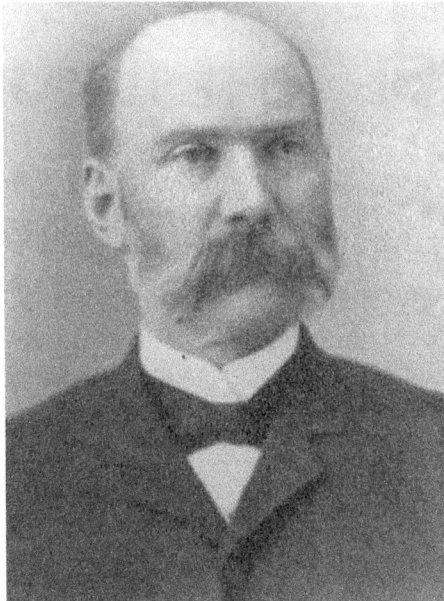

Joslin's father–Allen Lafayette Joslin (1833– 1911)

Part 8.
The Select Band

The Early Years of Medical Practice. Evolution or Serendipity?

"...Osler wanted to involve this select band of the brightest young physicians .."

A.McGehee Harvey

"Elliott Joslin, who of course, was famous for the obsessive zeal with which he followed all of his diabetic patients..."

D. Riesman

An early recognition of Joslin's prominence in the medical circles of Boston was the invitation to join the founding group of the Interurban Club. The origins and subsequent evolution of this group of men provide an interesting insight into the medical thinking and progress in America at the beginning of the 20th century.

The Interurban Club

On 28 April 1905 Joslin received an invitation from William Osler, the Professor of Medicine at Johns Hopkins in Baltimore. Acting on an idea proposed two years earlier by the surgical group in Baltimore led by Harvey Cushing, William Osler wanted to involve this select band of the brightest young physicians from four prominent cities to form a type of "travel club" which would meet regularly to discuss advances in the different centres, thereby forming a combined front to coordinate medical progress. Six young physicians were selected from each of the four cities: Boston, New York, Philadelphia and Baltimore.

180

A copy of the invitation was reproduced in the publication *The Interurban Clinical Club (1905–1976) A Record of Achievement in Clinical Science* by A. McGehee Harvey

One West Franklin Street,
Baltimore, Maryland.,
April 13, 1905.

It is proposed to start among a few of the younger men in the eastern cities an interurban club on lines somewhat similar to the Society of Clinical Surgery. The number of members will be limited. The objects of the club will be:

1. To stimulate the study of internal medicine.

2. By mutual intercourse and discussion, to improve our methods of work and teaching.

3. To promote the scientific investigation of disease.

4. To increase our knowledge of the methods of work in other clinics than our own.

It is proposed to meet twice a year to have demonstrations and discussion, but no set papers. The program of each meeting is to be supplied by the men of the city in which the meeting is being held.

It is proposed to hold the first meeting at the Johns Hopkins Hospital on April 28 and 29th. The rules to govern the club will then be discussed and adopted. You are invited to become a member and to be present on that date. Will you kindly let me hear from you as soon as possible in regard to your acceptance and also if you can be present at the first meeting?

(Signed),
W. Osler.

The assembled group met for dinner at the exclusive Maryland Club on the evening of 28 April 1905. A photograph of the 24 physicians reads like a "Who's Who" of prominent American medical minds of the period. That the choice was astute was to be proved by every member of the group, without exception, fulfilling their earlier promise and, in later

181

years, assuming leadership positions in prominent centres of medical teaching and practice.

Following the adoption of a Constitution the officers of the club were appointed. Joslin was nominated (later confirmed) as a member of the committee.

By a fortunate and interesting coincidence the initial meeting was held to coincide with Osler's final days in Baltimore (and in America). McGehee Harvey captures the drama of the moment.

"No one privileged to be present will ever forget the great teacher's last clinic – the amphitheatre crowded with students and physicians; the members of the newly formed club on the front benches, and in the pit the patient with Osler on one side and a perspiring student on the other.

The whole clinic was an inspiration, and left an indelible impression upon all, especially upon those who like myself have never had the privilege of sitting as disciples at Osler's feet........ He departed soon afterwards to take up the position of Regius Professor of Physic in ancient Oxford, probably the highest medical position in the English-speaking world."

Such was the reputation and the high regard in which William Osler was held by the medical community that simply being regarded as worthy of the invitation to join this select group would not have passed unnoticed in the upper echelons of the medical community.

Although Barnett did not elaborate on the significance of Joslin's membership of this club, he clearly recognised its importance in where Joslin may have been placed in the pecking order of prominent young physicians of that time.

With the exception of the First World War the Interurban Club met twice a year, once in spring and once in the fall till at least the middle of the 20th century. Its members are credited with having made some of the most important contributions and advances in medical knowledge and in the conduct of medical teaching and practice in the United States.

The club's constitution aimed for a membership of 24 but allowed a limit of 30. Upon attaining the age of 50 the member was put on an honorary list to make way for a younger man. In addition to William Osler, the first honorary member of the club, three other men were also invited to honorary memberships. These were E G Janeway of New York (later to become a dominant force in American healthcare, occupying a prominent administrative position in the medical division of the Surgeon General's office), S Weir Mitchell of Philadelphia, and R H Fitz of Boston. Fitz, whose earlier kindly guidance during his internship Joslin had never forgotten, was proposed as a member by Joslin and seconded by Richard Cabot. Cabot was the unanimously chosen President of the inaugural Council of the Club.

All the members of the club were involved in teaching clinical medicine. The interchange of methods of teaching was its chief aim and purpose, and this remained the dominant focus for years. The host city's physicians organised a programme to illustrate its methods of teaching and reported on results of their scientific projects.

At dinner of the first meeting day, always a Friday, the lessons of the morning and afternoon sessions were discussed. Also included for the dinner meeting would be topics "germane to the field of medical education or of clinical medicine."

According to McGeHee Harvey, "… It may be truthfully said that no one ever went away from a meeting of the Club without having learned something of value."

An outstanding example of an innovation in teaching clinical medicine, cited by McGeHee Harvey and which, over the years, I also found of great benefit, was the use of clinic-pathological conferences. This had originated in Boston at the instigation of Richard Cabot, and through the Interurban Club became a widely used teaching model throughout the country. It was a regular feature in the *New England Journal of Medicine*, a widely circulated and respected journal throughout the English-speaking world.

Richard Clarke Cabot (1868-1939)

Cabot, one of the most brilliant medical graduates of that time, was well known to Joslin. Although only a year older than Joslin, he had graduated from Harvard Medical School in 1892 (three years before Joslin), at the age of 24. During his internship at Massachusetts General Hospital in 1893, he had been awarded the Dalton Fellowship, the same as Joslin some years later.

Both had been guided by Fitz. It is tempting to speculate that Fitz may well have encouraged Joslin to emulate Cabot, pointing out the latter's dual contributions in clinical medicine as well as through his writings.

Cabot made seminal contributions to several areas of medicine at the same time as his pioneering work in establishing social workers as part of the medical team. Undeterred by the hospital authorities' refusal to fund the position, Cabot himself paid the first social worker's salary at Massachusetts General Hospital. In addition to books on medical topics, Cabot also wrote several books on ethics. At the age of 51 he was appointed Professor of Social Ethics while still holding the position of Professor of Clinical Medicine at Harvard University.

The distinguished cardiologist Paul Dudley White described Cabot as the greatest contributor to cardiology in his generation, citing Cabot's paper "The Four Common Types of Heart Disease" published in 1940, as a landmark in medical history.

His book on physical diagnosis published in 1901 went through 12 editions to 1938, and his book *Differential Diagnosis*, published in 1938, went through seven editions.

It is not difficult to see several parallels in the contributions made by these two outstanding men. Neither is it difficult to see one more similarity in the recognition–or rather the lack of recognition–afforded to them. Neither Cabot nor Joslin had a Boswell.

It is remarkable that Cabot's prodigious talents which were conspicuous in so many areas did not attract a single biography. Cabot's father, a well-known philosopher, was a friend and biographer of the celebrated Ralph

Waldo Emerson, who was one of Joslin's favourite writers and was quoted by him more than once, especially in his manuals. Emerson was related to Joslin through the Proctor branch of the family. A McGehee Harvey, himself remembered as one of the greatest physicians and teachers of his time, a successor to Osler as the Physician-in-Chief and Professor of Medicine at Johns Hopkins, and a member of the Interurban Club said:

" The finest and best result of the club and the one for which the members will forever hold the founder in grateful memory, is the friendships that have been fostered among the members in the years that have passed since Osler called them together. I feel I am not overstating the fact when I say that nothing in our medical life has been so delightful, so pre-eminently satisfactory as the close associations formed through the Club. They have grown stronger through the passing years and will continue to the end of life."

One example of the friendships and easy camaraderie which existed among the members, is an account of the good-natured ribbing Joslin received from some of the fellow members at the 100th meeting of the club. David Riesman, who edited the history of the club 1905–1937, said:

"Elliott Joslin, who of course, was famous for the obsessive zeal with which he followed all of his diabetic patients after he began practice in 1897, demonstrated this obsession by providing in the 100th meeting of the club a follow-up note on William Osler's patient with heart block presented at that first meeting."

Joslin had discovered the patient, Donald McCormick, some 37 years later in 1942, during a visit to Philadelphia in connection with the reprinting of the seventh edition of his textbook which had initially been released in 1940. Whether it was Joslin's well-known facility for remembering names or whether the patient himself (as some patients are inclined to do) mentioned his medical complaint is not stated, but clearly Joslin realised the importance of providing a follow-up, especially as McCormick had remained free of symptoms from the condition diagnosed and treated some 37 years earlier.

Unfortunately Riesman did not report Joslin's response, or retort (!)

Comments of a similar nature referring to Joslin's insistence on strict control of diabetes and regular reviews of patients were frequently levelled not only at Joslin but also members of his staff over the years. Alexander Marble, who was President of the Joslin Clinic in the late 1960s and early 70s, used to say that a certain degree of compulsiveness was necessary for the successful management of diabetes by the patient "as there are tasks to be attended to several times each day, seven days a week, 12 months of the year. Every year!"

Joslin remained a member of the Interurban Club till the end of his life.

Part 9.
1906

A Most Intense Decade: Joslin at Age 35 to 44

On the professional front during this time in his life, (and putting aside the activities at Buffalo Hill being pursued at the same time), Joslin was extremely busy. Barnett picks 1906 as the year which "might be thought of as the year that his career was launched..... By then Joslin had been in practice for eight years. He had been married for four years and had two children. "At this time, Joslin was juggling three roles.

Firstly, he was treating a wide variety of ailments. Secondly, he was a clinical tutor of medical students from Harvard Medical School. At this stage he was doing most of his hospital work at Boston City Hospital, one of his earliest appointments. Thirdly, starting in 1908, Joslin collaborated with a brilliant research scientist, Francis Benedict. This collaboration, which produced Joslin's most important research in diabetes, continued till 1917, ending, perhaps prematurely, due to his call-up for military service in World War 1.

Barnett refers to this triple role (medical practitioner, university tutor, and researcher), as a "triple threat" and ascribed to it the impact Joslin had on the medical hierarchy in Harvard Medical School, which considered the dynamic 40-year-old for the position of Dean of Harvard Medical School 1909–1910. This did not happen, and Henry Christian, a physician from Peter Bent Brigham Hospital, was appointed Dean from 1908 to 1912.

Although Joslin refused the position of Dean of Harvard Medical School, there is no information on any of the plans he had for his practice at that time. Certainly looking from the outside one would have been excused for thinking that there was no room for any more commitments. But that would be underestimating his capacity–and his ambitions.

What the intellectually syncretic Joslin had were plans to establish a private centre of excellence modelled along European, especially German lines, namely: outpatients to be treated through his office practice which he had already started in Bay State Road in 1906, inpatient treatment of more serious cases in hospitals, and finally, a research laboratory for tests on hospital patients but also, like the

European centres, conducting medical research.

Although his inpatients at this time were scattered between several hospitals, he was working towards establishing a substantial holding in the New England Deaconess Hospital. The facilities for treating patients in the office had been well established in his office in Bay State Road since 1906. However, the third prong of the three-pronged approach, namely, a research laboratory was little more than a dream.

The one aspect of Joslin's professional career in general, and diabetes in particular, which at this time he considered incomplete was first-hand experience in laboratory research on diabetes. Although this was not part of medical practice in America, it was very much so in Europe. The importance of laboratory research as an adjunct to a thorough understanding of physiological and, by extension, disease processes, had been impressed upon him firstly by Chittenden at Yale, and dramatically demonstrated to him during his visits to Europe, particularly Germany. He had never forgotten the gap he had felt in his own experience at the time when he had come across the brilliant Oscar Minkowski in Naunyn's department at the university in Strasbourg.

In retrospect, it is clear that Joslin had harboured ambitions of doing laboratory research on diabetes. The problem was what, how and where? The last element was being partly addressed by his arrangements at the Deaconess Hospital, where he had set up a laboratory for biochemical testing of blood and urine from hospitalised diabetic patients. This however was part of the clinical management of patients as opposed to investigating underlying physiologic abnormalities in diabetes. As it turned out the stars were well and truly aligned in favour of the ambitious charioteer! Only this time the spiked team of "three steeds" was different from Barnett's triple threat. Here Joslin needed to harness and manage the team of office practice, hospitalised patients and laboratory research.

1906 was also noteworthy for Joslin's hospitalisation with severe pneumonia, an incident of interest in more ways than one as will be seen later.

Francis Gano Benedict (1870-1957)

A year younger than Joslin, Benedict had been at Harvard around the same time and had studied chemistry.

His lifelong fascination with the subject had been kindled when, as a 13-year-old, he had gone to a lecture in Boston by Professor James Babcock on "4 Baskets of Coal". In the cellar of his home in Milwaukee, Wisconsin, the young Benedict had built a laboratory and, unsupervised, performed experiments. This clearly played a part in the young man's developing manual skills and a familiarity with gadgets. Years later Benedict would build ingenious devices for measuring heat production, not only in human subjects but also in animals large and small such as elephants and mice respectively.

Under the guidance of and as an assistant to Joshua Parsons Cooke, Benedict had studied chemistry, graduating with a Bachelor's and, a year later, a Master's degree before completing a Ph.D. at Heidelberg University in Germany in 1895. This experience had an enduring influence on the 25-year-old, who visited Europe regularly for the rest of his working life.

He returned to the United States and worked with Professor Webber Atwater, a chemical physiologist – the term biochemist was not in common use at that time – at Wesleyan University in Middletown, Connecticut. Benedict became a full professor in 1905. Encouraged by Atwater, he studied the physiology of nutrition. They collaborated in several nutritional studies and published "Experiments on the digestion of food by man" in 1897. Over a period of 12 years Benedict, with Atwater, conducted some 500 experiments on the metabolic effects of rest, exercise and diet. The results of the studies were published in six bulletins of the US Department of Agriculture Office of Experimental Stations under the title "Experiments on the Metabolism of Matter and Energy in the Human Body."

Atwater died in 1907. His death deeply affected his younger associate, at that time aged 37.

At around this time the trustees of the Carnegie Institute headquarters in

190

Washington were approached by the highly respected physicians William Henry Welch and John Shaw Billings to build a new nutrition laboratory in Boston. They had been impressed by the research into animal and human metabolism by the young physiologist then working with Atwater. They were worried that the death of Atwater might result in the bereaved young scientist being lost to the American scientific community. The Carnegie directors agreed and approved construction of the facility which was completed in record time.

In 1907 Benedict was appointed Foundation Director of the Carnegie Nutrition Laboratory in Boston. The building, in close proximity to the Harvard medical institutions, facilitated interaction between Benedict and many of the medical fraternity in several institutions including Harvard Medical School and Massachusetts General Hospital.

Also within a stone's throw of the new centre was the New England Deaconess Hospital. The chief physician to the hospital was none other than one Elliott Proctor Joslin!

If the proximity of the laboratory to Harvard medical facilities including the Deaconess Hospital was fortunate for Joslin's purposes, the possibility of a working partnership with Benedict was for him a heaven-sent opportunity! This, he had realised, was a unique opportunity to collaborate with a man who had a deep understanding of the underlying processes of energy utilisation within the human body.

Joslin, the physician whose entire professional dealings were limited to human beings, was strongly attracted to an association with Benedict for many reasons, including his wide experience and profound knowledge of comparative physiology, such as the deposition of fat (lipogenesis) in the goose! Little did he know of the other surprises Benedict had in store!

Benedict, a large man with a gregarious, generous disposition, willingly shared his time and expertise as well as equipment with Joslin.

The ambitious Boston physician could scarcely believe his good fortune.

Once again, with hindsight, it could be said that Joslin's instinct in refusing the position of Dean of Harvard Medical School, a largely administrative role, proved to be a master stroke, showing once again his uncanny instinct for recognising opportunities which suited his plans for his professional goals which, as was his habit, he kept to himself.

Benedict had exactly what Joslin needed: expertise, experience in laboratory research, and a wide range of laboratory equipment .What's more, unlike Joslin, Benedict was naturally gifted with a deftness when it came to instruments and tools requiring mechanical capabilities, a deficiency of which had been exposed and recognised in Joslin since primary school. By contrast, Benedict in his student and postgraduate years, had developed his mechanical talents to the extent where he could design and build any machinery needed for his experiments.

What's more, Benedict loved making gadgets. He had an interest in magic and used to design and make gadgets to use in his tricks.

Joslin was mesmerised, as much by Benedict's inventiveness and mechanical ability as by the tailor-made devices. As a young man Benedict had built instruments for measuring heat production not only in humans but, as it turned out, a fascinating array of creatures including mice, pigs, geese, elephants, and, to include cold-blooded animals in his work, even a boa constrictor! Joslin, himself inexperienced in comparative physiology, was speechless.

But this wasn't all.

Benedict's meticulous experimentation was matched by an equally impressive recording and cataloguing of details of his methodology and results. Like Joslin, Benedict had published his first paper while still a student.

Did Joslin and Benedict see in each other a kindred spirit?

Joslin's Collaboration with Benedict.

Between 1908 and 1912, Joslin and Benedict studied 24 diabetic patients in the fasting state with non-diabetic volunteers as controls. Joslin, with his habit of attention to detail, was deeply impressed with Benedict's faultless documentation of the different changes in the physiological parameters of fasting individuals.

A two-year study on the effects of a low carbohydrate and high fat diet, usually referred to as an over- fed state, provided valuable insight into how energy was used in the obese individual including obese diabetics. This work provided further insight into studies carried out by another of Joslin's contemporaries, Frederick Madison Allen.

Allen's work had demonstrated the need for further studies on the metabolism in diabetic individuals whose diet he had restricted to very low amounts of carbohydrate, protein and fat.

In 1908 Joslin carried out extensive studies in the fed and fasted state in 13 patients with diabetes. The patients were admitted to the Deaconess Hospital where Joslin's trained team of nurses weighed and measured the food for each subject. The results of this work were published as Carnegie Institute publication number 136 in 1910.

In 1912 a further study was published as Carnegie Institute publication number 176 on the study of 21 cases of severe diabetes.

The largest study of 113 cases was reported in the 1923 Carnegie Institute publication number 232. The delay was attributed (by Holt) to Joslin's military service in the First World War. The study had been carried out on these subjects without the use of insulin which had been discovered in 1921.

For his part, Benedict was equally fascinated by the dramatic changes in the amount of energy gained or lost by dietary manipulation of carbohydrate, protein and fat in patients with diabetes. He had studied metabolism in newborn infants, adolescents, starving people, athletes and vegetarians. Never in any of his subjects had he seen such dramatic metabolic derangements as were present in Joslin's diabetic patients.

Just as Joslin had been fascinated by Benedict's experimental subjects, it was now the physiologist's turn to glimpse the fascination of working with and on human subjects whose normal physiology had been changed by diabetes. Thus the research scientist and the physician researcher each found in the other's work unexpected excitement, pleasure, and knowledge. For just as Benedict, like many research workers unaccustomed to contact with patients, valued the experience, Joslin in turn was equally captivated by the experiments on animals.

Benedict made freely available all facilities, apparatus and machines Joslin needed to conduct the studies. This included several calorie metres and closed-circuit respiration apparatus with which he had studied animals and human subjects, modifying the machines as needed, depending on the size of the subject.

Besides the difference in the laboratory experience between the two men, Joslin will no doubt have noticed the difference in the reporting of medical case histories, mostly in the *Boston Medical and Surgical Journal*, and the meticulous recording of experimental data contained in the reports of Benedict's experiments. He was full of admiration of Benedict's record as a research scientist and made particular mention of it in his publications.

Although captivated by the work on animals, he never completely managed to be at ease with snakes (especially the boa constrictor) and alligators, or, for that matter, with the 1800 kg elephant! Joslin's contact with animals was restricted to the herd of cattle and a stable of horses he kept on his farm at Buffalo Hill. Whether or not Benedict, the gadget-maker and accomplished magician, ever played any pranks on Joslin using the animals and reptiles is not recorded.

Towards the end of his time with Benedict, Joslin grasped the very important association of undernutrition with a reduction in the metabolic rate. A high metabolic rate, he realised, bore a direct correlation with poorly controlled diabetes. His own experience of this critically important aspect of dietary restriction in diabetes was to remain a guiding light in Joslin's treatment of his patients throughout his working life, even though the centrality of diet in the treatment of children with diabetes was displaced by insulin discovered in 1921.

It was through Benedict's generous assistance that Joslin was able to fulfil his private ambition of doing laboratory research. It was through Benedict and his corporation that Joslin, over four years (1908–1912), had studied 24 diabetic patients in the fasting state and compared the results with a similar number of non-diabetics (controls). In1912 he had started a two-year study of low carbohydrate and high fat diet, which had been used by Allen in his experimental animals.

These studies further strengthened Joslin's belief that undernutrition was an important, even essential part of the management of his diabetic patients. He accorded, as was his custom, fulsome praise to all who helped him, including Benedict, but without providing any details. Several records of their work list Benedict as the first author and some covers of their three Carnegie Institute publications do not record Joslin as an author at all. If this caused any cooling off in their relationship, Joslin never mentioned it.

In the preface to the first edition of his textbook on diabetes published in 1916 Joslin said, "To Professor Francis G. Benedict of the Carnegie Nutrition Laboratory with whom I have worked so pleasantly since 1910, I am under obligation in every way; but I have not allowed him to read a word of what I have written because I wish to assume all responsibility for my mistakes."

In the second edition of the book, published a year later, he said, "To Professor G. Benedict I am under obligation in every way..."

There was no further collaboration between Joslin and Benedict after the First World War. When, in later years, Joslin planned a research laboratory for his own practice, there is no record of his seeking any advice or assistance from Benedict. Of course Benedict had been long retired by that time and there are no details on any continuing contact between the two men.

Joslin and Benedict, according to Holt, remained friends for the rest of their lives. Both were Harvard graduates and both were known for their capacity for hard work. Both may also have had French ancestors, Benedict's a little more colourful. A Franciscan monk, said to be related to Benedict on his father's side, in order to avoid religious persecution, escaped from the French authorities by hiding in a whiskey barrel!

It is clear, however, that Benedict was less driven than Joslin. He liked the good things of life, was an accomplished pianist and indulged in the hobby of magic. Unlike Joslin, Benedict retired in 1937, aged 67, and spent the last 20 years of his life on several pursuits including magic and lecturing on various subjects related to scientific work. One of the most frequently requested lectures was based on his publication, *The Physiology of The Elephant* published by the Carnegie Institution in 1936.

Benedict died in his summer home in Maine on 14 April 1957 at the age of 87. He said his favourite view was that of the Maine coastline which he could see from his home.

Joslin Brings the Laboratory to the Bedside.

By 1914 Joslin had fitted out a room at the Deaconess Hospital with respiratory equipment. He staffed this laboratory with nurses. He insisted, and saw to it, that they recorded, in exact detail, the food intake and fluid output. Barnett could not help pointing out the obvious, adding, "one might have thought that the nurses and patients were employed by the Carnegie Unit." He could almost have added, "and Joslin had Benedict at his elbow supervising the notations with the exactitude the chemist had taught the ambitious physician."

That the practice of bringing the laboratory to the ward was new to America is suggested by Joslin's comments in his final report on those years written in 1923:

"The cases whose metabolism is here recorded have been private patients of the writer and not patients taken from the public wards of a large general hospital. The experiments were performed <u>with</u> the patients rather than <u>upon</u> them because.... their cooperation was not only solicited, but also secured. The investigators and the patients considered themselves united in a partnership, having for its object, the accumulation of knowledge for the benefit of all diabetics, rather than for the given individual under investigation in particular. This altruistic principle was thoroughly appreciated by the patients."

The fact that Joslin sought to make these points places him in a position very different from most of today's investigators, whose work involves clinical or laboratory research without concomitant commitment to patient care. Although such participation in research would be difficult, even impossible, in today's medical setting with the supervisory powers of various committees, it was also uncommon in Joslin's day for an individual to have such wide-ranging interests, let alone active involvement in all of them.

The passage also reveals that Joslin felt the importance of establishing his ownership of the data because they were obtained from patients from his private practice.

It appears that he was now more than satisfied with his first-hand experience in laboratory research in diabetes. Not only did this time with Benedict complete what to him was, at least in his own view, a deficiency in his study of diabetes, the added involvement of his patients, including his own twist on what is today regarded as an essential part of clinical research, namely the experimental subjects' consent (signed and witnessed), will no doubt have been a cause of considerable satisfaction on his part.

A Durable Friendship

Joslin was aware that his experiments on his diabetic patients could have some relevance in the experimental work being done right next door in the Harvard Medical School laboratories by   Frederick Allen, and vice versa.

The locations of the three laboratories–Allen's at Harvard devoted to experimental diabetes in animals, Joslin's on his own patients at the Deaconess, and Benedict's joint endeavours with Joslin in the Nutrition Laboratories–was, from Joslin's point of view, almost too good to be true. Allen's studies on experimental diabetes in dogs, while metabolic studies in Joslin's diabetic patients were being carried out next door, was more than Joslin had ever hoped for. On top of this, having a physiologist of Benedict's calibre in-house was almost too good to be true!

Frederick Madison Allen 1879 – 1964).

Born in Des Moines, Iowa in 1879, Allen was a medical graduate of the

University of California and had served his internship at University of California Hospital in 1907 and 1908. He had also attended the University of Chicago medical school, and it was there that he had met up with physiologists Anton Carlsen and George N Stuart. Their work had a strong influence on the young graduate.

In 1909 Allen obtained a three-year research Fellowship as the Charles Follen Folsom Fellow, receiving $525 yearly to conduct research in the laboratories of Preventive Medicine and Hygiene at Harvard Medical School. The grant was also supported by $300 a year from the Proctor Fund which Allen knew, had been established by Ellen Osborne Proctor (1848–1902), the younger sister of Joslin's mother. She was Joslin's much-travelled spinster aunt who had helped him with his German and translated German scientific articles for him. Ironically, she herself developed diabetes and died from its complications at the age of 53. It was widely known that the research fund had been established through the efforts and persuasion of her nephew. Though never openly expressed, the pride felt by the ambitious mother for her only son's achievements was also shared by other members of the Proctor family.

Joslin, being Joslin, would no doubt have known not only of the arrival of the new recipient of the grant but, given his interest in the subject, also of the research project Allen had planned (which would have been described in his application for the grant).

The Eskimo Diet v the Hindu Diet and Allen's Triumph

In spite of their difference in age–Allen was 10 years younger–he and Joslin had one thing in common. They were both capable of working long hours without a break in concentration. Both were also gifted in their ability to keep methodical and accurate records of their work, such as the information (data) gained from the record of patients or laboratory animals.

Before insulin, the treatment of diabetes was limited to "medicines" including alcohol, opioids, arsenic and potassium bromide.

Like Joslin, Allen was a voracious reader, with a particular interest in anthropology. He had been struck by the fact that Eskimos seemed well nourished on a diet low in carbohydrates. He decided to use this Eskimo diet on his experiments on diabetic animals. To his delight, diabetic dogs, when fed a low carbohydrate diet, not only remained well but lost less sugar in the urine.

Allen had also read that in India adherents of the Hindu faith followed a diet consisting of large amounts of carbohydrate which was found to damage the pancreas, resulting in cases of mild diabetes turning into a more severe form.

Using the Hindu diet in his animals produced the same results. However, if the same animals were fed a diet rich in fat, the loss of sugar in the urine (*glycosuria*) was greatly reduced.

He concluded that patients should eat "according to the size of their pancreas", meaning that they should reduce carbohydrates and, if needed, increase their fat intake until their urine became free of sugar.

Between 1909 and 1912 Allen had operated on hundreds of animals in his laboratory to remove the pancreas, which made the animals diabetic. With his limitless energy and a prodigious capacity for working long hours, Allen got through a huge amount of work, including operating on 200 dogs, 200 cats, and a smaller number of rabbits, guinea pigs and rats. He recorded and catalogued his methodology and results in meticulous detail.

After the improvement with a combination of reduced starches and increased fat in the diet of diabetic animals in his laboratory, Allen took the critical step of treating human patients with the same diet. To his delight, the improvement in diabetes he had produced in the experimental animals was perfectly replicated in his human patients with diabetes.

Just when Allen told Joslin about this is not known, but given the close association between the two and the importance of the discovery, it is unlikely that Allen would have been able to keep it to himself for long.

Following the completion of the Research Fellowship at Harvard, Allen continued research at the Rockefeller Centre in New York, where he also had patients with diabetes in his care. In addition to the diet he had experimented with in Boston, Allen also insisted that all his patients, adults and children, engage in physical exercise every day, regardless of their physical state.

It was this insistence on exercise which seriously undermined Allen's popularity, and therefore his influence, on the treatment of patients, especially children, with diabetes.

Allen's Mistake: the Power of the Grapevine

What Allen had not foreseen was the reaction not only of the patients but also of some members of the medical and nursing professions to the effects of this dietary prescription, especially on children. In many of these patients, already weakened by the disease, the reduction in carbohydrates led to further weight loss and profound weakness. The parents of diabetic children were confused and alarmed at the effects of the treatment which they had expected would produce an improvement, not a worsening, of the condition. Allen's dogged insistence on patients exercising while on this restricted diet produced further weight loss and weakness, with some patients reduced to becoming bedridden.

Negative publicity travels faster than praise.

Allen did not have Joslin's gifts of rapport with patients or their relatives.

To compare Allen with Joslin at this point in their careers is a "no contest" from the very outset. Joslin, 10 years older, had much more clinical experience with clinical medicine and diabetes in particular. His report on diabetics in Massachusetts General Hospital had been published 10 years earlier. He had been trained by outstanding clinicians such as Reginald Heber Fitz. On the other hand, Allen was only 30 and had graduated from medical school a mere two years earlier. He had minimal experience in treating human diabetics.

He was simply not in the league of the experienced Boston physician. It is appropriate to quote Barnett's description which highlights the difference between the two men.

"Elliott Joslin's gentleman's upbringing left him both well-connected and well-schooled in the classics; he was able, for example, to read and write Greek. Frederick Allen grew up in much more modest circumstances near Chicago and went to medical school in San Francisco, graduating a year after the harrowing, but to a fledgling doctor, helpful, experience of the San Francisco earthquake in 1906. To earn money he practised in a frontier logging town as 'the' physician."

However, the main area in which Allen failed had little to do with his research or his competence as a doctor. A large part of his problem was quite simply that at his young age and with limited experience of handling the general public, not to mention the challenge of managing the parents of sick children, Allen had little if any appreciation of the importance of public relations. Quiet, reserved and at times moody, he did not mix easily and, usually being short of funds, was not known for sartorial elegance. His expression, frequently dour, did not help. Socially awkward, he had few friends. Barnett called him "a cantankerous loner".

Joslin's Support for Allen

Allen, however, had one reliable acquaintance who had befriended him shortly after his arrival in Boston. It was this friend who was to open doors for Allen, not only in the early years in Boston, but throughout his life.

This friend was none other than Elliott Joslin.

The association between Allen and Joslin, perhaps closer than previously recognised, was brought to light by Donald Barnett in his monograph on Joslin. Their association, in Barnett's view, was an example of "opposites attract!"

Frederick Allen's main literary contribution to medicine was the publication of the results of his experiments on hundreds of animals during his Research Fellowship at Harvard. Furthermore, he described clearly and in detail his operating method for isolating and removing the pancreas.

He also carried out one of the most complete reviews of the literature on his research topic, as well as a detailed exposition on diabetes as known at that time.

Allen's grasp of diabetes, not only in laboratory animals but in human beings affected by the disease, was extraordinary.

Therefore it was not surprising that the meticulously detailed documentation of the research and the exhaustive review of the literature produced a volume of 1179 pages containing more than 1200 references. The book was simply too lengthy to be accepted by any of the medical journals of the time. Ultimately, he borrowed $5000 from his father to publish it privately. In its preface he acknowledged "the good offices in connection with the publication" of Joslin, Joseph Pratt and Harvey Cushing. *Glycosuria and Diabetes* by Frederick M Allen, A.B, M.D. and published in early 1913 by W M Leonard of Boston was released for sale by Harvard University Press of Cambridge, Massachusetts early in 1913. (The sale price was not stated in the copy of the book I accessed online which, interestingly, was "a gift to the Library of the Harvard Medical School and the School of Public Health by Dr John Homans").

Allen's stay in Boston was not a happy one. From there he went to the Rockefeller Institute in New York, where he continued his research and also undertook treatment of patients with diabetes. In spite of his shortcomings he established a large practice and was regarded as one of the leaders in the field.

Mainly through Joslin's contacts and recommendations, Allen presented the findings from his experimental work on diabetes on more than one occasion. Also at Joslin's request, Fitz helped Allen with advice on clinical studies on diabetes. Allen stayed at the Rockefeller Institute for six years and gained increased prominence in treating diabetics. He never wavered from his belief in the use of restricted diet in patients with diabetes. In spite of the criticism of his methods of reduced food intake together with physical exercise, large numbers of diabetic patients were referred to him by many doctors. His reputation grew, and he was often referred to as "Dr Diabetes". His bedside manner remained a drawback. He was seen as inflexible and, according to some, short on charm.

If Allen felt he was losing ground with a patient, he would refer him to his friend Joslin in Boston. The personal approach to people in general and patients in particular by Joslin was noted by the patients, and more and more New Yorkers beat a path to the Boston physician's door. However, at no stage was there any strain in the friendship which existed between the two men.

Joslin supported Allen and the importance of his dietary approach to patients with diabetes throughout his life. Perhaps it was not widely appreciated by patients and parents of children with diabetes that dietary restriction as the treatment for diabetes had been practised, especially in Europe, for many years before any American physician used that method. Dietary restriction remains a cornerstone of the treatment of diabetes to this day. Yet there remain within the medical profession some who still question this aspect of treatment. Fortunately, the majority of practitioners maintain that dietary restriction is important. As recently as 2009 L D Lynn wrote: "No matter how one looked at this approach, all agreed that hundreds if not thousands of diabetic patients were kept alive long enough to benefit from the newly available insulin therapy, patients that otherwise would have perished before this great advance could be made available to them."

It is a little-known fact that Banting and Best, the Canadian co-discoverers of insulin, used Allen's operating method in their surgery on dogs to isolate insulin. The increasingly isolated and embittered pioneer physician would have seen some validation in that.

Allen died in 1964 at the age of 75, two years after the death of his steadfast friend and supporter, Joslin. As will be seen towards the end of the Joslin story, just as Joslin had been unfailing in his support for Allen, so was Allen in reciprocating the high regard and affection of his friend in Boston.

Part 10.
Writer

Joslin's Greatest Achievement?

"Reading maketh a full man; conference a ready man; and writing an exact man; and, therefore, if a man write little, he had need to have a great memory; if he confer little, he had need have a present wit; and if he read little, he need have much cunning, to seem to know that he does not".

Francis Bacon.

In the fall of 1916 Joslin produced what many regard as his seminal contribution to the field of diabetes.

Treatment of Diabetes Mellitus with Observations Upon the Disease based upon 1000 cases, by Elliott P Joslin M.D.; Assistant Professor of Medicine, Harvard Medical School; Consulting Physician, Boston City Hospital; Collaborator to the Nutrition Laboratory of the Carnegie Institution of Washington in Boston, was a 440 page book published in hardcover by Lea and Febiger, Philadelphia and New York.

The book was the first textbook on diabetes written in the English language.

It was dedicated by Joslin to his wife.

In 1918 he wrote *A Manual for the Mutual Use of Doctor and Patient*. The success of this book took the new author completely by surprise. The initial run, including two reprints, sold out in months. The second edition was published less than a year later in 1919.

From then on Joslin made it a rule to write a manual for each edition of the text.

Both the textbook and the manual were written with revisions and up- to-date information in succeeding editions for the rest of his life. Over a period of nearly 50 years Joslin wrote 10 editions of each. The 10th edition of the textbook and manual were issued in 1959 when the writer was 90 years old. The dates of issue of each edition of the textbook and manual are tabulated in a chart at the end of this chapter.

The Joslin Textbook

"..a pleasure and an inspiration.. "

E P Joslin.

The absence of such a reference book would generally be considered sufficient reason to write one. In Joslin's case, however, there were several reasons for doing so. He was deeply impressed by Allen's work, and this could have been the deciding factor in embarking on the project. Certainly his remarks in the preface of the book strongly support this view.

The "stimulating" condition referred to, as described below, was the practical simplification of treatment as suggested and practised by Allen. Joslin wrote:

"I would not have wished to write a book on diabetes three years ago; today it is a pleasure and an inspiration because the improvement in treatment is beyond question.

The introduction of fasting and the emphasis on physical exercise in the treatment of diabetes by Dr F.M. Allen, of the Rockefeller Institute for Medical Research has decidedly changed the outlook for this class of patients. "Fasting" is in itself a distinct advance, but the practical simplification of treatment which it entails is an almost greater advantage. Now, doctor and patient may know whether or not the treatment is successful. This condition is most stimulating. "

However, there was more than Allen's work which played a role in Joslin's embarking on these major writing projects which were to become an abiding commitment.

Textbooks on Diabetes in Joslin's Time: The European Influence

Books on diabetes had been written by men who wanted to share their observations in their own practices and laboratories. The best, in fact the only example of this in the United States, was Allen's *Glycosuria and Diabetes.* Although of interest to those engaged in laboratory research,

207

its huge volume of experimental information had limited value as a guide to doctors treating patients with diabetes.

Joslin had never forgotten the publication of Naunyn's *Der Diabetes Mellitus* in 1898. Although the German professor had published an earlier well-received book in 1889, which described his experience in treating diabetes with dietary restriction, it was the second, more complete text which interested Joslin. It was more clinical and therefore more useful for the practising physician.

However Naunyn's second book, like his first, was also in German and directed mainly at the European medical community.

Joslin knew of Apollinaire Bouchardat's *Diabetes Sucre* published in 1875.

Both the German and French physicians had been using strict dietary restriction for decades before it was advocated by Allen and Joslin. As already indicated, clinical observations by physicians in Europe, particularly by German and French physicians, of the benefits of restricting food intake, especially carbohydrates (starches), to reduce the amount of glucose being lost in the urine of diabetics had been known since the second half of the 1800s.

Apollinaire Bouchardat had noticed the improvement in diabetes through weight loss in soldiers as well as prisoners of war during and after the Franco-Prussian War, especially during the four-month siege of Paris in 1870.

The difference between the European and American approach to diet was that the former was based on clinical observation, as distinct from the American practice which was based largely but not exclusively on Allen's work.

Joslin's conviction of the benefit of dietary changes had resulted from having identified in Allen's work on laboratory animals one result which for him was a clinical pearl. This was that just as dietary restriction of starchy foods (carbohydrates) in the diet of Allen's diabetic animals reduced the amount of sugar lost in their urine, a similar diet had the same beneficial effect in human patients with diabetes.

He immediately grasped the significance of this finding and its application to the treatment of his diabetic patients. Even though he had used dietary restriction before this, as had others, especially in Europe, Allen's experiments were the first to use such large numbers of animals. They were the first such studies to be carried out in America.

Joslin had been convinced that dietary restriction had a definite role in the management of patients ever since he had visited Naunyn for advice on the treatment of diabetes in his mother in 1899. In the last manual for patients he wrote more than 60 years later, Joslin said that he had used dietary restriction from the time of his visit to Strasbourg in 1899.

One could speculate that he may have been hesitant to publicly endorse the European method without it being confirmed in studies carried out in America?

Allen's Experiments, a Tipping Point for Joslin?

Although in his private practice Joslin had been using a restricted diet for the treatment of his patients ever since his visit to Naunyn at the time of the onset of his mother's diabetes, he had also known of others in America using the same method. He spoke of how "Dr A.J .Hodgson, who has so long treated diabetes well, told me very clearly several years ago of the advantage of low diet."

However it was Allen's work which led to Joslin's openly declaring his support for the use of a restricted diet in the treatment of diabetes. What has perhaps not been sufficiently emphasised in the literature on diabetes is the critical step of applying the findings in *animal* experiments to *humans* with diabetes, which Allen did when he returned to treating patients with diabetes after completing his research on animals during his Research Fellowship in Boston. Joslin, using Allen's methods in his own laboratory studies, recorded the findings in two patients from his Carnegie Laboratory ledger.

Case #740, a 20-year-old man with diabetes was treated for one year with an undernutrition diet including fasting. The young man wrote back to say that he had noticed a marked improvement and was well enough to go back to work one month after discharge.

Case #1025, (who was also included in his textbook), was another 20-year-old, this time a woman, who after a short period of starvation, was able to overcome a serious chemical imbalance (acidosis) during her 12-day hospital admission.

Barely able to contain his exultation, Joslin, in the preface to the first edition of his textbook, stated that it was "a pleasure and an inspiration because the improvement in treatment [with diminished food intake–starvation] is beyond question. The introduction of fasting and the emphasis on physical exercise in the treatment of diabetes by Dr F.M. Allen has decidedly changed the outlook for this class of patients". Aware that in spite of his remarkable findings, Allen was never accorded the recognition, let alone plaudits, for his contribution to the treatment of diabetes, Joslin was keen to support his young colleague.

Unfortunately, the death rate in spite of the improvements described above was high. Both the patients from his Carnegie laboratory ledger y lived for only one year after the diagnosis of their condition. It must also be remembered that the markedly reduced food intake produced weakness which often rendered the patients unable to attend to even their most basic needs. In this difficult and challenging situation it was Joslin's personality that was noted by onlookers. Barnett mentioned a conversation with Dr Priscilla White, stating "how awed she was over EPJ's equanimity and the steady kindness he showed the many starved and often fatally ill patients on the wards in 1921- 22."

The prominence Joslin gave to Allen's work is seen in the preface of his book, as well as in the detailed description of the method in the text. Indeed, he went so far as to call this period–prior to the discovery of insulin–"the Allen Era," in the history of the treatment of diabetes. High praise indeed given that the preceding period, "the Naunyn Era" was named after one of Joslin's heroes.

There were two other factors which may have played a role in Joslin's producing a text on diabetes. The first was the body of knowledge accumulated from his own practice. As indicated in the title, Joslin had based the information he presented in this volume on 1000 patients he himself had seen and cared for during the previous 16 years. During his internship Joslin had learned that accumulated data from a large number of patients was useful in understanding the manner in which a particular condition affected the afflicted – referred to in medical jargon as the natural history of a condition, in this case diabetes.

The second reason for his being persuaded was a personal one. Joslin's mother had presented with diabetes in 1899. Following Naunyn's advice, Joslin had treated her with strict dietary restrictions. The first time he stated this emphatically was in 1923. It was the opening sentence of the preface to the third edition of the textbook.

"In the early months of the century Naunyn taught me with Case No.8 that his methods enabled a diabetic of 60 years to live out the full expectation of life. (The diabetic of 60 years refers to the age of the patient at the time of the discovery of diabetes and not the duration of the disease. He did not divulge the identity of the patient. That was to happen nearly 40 years later!)

This very basic aspect of the treatment of diabetes is also one of the most challenging. Difficulties encountered by the individual in adhering to the restricted diet 24 hours a day, seven days a week, 365 days a year are best appreciated by those who have to suffer this fate and those who care for them. In supervising his mother's diet, Joslin had the advantage of having a patient in-house. In the final manual he wrote Joslin said, "I never knew her to break her diet." That she lived beyond the age expected of her non-diabetic peers demonstrated for him all the proof he needed to be convinced of the efficacy of dietary restriction in the treatment of diabetes.

At that time dietary restriction was the only treatment available for treating diabetes. Insulin had not been discovered, and development of the many tablets now available to lower blood glucose was about 50 years into the future.

Joslin, the Canny Merchant and the Benjamin Franklin Connection

Whether or not Joslin also recognised that he had identified the hitherto untapped market for a textbook on diabetes written in English is open to question. Like most, if not all of his decisions on his medical practice as well as domestic plans, Joslin appears not to have discussed them with anyone. Or if he had, he, (and they), certainly had not written about them.

What is clear is that he now realised the need for an English-language textbook on diabetes because he could point to Allen's experimental findings confirming the usefulness of undernutrition in its treatment. He had seen evidence of this in his own patients, but clearly did not consider that as being sufficient to make the claim in writing.

As was one of his well-known habits, no sooner had he made the decision to write, he wanted the task completed!

And Joslin proceeded to do just that!

At this time Joslin, in his mid-40s, was well known, liked and respected. He was wealthy, and although holding several appointments including academic ones, had always kept his private practice at the centre of his professional life.

He had started his own register of diabetic patients in his practice soon after his graduation, even when he was an assistant to Putnam. From around 1910, according to one of his assistants, Joslin saw most of the diabetics himself, leaving non-diabetic patients largely to his assistants. It was therefore not surprising that he was recognised as one of the few physicians with a medical practice dominated by a single disease.

By 1915, he had seen in excess of 1000 patients. Unfortunately this included 400 deaths. To be prepared to write a monograph based on his own clinical experience, especially with such a high mortality rate (40%), required a strength of conviction seen in few men.

In late 1915 the intellectually syncretic clinician, avid correspondent, accomplished writer (and the ex-editor of the Leicester Academy student newspaper!) made the decision to go into print.

The choice of the publisher was predictable. Joslin chose the long-established, family-owned firm of Lea and Febiger of Philadelphia, acknowledged leaders in the business of publishing medical books.

With his keen sense of history, Joslin may also have chosen Lea and Febiger because of the connection between Lea, the senior partner, and Benjamin Franklin (*yes, the Benjamin Franklin!*).

The history of the company records that the business had been acquired through the marriage of Lea to a daughter of Carey who had established the original printing firm. Carey had learnt the trade of printing from Benjamin Franklin, better known as one of America's Founding Fathers but who was a printer by profession. Franklin had conducted much of his business in Paris, where Carey had worked with him.

I obtained from the archives of the Historical Society of Pennsylvania a copy of the memorandum of agreement for the publication of Joslin's textbook. It states (in part):

"MEMORANDUM OF AGREEMENT made this 18th day of January, 1916 by and between Elliott P. Joslin, M.D. Boston, Mass. and Lea and Febiger publishers for themselves and their assigns, that Dr E.P. Joslin shall write and prepare for the press, a work on the Treatment of Diabetes Mellitus to make a volume of about 300 pages, the same number of pages to include engravings selected from among those already in the possession of Lea and Febiger and a reasonable and sufficient number of new cuts which shall be prepared by Lea and Febiger from engravings, photographs, drawings or prints to be furnished by Dr. E.P. Joslin.

The said work is to be completed and ready for the printers by February 1, 1916, except in case of illness of Dr. E.P. Joslin.

Lee and Febiger shall print and publish the said work wholly at their own expense, in such style as they deem best suited to the market, and shall pay to Dr. E.P. Joslin a royalty of (10) per cent on the catalogue (retail) price and cloth binding for each copy by them sold, and Lea and Febiger shall render annual statements of account in the month of January, and make settlement in cash 30 days after the date of such statements……..

… The royalty shall be estimated at 10% of the actual price received for each copy.....

.. Should further editions be called for, it is agreed that Dr E.P. Joslin shall revise and bring the work up to the then existing state of the science and when called upon, so to do by Lee and Febiger..."

It is clear that Joslin had already completed the text before approaching the publisher, because in a letter on an unrelated matter to Simon Flexner (Director of the Rockefeller Institute for Medical Research) in March 1916, he mentioned that he had delivered the manuscript to the publishers. The publishers were also prompt in producing the finished product and submitting it in November 1916 to the *Canadian Medical Association Journal* for its book review section.

(It is said that Joslin's military call up caused him to miss the publisher's deadline, and the final proofreading was left to his secretary, Helen Leonard. Although not stated in the agreement signed by Joslin, the publishers had not foreseen war as a reason for the delay.)

Anticipating what might be regarded as its chief criticism, the author was ready with an answer.

The troubling detail was that 400 of the 1,000 cases mentioned in the title had died, a damning outcome which would have been a daunting statistic for any doctor and one which he may, understandably, have been reluctant to disclose. Yet in the preface Joslin simply stated, "For the benefit of my patients, it has seemed well worthwhile to summarise my work with them during the last 18 years, and *I have honestly tried in these pages to let the 400 fatal cases tell their useful lessons to the 600 living.*"

He made no attempt to defend himself or the medical profession for the high mortality rate which in the modern era would be alarming to say the least. In fact he did the very opposite, diving headlong into singing the praises of the practical and simple treatment of diabetes with the combination of diet and exercise, the efficacy of which had been demonstrated by Frederick Allen firstly in the laboratory in animals and later in diabetic patients in hospital.

The recognition of the alarming increase in the incidence of diabetes today–the trend had been noted by Joslin even then–makes his comment in 1916 on the number of individuals so affected thought provoking, to say the least. "In the United States there are, I suppose, more than half a million individuals with diabetes," he said.

In 2017 The Centre for Disease Control and Prevention (CDC) put the incidence of diabetes in the United States at more than 100 million, a 200-fold rise.

The World Health Organisation estimated the number of diabetics worldwide to be in excess of 400 million in 2014. Interestingly, the first two tenets of treatment on the WHO website are diet and physical activity (followed by medication and regular screening and treatment for complications.)

So dietary restriction, as advocated in the early years by many physicians including Joslin, still occupies a central position in the management of the condition.

The mental toughness and courage of the writer is obscured by his optimism and enthusiasm. As if this weren't enough, he used positive reinforcement to remind his readers that "*Tuberculosis gave consumptives and the rest of us fresh air. The modern treatment of diabetes is giving the community very definite ideas about diet and the desirability of maintaining the body in the best possible physical condition. Between the consumptive and the diabetic we have little excuse to be ill.*"

Given the rising incidence of obesity and diabetes in the world today, Joslin's exhortations on avoiding obesity uttered more than a century ago, although just as relevant today, remain largely unheeded.

Joslin was always humble and never given to self-promotion, let alone self-praise. He was also conscious of his position in the medical hierarchy, which included physicians not only in the United States but more importantly, in Europe. He was quick to acknowledge the wider experience of men like van Noorden in Germany whose medical opinions were based on having seen some 20,000 diabetic patients in the early 1920s. In those years Joslin's practice had around a quarter of that number.

Whether or not he ever realised the long-term effects of the rules he established within his practice is unclear. However, it is a fact, now of historical significance, that an outstanding contribution of his practice to the understanding of diabetes resulted from the careful record-keeping which he established and upon which he insisted when others joined his practice. It is from these records that the Joslin Diabetes Centre, upon reviewing its files, determined that during the first 100 years of the medical practice started by Joslin some 200,000 diabetics had been seen there, investing it with a status recognised and respected throughout the world.

The acknowledgement in the book's preface of contributions by his colleagues reveals the breadth of Joslin's contacts. An avid correspondent, he would in today's jargon, be called an expert networker. Starting with his local contacts going back to Graham Lusk, whom he had first met during his extra year at Yale, he included other American colleagues as well as European authorities, Naunyn and von Noorden in particular. Nor did he forget Benedict or his own assistants, Goodall, Stanwood and Brigham. Nurses, whose role in the management of diabetes had been emphasised, indeed championed by Joslin from the very beginning of his interest in the condition also received special mention.

The retail price of the initial run was $4.50 per book. The contract specified that the author would receive royalties at the rate of 10% of the retail price! The agreement included a clause that the account was to be settled by the publisher on 31 January each year.

Initially, 2000 copies were published. Clearly there were some spares, Records show that 1000 copies had been sold by 31 July 1916, 500 by 9 November, 500 by 16 October 1917, and 18 by 25 November 1917. Thus the entire stock sold out before the end of the year. However, given the rate of return at $.45 a copy I was not surprised, upon looking at the entries in the publisher's ledger, to find the princely sums of around $12-$20 being remitted to the Boston physician on 31 January each year!

In conversations with me during my time with Dr Priscilla White, she told me that the fact that Joslin was wealthy without relying on his income from medical practice was well known. Clearly, the contribution to his wealth from the sale of his book would not have been significant.

What the book did, however was establish Joslin's credentials well beyond Boston, resulting in a sharp increase in the number of referrals to his practice which would undoubtedly have caused an increase in the income from his practice. Records of the number of patients seen confirmed a sharp increase after the publication of the book in 1916.

The success of his textbook clearly took Joslin by surprise, as it did the publishers. More out of courtesy than any real expectation, Joslin was approached to decide whether he wanted to revise his work prior to the first reprint. After all, it was less than 12 months since the first publication.

They were wrong!

There was a prompt reply from the Boston physician. Yes, he did! And, no, it will not be a reprint but a new edition!

Having almost rushed to proclaim that "advancing the treatment of diabetes, which began with the introduction of fasting by Dr. F.M. Allen", Joslin wanted to present further statistical evidence from his own patients in order to show that the improvement claimed was real.

The Buoyant Author

The second edition, published in 1917, stood up to its claim made in the title *The Treatment of Diabetes Mellitus with Observations upon the Disease based upon 1300 Cases.*

In the preface Joslin wrote that the book had been "largely rewritten, using as a basis the experience gained in another year of study of new and old diabetic cases…61 tables in edition one had been revised and 59 new tables and 10 illustrations added."

Although clearly exuberant, he was also cautious.

He turned to his first mentor, Reginald Heber Fitz. Ever gracious, Fitz who had been delighted with the publication of Joslin's book, gave him at least two pieces of practical advice.

Firstly, he reminded Joslin of the value of case reports, a lesson he had learned as an intern when writing his paper on patients with diabetes admitted to Massachusetts General Hospital, a project which had been suggested to him by Fitz. This resulted in Joslin's adding a case ndex. The case index, was nearly as long as the general index and had Joslin included the 25 cases mentioned in the tables, it would have been longer. Fitz suggested that Joslin compile the list as he went along. Joslin never wrote about his techniques of writing, and it is entirely possible that he was doing this anyway but, given his respect for Fitz and his own nature, would not have said so.

Upon seeing this feature, any practising physician would recognise its value as a journey through the clinical spectrum of diabetes, which is the way problems in diabetes are often brought to the attention of a doctor by the patient. It was the first time I had come across this in any textbook and, given its usefulness, surprised that it has not been used in other textbooks on the subject.

(I had to admit to wistfulness at this as another example of the wide experience and profound knowledge of physicians at MGH of the early to mid-1900s. They were men of exceptional ability. I still remember many of the practical lessons learned from the staff at the MGH during my time there in the early 1970s. It was not uncommon to see, seated in the front row attending the Saturday morning clinical conferences, men and women who were world authorities on different medical subjects and authors of textbooks used throughout the world.)

The second suggestion, which again showed the guiding hand of his teacher, was to emphasise the different practical aspects of treatment suggested to diabetics in Joslin's "primer", *A Diabetic Manual For The Mutual Use of Doctor and Patients*, which had followed the publication of the textbook's initial edition. In the second edition of the textbook, Joslin emphasised these in bold print. The highly experienced Fitz clearly recognised the need for practising physicians to be aware of the practical day-to-day aspects of treating diabetes!

The success of the first edition had emboldened the Boston physician to champion the improvement in the treatment achieved by reducing food intake and engaging in regular physical exercise. In fact, he placed exercise above reducing the amount of food eaten in his instructions to patients.

" It is better to discuss how far you have walked than how little you have eaten," he wrote.

He repeated the observation made by Dr Sabine, one of his friends who was a general practitioner in Brookline, that patients who preferred a camping trip as part of their annual holidays generally enjoyed better health than those who went on less active pursuits. Joslin himself made the comment that when a man's promotion at work brought him indoors (into an office), he became a candidate for diabetes.

However, it is equally clear that at that time the distinction between childhood diabetes and diabetes in adults was not fully appreciated. Treatment with dietary restriction of starches together with an emphasis on physical exercise is the standard treatment of adult-onset diabetes even today, but has to be changed, often quite markedly, by reducing exercise in children who are debilitated by the condition, especially before treatment is started.

Emphasising the need for education of the patient, he reminded them that "a patient is his own nurse, Dr's assistant and chemist." He called this a triple vocation and advised "diligent study."

"You are all living so much longer as a result of better treatment and new discoveries. Therefore, face the facts, accept the situation, study the disease and become the master of your fate," he urged.

It would appear that the publishers had not expected Joslin to pen a second edition so soon after the first, especially as Joslin had told them of his plans to write a manual for patients with diabetes. Pointing this out to the author, they reminded him that since supplies of the first edition of the text had been exhausted before Christmas, it would be prudent to work on that before embarking on writing the manual for patients.

Once again, demonstrating his work ethic and capacity for burning the midnight oil even after his exhausting day-time schedules, Joslin completed the second edition within the first three months of 1917. This time Lea & Febiger, instead of the 2000 copies published for the first edition, started with 3000 copies. The entire stock was sold out by December 1918.

In a typically self-effacing and modest recognition of the success of the first edition Joslin said, "The more than kind reception accorded the first edition has led me to take even greater pains with the second. The book has therefore been largely *rewritten…..*"

He included the latest concepts of diabetes and also incorporated answers to questions raised by doctors and patients who had read the first edition. In addition he provided a follow-up on the patients he had referred to previously.

Taking a broader view, Joslin said "The treatment of diabetes today is a serious problem, not only for the patients themselves but for the nation at large". He did not mince his words, declaring that "no student of diabetes will gainsay the statement that the diabetics in the United States alone waste food sufficient to supply the needs of many thousands of individuals the year round. If this book helps to avert this waste, particularly at this time, [he was referring to the first World War 1914-18] and also benefits some of these patients, it will have accomplished the purpose for which it was written."

Sales of the second edition were steady, ranging from 500 to over 1000 per year.

Succeeding editions of the textbook chronicled the evolving changes in the understanding and treatment of diabetes. Joslin's opinions on the relative importance of different issues were reflected in his writing. Often he foreshadowed these in introductory remarks contained in the preface. In dedicating the textbook to different individuals prominent in research or other aspects of diabetes, he not only publicised but gave due recognition to these men who were almost always younger than he was. Given Joslin's prominence in medical circles, not only in the United States but in Europe as well, such recognition was high praise and much appreciated by those so honoured.

Basic lessons for patients were often emphasised in the preface. Thus, even in the first edition Joslin stated that "*any method of treatment, to be of maximum service, must be simple alike for physician and patient, for the practitioner is a very busy man and the patient must clearly understand the reasons for a Spartan life.*"

"Who Wants a Vacation?"

The period following the interruption of Joslin's practice by the First World War was initially dominated by activities relating to his restarting his practice. The second edition of his textbook had been written within a year of the first edition. Just when he had planned to write the third edition is not clear. What is obvious, however, is that Joslin recognised the magnitude of the effect insulin would have on the life of the diabetics, and realised that it was essential to present this in both his publications, the textbook in 1923 and the manual the following year.

The deep impression made on Joslin by the dramatic effects of insulin, especially on diabetic children, is best described by him in the preface.

"Who wants a vacation when he can watch mere ghosts of children start to grow, play and make a noise and see their mothers smile again, and read in the paper that this young colonel, with the Victoria Cross, after 10 years of faithful dieting has nearly won the local golf championship."

The third edition, issued in 1923, deserves special mention for several reasons. Firstly, it was in 1923 that insulin became generally available for diabetics in America.

Secondly, its dedication to "Banting and Best and the Toronto Group of Insulin Workers" marked the beginning of Joslin's association and friendship with the two Canadians, especially Best, which was to endure to the end of Joslin's (and tragically, also Banting's) life. Banting died in a plane crash in 1941.

Banting and Best were the only ones to whom Joslin dedicated two editions of the textbook, the second being the eighth in 1946, the 25th anniversary of the discovery of insulin. The fact that Charles Best had become particularly fond of his ageing mentor, with whom he had kept closely in touch since their first meeting in 1921, may also have been a reason for this gesture by Joslin.

The preface begins with a short but moving reflection – almost a soliloquy – on the personalities who bestrode the medical stage in the early years and whose names were part of the history of the condition. Many had influenced Joslin through their writings and, in later years, personal contact. He mourned them as "the other diabetic saints," saying "how they would have enjoyed this year." He named Cantani, Kulz, Lepine, and Bouchardat.

Joslin had always admired Bouchardat, referring to him as the "Prince of Physicians". The French physician, regarded by some as the father of diabetology, had devoted his life to the study of the subject and the care of diabetics. Joslin never failed to visit Bouchardat's grave in the Pere Lachaise Cemetery whenever he visited Paris.

(*The grave of Claude Bernard, the celebrated French scientist, is located in the same cemetery. However, perhaps the most famous French physician, Jean Martin Charcot, is buried in the cemetery at Montmartre.*)

Bouchardat practised at Hotel Dieu, a hospital in Paris, which dates its beginnings from the sixth century. The hospital, still in operation at the same site across the road from Notre Dame, has a room in its attic where my wife and I have stayed during our visits to Paris. After-hours access to the room is by sharing the emergency ward elevator, often carrying a patient to the operating theatre!

The third edition is also remarkable for a 100-page essay on insulin by Joslin. It includes in detail his experience with the new preparation, and demonstrates a remarkable grasp of the finer points of the practical aspects of insulin use, ranging from methods for preparing and drawing up the solution in the glass syringe to adjusting its dose, depending on type (protein, fat and carbohydrate) and amount of food eaten and physical activities undertaken by the patient.

Later Editions of the Textbook

The only other individual to whom Joslin dedicated one of his textbooks was the New York banker and philanthropist George F. Baker. Baker had financed the Baker Building at the Deaconess Hospital allowing Joslin to establish a laboratory for studies on, and services for, his diabetic patients. Joslin was the first Director of the Baker Research facility.

The dedication in the fourth edition of the textbook, published in 1928, says:

"George F. Baker, banker and philanthropist,

Who by efficient length of days, a stimulus to the middle aged. Founder of the George F. Baker Clinic for Chronic Disease at the New England Deaconess Hospital, Boston, Massachusetts."

Joslin's early recognition of diabetes as a public health problem stemmed from his observation of diabetes in his own hometown of Oxford in the early 1900s.

"For the government the extent of the diabetic situation is serious," he stated in the preface to the eighth edition published over 70 years ago, drawing attention again to the increasing number of diabetics in the American population even then. He did not mince his words, and bluntly foreshadowed the financial burden the government could expect! Today diabetes is prominent in the costlier categories of healthcare which are a continuing challenge for providers of healthcare and ultimately, the government.

Perhaps inspired by the dramatic experiments in Toronto, the fourth edition released in 1928 included an excellent section on experiments carried out on dogs by Professor Hedon and reported in a French medical journal in 1924. An additional feature of this edition was the emphasis on children with diabetes and diabetes in pregnant women which were both accorded separate sections. Diabetes in pregnancy was a single author contribution by Dr Priscilla White, who would later become a world authority on the subject.

It is also interesting to note that compared to the first edition issued in

223

1916, knowledge in various fields related to diabetes had led to such an increase in information that the size of the 1928 edition was more than double the initial publication.

The fifth edition (1935), and the sixth did not have a specific dedication. In the fifth edition he noted that he had "about 300 doctors, 1000 children and in all some 13,000 cases" attending his practice. That number of doctors as patients attending a physician's private practice would be considered an exceptionally large number, even by today's standards. The fifth edition also saw, for the first time, his first three associates, Root, White and Marble as co-authors. On the title page below Joslin's name complete with his academic and clinical appointments are listed the names of the associates in smaller type under the heading "with the cooperation of the". The spine of the fifth (and the sixth) editions continued to carry only Joslin's name. From the seventh edition published in 1940 through to Joslin's last textbook released in 1959, the co-authors received equal billing on the title page and the spine.

A natural progression of the increased scope of diabetic complications, dominated by damage to arteries in the legs and in the eyes and kidneys, was recognised by Joslin several years earlier when he had started to add specialists to his team, starting with the surgeon Leland McKittrick in 1926.

However, perhaps displaying a characteristic of an ageing warrior, he was not giving up easily. In the preface to the fifth edition he said, "To practice diabetes today one must be, first of all, a general practitioner,.." Then relenting, perhaps reluctantly, he added, "although one longs in addition to have training in a dozen specialities."

However, he did acknowledge the advantages of specialisation (within the sub-speciality of diabetes) by recording the contribution of an earlier assistant.

"My former assistant, Dr William R. Jordan studied the nerve complications of our diabetics and revealed much that we have overlooked."

Interestingly, my copy of the fifth edition belonged to a Dr Cushing (not related to Harvey Cushing as far as I could determine). Whether she was one of the 300 or had simply bought Joslin's book for her library is not known.

Though not specifically dedicated to anyone, the sixth edition may as well have been dedicated to the Danish chemist Hans Christian Hagedorn (1888-1971) because of the opening sentence in the preface.

"Protamine Insulin necessitated the revision of this book. Of its value, my associates and I are convinced, because we see in protamine zinc and other insulin compounds, which will follow in its train, the beginning for the diabetic of a new and better epoch – *The Hagedorn Era*."

In 1936 Hagedorn had discovered that the effect of injected insulin could be prolonged by the addition of a protein called protamine. Later, combining the new preparation with zinc prolonged the effect even further to 24 hours from the original 2–4 hours. This was a major breakthrough for patients with diabetes because, instead of having 4, 5 or 6 injections every day, they could control their blood sugar levels with a single injection each day.

Later in this edition Joslin also made an interesting remark regarding his friend Fredrick Allen. Often described as dour, it appears that even Allen's written expression was known for an economy of words which may explain some of his difficulties with communicating with patients. Commenting on Allen's writing Joslin said, "Dr F.M. Allen with his gift of terse expression…" (p332).

The frontispiece to the seventh edition is a photograph of a plaque stating in part, "but our minds linger as well on the animals who gave up their lives not for their masters whom they loved but for diabetics whom they did not even know." And what could well be regarded as a dedication, "To those who give their lives for the welfare of mankind."

In 1940 Joslin, entering into his 70s, looks back on his career, beginning his preface with "This book records the facts which have helped me treat 19,000 diabetics .. over a period of 40 years."

Then, perhaps for the first time, an admission. "It is easily seen that this expansion has necessitated too much detailed knowledge for me". He goes on to speak of his associates who "during the last 15 to 19 years have stamped their identity upon diabetic progress in this country". He was referring to Root, White and Marble – in that order!

(During my time in Boston I noticed a sense of competition between at least some of the members of the staff in their association with Joslin. White, in a conversation with me said, "I started with Dr Joslin before Dr Marble. Only Dr Root got to work with him before I joined.")

The seventh edition also contained one of the few instances of his acknowledging his son – "for the last five years my son, Dr Allen P. Joslin has borne much of the burden and heat of the day's work in office and hospital...."

Lastly (what made my heart warm,)... *And I cannot overestimate the stimulus we have all received from the group of graduate physicians who have held Fellowships in our clinic.* " I hasten to add that I cannot number myself in that select group who knew him but, as stated in the preface of this work, I believe that every Fellow, past and present, of the Joslin Clinic holds that association as a special and unique period in his or her postgraduate career.

Towards the end of the preface he finishes with his usual reference to the classics or philosophy, in this case the latter. "Josiah Royce [a Harvard philosopher] believed in "the fecundity of aggregation," and we trust this volume illustrates his concept. It represents the efforts and contributions of patients and doctors, of collaborators whose names appear in the text..."

In permitting the participation of others was he sensing that it was time to loosen the reins of the steeds he was controlling in pursuit of his personal goals and ambitions?

Little did he know that the Gordian knot of his destiny was still firm and would be tightened even more.

The eighth edition is unusual in that it included, for the first and only time, an additional name in the list of contributing authors. Dr C Cabell Bailey was listed along with Root, White and Marble.

"Progress in diabetes has always started in the laboratory," wrote Joslin in the preface to this edition. The new contributor was the sole author of a chapter on experimental diabetes. Bailey also revised several other sections which resulted in this edition being longer than any other at 861 pages. Bailey did not stay with Joslin for very long, returning to his home state in the south of the United States. However, he retained his relationship with Joslin and his associates in Boston, even after Joslin's death.

In the later editions increasing contributions from his associates, especially White, Marble and Root, assisted the ageing Joslin. However he maintained firm control of the project through to the 10th edition, published in his 90th year. But even greater than the contribution of his medical team was the overall guidance and editorial assistance of Anna Holt who, having retired several years earlier, returned to help with the final (10th) editions of the text and the manual. This is described later in this account.

Seeking Joslin: the Joys of On-line Search

And for the little, little span
The dead are borne in mind,
Seek not to question other than
The books I leave behind.

Rudyard Kipling.

Now in its 14th edition, the first edition of Joslin's textbook is considered a classic .It is much sought after and difficult to obtain. I had the advantage of the efforts of my friend and fellow bibliophile Professor Milton Roxanas of Sydney University who located a copy online. Interestingly, the book belonged to a fellow-physician who lives in Chestnut Hill, a suburb of Boston located almost next door to the Joslin Diabetes Centre. Even allowing for inflation over the last 50 plus years, (the original price was $4.50), the $250 I paid is still considered a steal by book collectors. (My copy is not for sale!)

Finding an original copy of the second edition was nearly as difficult as the first. When I examined the book online, my heart sank at a handwritten note in lead pencil on the flyleaf, "classic." A handwritten invoice ($80) with the rubber stamp of the bookseller who like the physician from whom I had obtained the first edition, was also from Chestnut Hill, Boston.

The reason for getting the second edition was my curiosity about the short time interval from the issue of the first. Like the publishers, I wondered about Joslin's reason for doing this. Displaying an uncanny instinct for anticipating the question, Joslin did not keep me waiting! It was answered in full in the second paragraph of the preface.

"In the additional 120 pages and more of the new edition, for much in the former edition has been condensed, I have incorporated answers to questions raised by doctors and patients since the previous publication as well as the conceptions of diabetes now uppermost in my mind... A Case Index to supplement the General Index and a record of the subsequent history of nearly all cases mentioned in the earlier edition increase the value of the volume."

In retrospect, the significance of the 1916 and 1917 editions was possibly diminished by events beyond Joslin's control, the unforeseen interruption stopping him mid-flight, so to speak. Along with thousands of young men and women in the United States, Britain and Europe, he had to put his life on hold to serve in his country's armed forces.

Over a ten-year period I managed to acquire all 10 editions of the textbook. Some, like the first and second editions, were owned privately, some were from libraries, usually donated by families of doctors. Some, unmarked, invited speculation as to the previous owners. All except two copies were obtained from sellers in the United States. There was a copy from Argentina (in English), and one from the medical library of the University in Heidelberg in Germany. On the flyleaf of this last one was a faded scarlet stain. I dismissed the idea of it being a bloodstain, the result of a duel fought by aspiring physicians fancying their prowess as swordsmen–a practice for which the university town was well known in those years!

Part 11.
Teacher

The Joslin Diabetic Manual – Encore or Main Event?

"Tis not knowing much, but what is useful that makes a man wise."

Thomas Fuller 1732*

In the entire spectrum of common chronic afflictions visited upon the human race, diabetes occupies a unique position. This is because the patient has to treat himself with a combination of diet and medication, either or both of which may need to be changed–often more than once a day–by the patient. The need for an instruction manual, therefore, is self-evident.

A case could have been made for Joslin to write the manual before the textbook. It is entirely possible that he had done this but chose to release the textbook first, perhaps because he recognised that it was an important first. Certainly the textbook generated great publicity for him beyond Boston and the neighbouring cities where he was well known already. "Any publicity is good publicity" is a common commercial slogan, and the publicity generated by Joslin's first book may well have paved the way for more successful marketing of his second offering.

*This aphorism was used by Dr George P Kozak, (a senior physician at the Joslin Clinic during my time), as the epigram in the introduction of his book *Clinical Diabetes Mellitus* published in 1982.

A Memorandum of Agreement in Time of War

A copy of the original contract bearing the signature, "Elliott P. Joslin", as well as the signatures of his two faithful secretaries, Marjorie Wood and Helen Leonard, dated July 19, 1917 formalised the agreement between the writer and Lea & Febiger for Joslin to prepare "a manual of directions for diabetic patients." The contract specified that the said work be "complete and ready for the printers preferably, by October 1, 1917 but not later than December 1, 1917".

To meet the deadline, Joslin had to seek the help of his secretary due to his unforeseen call up for military service. He was ordered to report for duty on 6 February 1918. Unable to do the final revision himself, Joslin left the task to her.

In the preface to the manual he acknowledged her contribution with "I'm especially grateful to my publishers because of their continued courtesies, and to my secretary, Miss Helen Leonard, upon whom has devolved the final revision of the proof."

Publication of the manual was completed and was ready for issue in November 1917. Its sales, at 45 cents a copy, followed the pattern of Joslin's first book. By June 1918 the initial run of 2000 copies had been sold. At this time Joslin was still in the army. A further 2000 were sold between June and December 1919 when the publishers produced a run of 7500 copies, the largest single lot up to that date. Looking through the records in the Lea Febiger archives, one can see that the manual retained its readership with yearly sales of around 7,500 copies.

The Power of the Joslin Pen

First and foremost Joslin was known for his facility of language, written as well as spoken. The tone of his delivery was almost conversational. Often this meant leaving scientific explanations in the background while giving prominence to encouragement and reassurance. Joslin's language was simple, direct and free of medical jargon. During a visit to the Joslin Clinic some years after completing my Fellowship, while visiting the Marble Library, I recalled seeing a manual written by another physician (many years after Joslin had popularised this aid to diabetic care) and noticing a note in the margin in Joslin's handwriting. "Too many long words," it said. He had put a circle around gluconeogenesis, a biochemical term used to describe a process by which the body produces sugar (glucose).

Although he did not resile from describing the discomforts and concerns suffered by the patient and, in the case of children, their parents, Joslin was adept at providing reassurance. He pointed out that diabetes was "not painful, unsightly or infectious." He adopted a simple and unsentimental approach to convince the patient that his (Joslin's) optimism was based not on reassurance alone, but on a clear and logically sound pathway to achieving control of the condition.

The manual offered meaningful hope for survival. It proved especially useful for parents of diabetic children. Before the discovery of insulin, children who developed diabetes usually did not survive more than two years. Even minor infections like a cold frequently led to an accumulation of certain chemicals in the blood (acidosis) which was fatal. The anxiety, apprehension and fear which beset any human being suffering from a potentially fatal condition, which is not fully understood and has no known cure, is an unbearable burden, especially for the young and their parents.

This was the challenge that faced the doctors of that time when called upon to treat especially children so afflicted.

Dr Joslin, A Human Being First and a Physician Second

What Joslin was able to achieve through his method of communicating with the patient and those involved in caring for him or her was to be able to present the condition of diabetes as being a condition which was *relatable*. The value of this can only be appreciated by those who have experienced the sense of isolation when afflicted with a condition, even when effective treatment is available. The burden was much more profound in the case of diabetes before the discovery of insulin. Repeatedly I came across accounts, not only by his colleagues but by patients and their relatives, of Joslin's personal approach which was dominated by compassion. A mother spoke movingly of his deep empathy. That this view was also held by his colleagues is supported by the large number of doctors who referred themselves to him to care for their diabetes.

Barnett's detailed description of one of Joslin's patients would strike a sympathetic chord in anyone who has been involved in the life of young people so afflicted. The account contained in his book on Joslin is presented here in brief.

It is the story of Frances Putnam, the daughter of James Putnam, the senior physician Joslin had joined as an assistant in 1898. Frances was born on 20 October 1897. The young graduate was very taken by the child's good nature. He had given her a charm engraved with "from your would-be admirer, Elliott Joslin."

Tragically, in 1912 Frances developed diabetes. By this time Joslin's reputation in managing the condition was well known. But it was before insulin had been discovered. The Putnams brought their child to him. There is a memorable account in Frances's mother's diary of Joslin's compassionate care of their daughter who died within a year of contracting the condition. She noted that Joslin was "a human being first and a physician second". She spoke of "the look of compassionate concern on Dr Joslin's face."

Putting the Patient in Charge – Another Joslin Initiative

To emphasise the unique role of the patient with diabetes in his day- to-day management, Joslin placed the responsibility squarely upon the patient's shoulders even before starting the first chapter. In his dedication he declared,

To the diabetic patients of the United States of America.

"Upon each one of you rest responsibilities of saving food both by your own example, shown in the careful treatment of yourself, and by instruction of those about you in food values."

To hammer home the point, the frontispiece contained a photograph of three lumps of sugar obtained after evaporation of urine samples of patients in his practice identified by their case numbers. The first was a heap of sugar cubes weighing 680 g which is the amount of sugar lost through the urine of a severe diabetic in a single day. Joslin calculated that losing this amount each day would lead to a yearly loss of 516 pounds (1 1/2 barrels) of sugar a year! Next is a smaller heap of sugar from a moderate diabetic losing 240 pounds (2/3 barrel a year,) while the third was from a mild diabetic losing 140 pounds/year.

I have not counted the number of lessons imparted even before the reader has reached the opening chapter.

Ever the diplomat, Joslin was only too aware of possible criticism by members of his own profession that he was advocating self- doctoring and encroaching on the hitherto exclusive domain of the medical profession. Hence the title *A Diabetic Manual for the Mutual Use of the Doctor and Patient.*

When encouraging the patient that "he is his own nurse, doctor's assistant and chemist", he hastened to add that "if he tries to be his own doctor, he will come to grief ".

The knowledge of diabetes at that time was limited as indeed were its manifestations because, as already stated, often patients did not survive beyond a few years. Thus the burden of complications of the disease which are seen today because diabetics now live longer was not known at that time.

Joslin therefore devoted a large part of the manual to details of the dietary needs and restrictions. Starting with the importance of using scales to weigh the food, he explained how to calculate the caloric value of commonly used items. Sample diets were described including a seven-day menu plan.

Emphasising that education through self-management was worthwhile for patients, he stated that "to acquire the requisite knowledge for this triple vocation (nurse, doctor's assistant and chemist) requires diligent study but the prize offered is worthwhile for it is nothing less than life itself."

Joslin's ability to persuade his readers to his viewpoint was not only because of their own, but also due to their doctor's regard for his reputation as a leading authority on the subject. A good example of this is found in the preface to the sixth edition.

"A knowledge of the disease," he said, "is a great asset to the diabetic."

He then followed it with actual examples from his patients.

In this instance he revealed that he had in his care at that time 300 doctors.

(There are few greater compliments to a physician's expertise than having his colleagues seek his advice on their own or their families' health problems).

He compared the survival rates of the doctors with patients less familiar with diabetes and revealed that not one doctor had died from diabetic coma. He used this to stress to all diabetics the importance of learning about their condition. Hence the need for a manual on the subject.

The manual, true to its title, was a guide for the treating doctor as well. It is thought-provoking that the writer in the early 1900s advocated a team approach to the treatment of diabetes. The team he suggested, and which he had used in his own practice for several years, would be considered modern, even today. Indeed, Joslin advocated including chemists in the treatment team, an innovation not seen in the treating teams in most parts of the world even now.

Nurses trained by Joslin, the best known being Harriet McKay, became an integral part of the group. Their training was so thorough and their experience so broad that Joslin nurses were sought after in places distant from Boston. Indeed the request was most commonly from doctors who considered themselves inexperienced by comparison with Joslin-trained nurses in the treatment of the everyday problems of diabetes. One example of this as early as 1918 was when Joslin's colleague Frederick Allen was treating Elizabeth Hughes, the 11-year old daughter of the prominent US Supreme Court judge, Charles Evans Hughes. A Joslin nurse supervised Elizabeth's day-to-day care.

Information in the manuals as indicated by the contents listed in the beginning gave the reader access to any information needed for a particular problem. A clear description of diabetes was followed by sections on recent improvements in treatment which would engage the interest of patients in particular, but given the frequency with which health professionals are asked about "the latest", the information was also valued by members of the medical team.

A chapter on the history of diabetes may not be of great interest to a diabetic, especially one who has only recently developed the condition and is turning to the manual for information. He may not have any interest in, or patience with, a history lesson.

The very next chapter, however, has the reassuring title of "Questions and Answers for Diabetic Patients." This was a direct result of Joslin's experience acquired over many years. He had a gift for sensing the patient's needs as well as anxieties, most commonly expressed through questions or enquiries into their own symptoms and the possible relationship of these to diabetes. Here, along with his own contribution, he'd include a separate section written by one of his teaching nurses. It was interesting to see the difference in the kind of questions patients posed to the nurse as opposed to the physician.

Patients told me that this was the first chapter they turned to upon acquiring a copy of the book and almost always found answers. Many felt reassured that their problems were not as uncommon as they thought.

The chapter is a thought-provoking discussion on a wide range of topics which, in the view of patients, are related to diabetes – *their* diabetes. Photographs and diagrams illustrate the practical aspects of treatment such as how insulin should be withdrawn from a bottle, how gas bubbles could be expelled from the syringe, and the angle at which the needle should be placed before piercing the skin. Line diagrams showed the different areas of the body where insulin was to be injected.

Concise, clear answers free of medical jargon were one of Joslin's many gifts and are repeatedly demonstrated in his writings in the manuals.

Therefore, it is not surprising that he was respected, some used the word revered, not only by patients, but in the case of children, their parents as well.

Joslin the Showman: Director, Producer &Choreographer

Joslin frequently involved his patients in the manuals. Although their actual identity was kept from the reader, many were featured complete with photographs. He always made a point of stating that this was done with the patient's permission.

A good example is an eight-year-old called Barbara whose photograph appears in the fourth edition. "How Barbara felt after taking insulin" is the caption of the photograph of the child doing a handstand! Joslin made this point because, unlike the needles of today which are manufactured by sophisticated methods and machinery, needles in the early to mid-1900s had a wider bore and sometimes had to be sharpened by the user. *Injections caused pain,* a daily challenge for the parents who had to give them, often more than once a day.

Over the years "giving my injection" was the most frequent complaint made to me not only by the young but also adult diabetics. Therefore Barbara was a boon for Joslin. As evidently were her parents.

Joslin the showman – even the prim Miss Anna Holt, his memoirist, described this trait in him – excelled himself by having little Barbara demonstrate self-injection of insulin before a combined meeting of doctors of the New York Academy of Medicine, the Philadelphia Paediatric Society and the New England Paediatric Society at the New England Deaconess Hospital in 1927.

The returns for the Boston physician from such a demonstration require little elaboration. Certainly the publicity did no harm!

What should also be observed, however, is the empowering effect this had on the patient and her parents, and through them on other diabetics.

(It must be remembered that American medicine permits direct access to medical specialists without referral from another practitioner as is the practice in some other countries including Britain and Australia.)

Another of Joslin's habits in writing his manuals was that of including details of a patient's treatment in summary form. Thus, under Barbara's photograph doing a handstand, the caption read:

How Barbara feels after taking insulin.

Case number 4702. Age at onset:8 years; duration to February 1929, 3 years, 9 months. Recent diet: carbohydrate 75 g, protein 70 to 75 g, fat 110 g. Insulin 20 – 0 – 15 – 5 units.

(Insulin was described according to the number of units being taken: before breakfast, 20 units, nil before lunch, 15 units before the evening meal and 5 units at bedtime.) This form of shorthand provided the essential facts of the patient's diabetes treatment for herself as well as her doctor.

This was the form for describing the main features of a patient for Joslin's early morning meetings which all members of the staff were expected to attend at 8 AM – sharp! The practice was continued long after Joslin's death.

Then, perhaps to jolt the reader back to full attention, there is a captivating photograph of a patient holding a docile looking pet lion! The caption reads "If a diabetic child can control a lion, she can certainly control diabetes." He could change tack from the precise, even didactic form of writing, to musings and introspection.

The Pepys of Diabetes?

The fullness of the description of diabetes, especially in his manuals, reminds one of the value of the small detail in presenting a full picture. Having studied classics at Yale, Joslin retained an interest in literature throughout his life.The value of the complete essay was evident in all his writings. The mastery of the finer details is a true indication of the physician's competence. Little wonder that even modern writers on diabetes have referred to Joslin as the greatest diabetologist of the twentieth century.

Samuel Pepys (1633-1703), the renowned English diarist, is owed his fame because he recorded his times in great detail. This allowed readers in later years to view life in Pepys' England without the gaps they encountered in descriptions which presented only the main features – the highlights. Although the Pepys diaries covered a period of only 10 years, the inclusion of the minor details permitted a more complete picture of that period than many other descriptions.

It was the same with Boswell's biography of Samuel Johnson, best known as the author of the first English dictionary. The accuracy of Boswell's description was such that it permitted later (medical) scholars to make the diagnosis of Tourette's syndrome, an ailment which troubled

Johnson, and which explained some of the good doctor's "idiosyncrasies"!

The user-friendly arrangement of topics in Joslin's manuals almost made an index unnecessary. However, true to form, Joslin did not leave any stone unturned in ensuring that each manual was complete with a comprehensive index. Thinking (rather foolishly as it turned out) that there could be nothing in the index of a diabetic manual primarily designed for patients which I (being a specialist in the field !) would not be able to answer, I went through the index of the 6th edition. I was doing well–but not perfectly–until I got to Z and was completely stumped by zweiback. In the end, I had to admit that in any little games I played, Joslin invariably got the better of me. I suspect I was not the first one to have tried this. (Zweiback is a rusk or sweet biscuit popular in European countries).

Practical management ranging from measurement of sugar in the urine and blood to everyday problems such as dental hygiene were described in clear and simple language. Advice and instruction also included warnings of the dangers of practices or products considered incorrect.

Joslin did not hesitate to criticise a treatment if he did not agree with it. For example, when discussing recipes he stated, "Many books have been written containing recipes for diabetic patients. With modern methods of treatment, however, *most of these rules are worthless* for severe diabetic patients because of their high content of protein and fat." Instead, he suggested that "in general such patients prefer, and should be encouraged, to take simple natural foods rather than artificial ones." If he suggested a proprietary line, the footnote would provide the name and address of the store which stocked the item.

Even if diabetes did not have any particular influence on certain complaints troubling a patient, the fact that the responsibility of care was, in the first place, the patient's own, is a burden often not fully appreciated. Anything which troubles a diabetic patient is usually, and not always correctly, considered to be related to his sugar. Only those experienced in its management, either as parents of children with diabetes, or adult patients themselves, realise the need for answers to queries which may be considered trivial to the unacquainted. Therefore the management of diabetes, especially in children, was challenging for many medical practitioners then and even now.

Joslin addressed diabetes not only with the mind of a doctor, but when addressing a patient or his parents he spoke from his heart. His compassion endeared him to patients as well as their relatives. Nor did it escape the notice of any onlookers including his staff.

The later editions were written in most, if not all, instances to mark, champion, or celebrate significant advances in the treatment of diabetes. It is the experience of most physicians in practice that patients are reassured if their doctor is keeping up with medical and scientific advances. The latest or research related treatments are understandably of great interest not only to patients but, especially in the case of children with diabetes, their parents. Reading any of Joslin's manuals for patients displays this sensitivity in him in a manner which sets an example for anyone writing for the lay public.

In addition to the popularity of the manual in the United States, Britain and Europe, translations into Spanish spread his fame in South America. The connection with that country was immeasurably strengthened by the assistance Joslin gave to a young medical researcher called Bernardo Houssay. Dr Priscilla White told me that the brilliant investigator had difficulty having his work published in the United States until Joslin had intervened. Liked and respected by the medical and scientific community in Boston, Joslin had little difficulty in having a word with the editors of medical journals which in many instances had carried articles written by him. Houssay's publications were well received and led to worldwide recognition of his contribution. He went on to win the Nobel Prize for his work on the pituitary gland and its connection to diabetes.

White said, "Houssay never forgot what Dr Joslin had done for him."

A manual was published to follow each edition of his textbook, usually within one year. He continued this together with his many other activities for more than 40 years.

If writing the first textbook on diabetes spread Joslin's name in the medical fraternity, his manuals for patients reached an even wider audience.

As already noted, Joslin timed the issue of new editions to coincide with significant events in the treatment of diabetes. A good example was the sixth edition, published in 1937. Its preface stated,

"Insulin rescued the diabetic and set him on his feet, but *protamine* insulin has given him an opportunity to live almost like a normal individual."

Keeping the Reader Interested

Mystery, it is said, is the charm of life. Joslin certainly believed this, or at least he used this to tantalise or keep the reader guessing.

Epigrams introduced many chapters. They were drawn from his wide interests in the classics, philosophy and history in which his interest continued throughout his life.

However not all epigrams were from his own collection. I was intrigued to read in the second edition of his textbook a reference to "my friend who supplies me with epigrams". Having looked at the acknowledgements and footnotes in all 10 editions of his text as well as the manuals I did not discover the name of the "friend".

In the second edition of the manual, published in 1919, Joslin concluded his preface with acknowledgement of the assistance of his secretary Anna Holt and the assistant at that time, Dr Albert Horner, and "to that one rare friend who offered criticisms..." Another secret he kept from his readers – and me!

Elsewhere in this work I have referred to the epigram attributed to James Phinney Baxter, Joslin's uncle, a connection not mentioned by him. One explanation for this may be that Baxter was firmly against vivisection, which was contrary to Joslin's attitude to the use of animals in experiments to benefit humans. After all, it was through experiments carried out on dogs that insulin was eventually discovered. Joslin devoted a good deal of space in his writings to this subject. He also had a plaque designed featuring animals used as experimental subjects.

Then there was the mysterious "H.R.A", again acknowledged in the preface of several of the manuals for contributing to the chapter on diet and exercise. I asked Donna Younger about this but she was also in the dark.

Repeatedly I found myself engaging in this kind of exercise of searching for his secrets, only to discover that he was always a step ahead, keeping my interest/curiosity alive but at bay! Was this one of his techniques for keeping a tight rein on his staff, I wondered?

I now understood what Priscilla White might have had in mind when, during a conversation with me at the girls' summer camp in Oxford, she said of Joslin, "He could have been anything."

It was during this time that I spent with this remarkable physician, renowned for her pioneering work of management of the pregnant diabetic and the care of babies and children born with the condition, that I learnt many things about Joslin whom she clearly admired and to whom, according to Barnett, she was fiercely devoted. In her own words, White had a father-daughter relationship with Joslin.

(Permitting myself a slight digression, Priscilla White had about her an aura recognised by all who associated with her, however briefly. In an age when women weren't admitted to the Harvard Medical School, undeterred, she went to Tufts, graduated near the top of her class, and went on to become a world authority on diabetes. White's contributions to the treatment of many aspects of diabetes remain pertinent to the present day. Hers is a story waiting to be told.)

The Teacher Who Respected His Patients and Their Intelligence

Joslin encouraged his patients to read about scientific advances. Quoting the great French physician Louis Pasteur, he said. "Chance favours only the prepared mind." Only, in this case (9th edition, page 41), the quotation was in French! Was that to keep the reader interested? or awake!

Photographs of eminent scientists and physicians provided added interest to readers of the manuals. Thus portraits of Frederick Banting and Charles Best appeared in several editions.

Some of the writings in the manuals are little short of brilliant in the exposition of the subject matter through the simplicity of his prose and conciseness of description. One would be hard pressed to find a more complete description of the history of diabetes than the one written following the development of protamine zinc insulin in 1937. Starting with ancient history in India and Rome, he quickly moves to the salient developments in Europe and England before describing the important part played by the pancreas as revealed by Banting and Best of Canada.

He never forgot the contribution of Fredric Allen of New York, whose work on undernutrition averted death for many diabetics (albeit at the cost of marked weakness from weight loss) before the discovery of insulin. Joslin never joined those who criticised the dour and unpopular Allen, but demonstrated the courage needed when supporting one not widely respected. Both remained steadfast in correctly attributing the success of undernutrition to avoid death as was seen most spectacularly when insulin became available for these patients.

He brought the patient up to date with the latest advances in insulin production such as from the addition of a protein (protamine) as described earlier.

Joslin recounted many stories of the dramatic rescue of patients by insulin. He went to great lengths to present the story of Richard Minot, one of his patients and a Harvard professor whom Joslin treated with one of the earliest batches of insulin. Minot went on to prominence in the life of the Harvard research community, culminating in being awarded the Nobel Prize for Medicine and Physiology in 1934 as a co-discoverer of the treatment of pernicious anaemia. One of the nominators of Minot for the prize is recorded in the Nobel archives as "Elliott Joslin, Boston." Barnett called Minot Joslin's prize patient. The medical scientist's photograph featured in the frontispiece of Joslin's last manual, published in his 90th year in 1959.

Many other patients, some named and some unnamed but identified by their case numbers, were also praised by him. Some are mentioned to emphasise a point he was making by way of instruction.

Indeed, one could argue that if Joslin had a favourite, it was the individual with diabetes.

I did not find a single instance in the manuals of the writer talking down to patients. I wondered about this when I noticed that he often used French or German terms without providing their meanings, but guessed that his response to any question on the matter was likely to be countered with a comment like if a person can control his diabetes, he can use a dictionary (as he did on a photo of a patient with a lion's cub.)

Although a very private man and less forthcoming about himself Joslin, unlike other citizens of New England who are known for their reserve, was unusually generous with personal details. On one occasion he confessed, "I fear I am a little hard-hearted towards my over-weight friends". (He was never hard-hearted towards patients.) He then revealed that "a New England conscience compels the disclosure that my grandfather weighed 300 pounds..." Such passages, which read more like conversations with the reader, undoubtedly proved appealing to an increasing number of diabetics. Joslin often quoted from letters written to him by patients. In turn, when I looked through his records, I also found very personal touches in his replies to them.

After providing the results of any laboratory tests done during their visit, Joslin would emphasise the aspect of management successfully carried out by the patient. At that time the term positive reinforcement was not in common use. Yet his approach to patients demonstrated it frequently.

Another of Joslin's customs when writing to patients was enquiring after other members of the family: he was always on the lookout for diabetes in more than one member of a family. On such occasions he would enclose a stamped, self-addressed envelope to encourage a reply. Donna Younger told me that any unsolicited mail from a patient including Christmas cards, was acknowledged with a handwritten note from a staff member. Even after all the years since Joslin's death, she rolled her eyes and could barely keep a tinge of exasperation from her voice when telling me about this, adding that the younger members of the staff – she was the youngest when she joined in 1961 – were co-opted into stuffing Christmas cards into envelopes at Christmas time.

The overriding impression on reading his letters to patients was that they were from a kind and caring man who happened to be a knowledgeable physician.

(Writing to patients after each visit was still the norm at the Joslin Clinic in my time there. It was different from the custom in Australia where letters were, and still are, written only to the general practitioner caring for the patient. I recall one of the physicians on the Joslin Clinic staff receiving a curt note (which he showed me) from the Medical Director, Dr Robert F Bradley asking for the letters to patients seen by that staff member earlier in the week "to be completed and brought to my office within 24 hours."

The Manuals an Enduring Legacy

The Joslin manuals were much more than instruction guides. They were a reliable source of information of new developments in the treatment but also in the understanding of diabetes from medical research. His reading and contact with workers in the field of diabetes research not only in the United States but also in Europe and England was described in simple non-technical terms. The work of a medical researcher Mervyn Griffiths in Canberra–he referred to Australia as "far-off Australia"–was mentioned in several manuals. Joslin himself had continued to contribute to the medical/scientific literature for several years, even after starting in private practice, as he had continued to hold academic appointments in Harvard Medical School

Through the manuals Joslin reached out not only to his own patients, but the wider community of diabetics. Specific mention of patients, especially if accompanied by a photograph, was a special honour for not only the patient but also his/her parents. Would such parents ever begrudge making a donation for diabetes research aiming to improve facilities for treatment, especially if a written request came from Dr Joslin accompanied by a stamped, self-addressed envelope?

The manuals drew patients into the inner fold of diabetic management. Joslin's encouraging manner, accompanied as it was with practical advice and treatment-oriented habits, created a sense of independence and self-reliance in the patient and his/her parents. He never evaded difficult questions, and acknowledged the gaps in understanding the diabetic process at that time. His advice to patients before the discovery of insulin illustrates not only his aptitude for treating a difficult disease but also his empathy for the afflicted and their relatives. One patient wrote of Dr Joslin's profound compassion during the failing treatment of a child with diabetes before the discovery of insulin. Priscilla White, who had worked with Joslin in the pre-insulin era, said she was "in awe" of Joslin's capacity for compassion towards suffering children and their parents. As noted previously, before insulin a child with diabetes usually survived for an average of two years – just a minor infection like a cold being enough to precipitate diabetic coma and death.

Acts of kindness towards their children are seldom forgotten by parents.

My Collection of Joslin's Diabetic Manuals

Over many years I managed to locate and acquire all 10 editions of the manual. All were original Lea & Febiger prints except for the first which was being offered for the price of $1000. I had to be satisfied with a reprint.

All the original editions were owned by men, women or children with diabetes. Some had been donated to libraries.

One was a gift from a daughter to her father, and on the fly leaf a touching note: "To Dad, in the hope that this will persuade you to care for yourself." What stories may lie behind that hope or encouragement?

Another had a postcard addressed to a young woman in Maine (Massachusetts) expressing good wishes for a recovery from her "condition." In those days—and in some communities even now— illnesses such as diabetes and tuberculosis were taboo subjects.

There was a pressed flower in one, with a note from a mother to her daughter in college, dated 1939.

"Write or send a copy to Mr Eaton" was jotted on a piece of yellowed paper in the third edition. Was this a doctor, and was Mr Eaton one of his diabetic patients?

Or did the manual belong to one of the 300 doctors who had diabetes and attended his practice as mentioned by Joslin?

It is interesting that the manuals in several cases were owned by individuals from distant parts of the United States, including the West Coast. One was obtained from a second-hand book dealer in Germany. Clearly the Boston physician's reputation had spread not only to all corners of the United States but also beyond its shores.

It was remarkable that at least three of my copies were dated by their owners in the 1980s. All were the last edition, the 10th, originally published in 1959. In spite of the many advances in the treatment of diabetes, clearly the Joslin manuals still had useful and practical information for patients several decades after the "Dean of Diabetes" had ceased to impart his wisdom in person!

Most editions were reprinted several times. That he did not lose his touch is revealed by the final edition (the 10th) released in 1959, being reprinted three times (1960, 1962 and 1963)!! Joslin had turned 90 in 1959 but his it is clear that his advice continued to resonate with many patients long after his death.

The manuals also have an enduring benefit for students of the history of diabetes. Also, and not surprisingly, they contain several essays of sublime quality.

If, as Barnett said, Joslin was like a missionary who carried a message of hope for diabetics, *A Diabetic Manual for the Mutual Use of Doctor and Patient* was the document he left them as a guide – and as his gift. It might also be said that his manuals were his legacy.

Dates of Issue of Joslin's Textbook and Manuals

Edition	Textbook: date of release	Manual: date of release	Comment
First	1916	1918	Joslin on military service 1918. Secretary proof reads the manual.
Second	1917	1919	Textbook revised and rewritten in less than 12 months after 1st ed.
Third	1923	1924	First text and manual after discovery of insulin. Joslin is effusive in textbook but cautious in manual.
Fourth	1928	1929	Joslin gives seal of approval to insulin for patients in manual.
Fifth	1935	1934	For the first time three senior associates acknowledged as co-authors in textbook.
Sixth	1937	1937	Dr Allen P Joslin (son) acknowledged for the first time–in the preface of manual.
Seventh	1940	1941	Uses (uncle) Philip Feeney Baxter's Persian poem as an epigram in manual.
Eighth	1946	1948	Final proofreading of the manual August 21, 1948-"Saturday afternoon." Sentimental at 79?
Ninth	1953	1953	The first backward glance? Reflects on his 50+ yrs. of practice in preface of the manual.
Tenth	1959	1959	Comes clean on identity of Case 8 in manual–after 60 years!

The "Off-Duty" Joslin: Customs and Habits

What has not been stated in any writings on Joslin is that he himself followed much of the advice he was giving diabetic patients. Although not a diabetic, Joslin, perhaps preternaturally disciplined, never carried excess bodyweight. He also practised what he preached on exercise, and for him regular exercise took the form of walking daily. Even in his late 80s, when he had moved to an apartment in the Longwood Towers situated a few hundred yards from the clinic, he walked to and from work daily. Horse riding on his farm in Oxford, where he spent most weekends, remained an activity pursued to the end of his life. So, to apply one of Joslin's favourite analogies for patients to himself, of the team of three horses – diet, exercise and insulin – for the diabetic patient to manage, Joslin faithfully managed two of them throughout his life! One could speculate that his mother's adherence to her diet and maintaining her lower body weight throughout her years of treatment by her son was an example for the treating physician as well!

Little is known of the personal habits of Joslin's father, but it is tempting to speculate that the Proctor genes were evident in the strong personality of Sarah Proctor Joslin's only son.

Although he never promoted himself in any way and was known for his reserved manner and humility, Joslin's abstemious nature was well known to those close to him. Nearly every description of him (published and verbal) by his colleagues included comments on his personal habits of strict self-discipline.*See note on the next page.

His abstention from cigarette smoking and alcohol was life-long. I was told (by Leo Krall,) that in his later years, when walking to his office from the Deaconess Hospital after doing his morning rounds of patients,if he saw a cigarette butt on the pavement he would stop and, looking over the group of younger colleagues, address one who smoked. "You smoke, you pick it up!"

By contrast he was unfailingly kind and compassionate towards his patients. In one of his manuals he described a touching incident recalled from patient interviews. Coming upon an unprepared patient who could

249

not recall breaking his diet until prompted (and then he did!), Joslin said, "I always pity him and on very exceptional occasions am able to recall with satisfaction after the interview, Solomon's soliloquy in Proverbs 16, verse 32 ."(Joslin manual sixth edition, page 61.) This verse praises self-control and speaks of one who is slow to anger.

Joslin's piety, which like most of his personal life remained private, was well known to those close to him, especially Anna Holt. She spoke of his lifelong habit of never retiring before he had read the Bible and prayed.

*The only recorded lapse in Joslin's self-discipline was his remark in the eighth edition of the diabetic manual published in 1948. It said, "I remember I gained 17 pounds in 17 days following pneumonia in 1906 and then called a halt to overeating." Given that the first manual was published in 1918 one can only speculate on Joslin's reasons for withholding this information for 30 years.

Part 12.
War

Joslin's Practice and Commitments Pre-World War 1

The publication of Joslin's textbook in 1916, followed by a second edition the following year, was during a particularly busy period in his academic, professional and personal life.

The 47-year-old popular Boston physician's practice was flourishing, with patients in several hospitals including the New England Deaconess where he was the principal physician, as well as in several of the smaller hospitals scattered over the city. Prominent among these small institutions were Corey Hill and Faulkner Hospitals.

At the same time he had a busy schedule of bedside teaching for medical students at the Harvard Medical School, serving on various committees including one associated with the medical library, and giving public lectures on common medical topics such as pneumonia.

In the archives of the Massachusetts General Hospital I found old newspaper clippings advertising free public lectures at the Harvard Medical School, the topics ranging from pneumonia to gastric acidity. Joslin's name was featured as a lecturer frequently but the topics were various common ailments. Diabetes did not feature as a topic.

In 1898, the date of Joslin's first appointment to Harvard Medical School, his position was Assistant in the Department of Physiological Chemistry. Doubtless Joslin would have recalled the advice of Professor Russell H Chittenden ,(which he had followed), suggesting that after finishing college at Yale he spend an extra year studying physiological chemistry in the Sheffield School of Engineering which Chittenden had started in order to train young men planning a career in one of the sciences, especially medicine.

In 1900 Joslin became Assistant in the Theory and Practice of Physic. Physic is an old term for the body of knowledge in the field of medicine and is still used by Harvard Medical School. The Professor of Medicine at Harvard during my time in Boston in 1969 and 1970 was the highly respected and distinguished George Thorn, whose official title was Professor in the Theory and Practice of Physic. Thorn was also the editor of the textbook of medicine, originally edited by Harrison, which was the textbook I had used in my senior years at the Sydney University Medical School.

Joslin had also continued his association with Benedict at the Carnegie Nutrition Laboratory, and was still involved in conducting metabolic studies on severe diabetics in association with him.

His family of three children, now aged twelve, ten and eight years, saw little of their father whose day invariably began before sunrise and often ended close to midnight. One of his younger associates recalls that around midnight Mrs Joslin would tap her heel on the floor above her husband's office to call time.

This period also saw the aspiring country squire increasing his landholdings in Oxford. He had continued to add to his original parcel of land until he reached his goal of 300 acres. The land was then divided into various areas including fields for agricultural produce, a poultry farm and stables for horses. Recreational areas including a croquet lawn and tennis court were established in the grounds of the three-storey country home.

Given this scenario of home life and professional commitments, it is not difficult to understand that Joslin's interest in world affairs was, at best, limited to newspaper headlines and conversations with colleagues and patients.

Some events, however, are bigger than an individual's interests and preoccupations.

6 April 1917. Woodrow Wilson Declares War on Germany

The United States had resisted joining the war in Europe between Germany and the Allied forces of Britain and France, maintaining that America had no quarrel with either party. Eventually the threat of German U-boat attacks disrupting American commerce and threatening its security started to sway public opinion. The release by Britain of the Zimmerman telegram (which had been intercepted and decoded by Britain) revealing, the urging by Germany for Mexico to attack the

United States, allowed Woodrow Wilson, the American President, to prevail upon Congress to abandon its favoured position of neutrality.

On 6 April 1917 Woodrow Wilson declared war on Germany and America joined World War I.

The First World War had started in 1914, and doubtless Joslin would have seen posters urging young men and women to join the war effort. The most memorable poster, "Uncle Sam Needs You", with the model's finger pointing at the viewer, was based on a British poster featuring the English war hero Lord Kitchener and the slogan "Your Country Needs You". This had proved so effective in attracting volunteers to the British forces that the Americans adopted the same approach with a local model.

And so it was that Joslin, one day in late January 1918, in the midst of his frantic professional and family activities, received a short letter from the Government of the United States of America spelling an abrupt cessation of all his activities and postponement of all his plans.

He was ordered to report for military duty at 9 am on 6 February 1918.

Joslin's Military Service

Upon receiving his call up Joslin closed his office practice, leaving detailed instructions with his then assistant, Dr Albert Horner, for the treatment until discharge of patients in the various hospitals.

The project at the Carnegie Institute, which had been completed but was not ready for publication, was of particular interest to Joslin because it involved the largest number of his patients studied up to that point. Joslin notified Benedict of the sudden change in his plans and they decided to postpone publication till his return. The findings on 113 patients were eventually published as Carnegie Institute publication number: 232, five years later in 1923.

Joslin's initial placement was at Fort Devens, Massachusetts. The camp, named after Major General Charles Devens, who was from Massachusetts and had served in the Union Army during the Civil War, was situated in Ayre and Stevens, two small towns in Middlesex County, some 36 miles west of Boston. It had originally been the site of Camp Stevens, which had been set up during the Civil War as a training camp for volunteers. During World War I the Federal Government again used Ayer to establish Fort Devens in 1917 to train New England soldiers. The small town with a population less than 1000 at that time was suddenly home to troops numbering close to 100,000.

Following a period of orientation and training, Joslin served as Head of Medical Service in Fort Devens. Six months later he was assigned to the medical service in the army facilities situated in Mesves-sur-Loire in France. Shortly after joining the services he became the Medical Consultant with Howard Collins as his surgical counterpart. The following year, 1919, Joslin was promoted to Lieutenant Colonel.

Assigned to the medical corps, Joslin suddenly found himself in very strange surroundings. In addition to the different routine of military service, medical practice, for practical purposes, was more an exercise in working as part of a large team of doctors. The large patient population presented its own challenges such as transport, as well as issues of public health such as hygiene and sanitation. All this was an entirely new experience for him.

To say that Joslin's entry into the Armed Forces was eventful would be an understatement, for destiny would deal an unforeseen and unspeakably cruel blow to the young American servicemen including the Boston physician.

It was something that neither Joslin, nor indeed the US Army, had foreseen.

The Unexpected Enemy. How the Influenza Epidemic Decimated US Troops, 1918–1919

"The flu depleted and demoralised troops, and may have diverted military and political leaders from fighting the war to combating disease. It ultimately killed more military personnel than did enemy machine-guns and artillery."

"The influenza epidemic in the US military therefore provides a cautionary tale about the power of war to change the health environment and the power of disease to influence the conduct of war."
Carol R Byerly, Public Health Report 2010, 125- (supplement: 3), 82–91.

Within days of Joslin's reporting for duty the first casualty, not from army duty but complications of influenza, was reported in the southern part of the United States. The epidemic of influenza which had started in the fall of 1918 was to dominate the medical care required by the troops. In addition to treatment – preventive vaccines had not been developed at that point – a large part of medical care consisted of instituting basic principles of sanitation and hygiene, segregation of the infected as much as was practicable, and education of all those who were fit enough to take part. The sheer numbers of patients requiring medical attention was almost overwhelming. Joslin, like other physicians and surgeons who were more accustomed to providing individual patient care, found himself in a position which was entirely new as far as the demands on his expertise were concerned.

The rapidity of the spread of influenza, facilitated by the crowded conditions in the army camps, reached epidemic proportions in a matter of weeks. The epidemic which had to be managed by the Army and Navy medical officers is recorded in the annals of war history as the worst of its kind. If Joslin was out of his depth, so were his fellow medical officers. The doctors and their patients saw little military action. The war effort was more an exercise in the logistics of transporting large numbers of flu-stricken soldiers and not wounded servicemen as both parties had anticipated. Neither the doctor nor the patient had the luxury of individual care as was the norm in private practice, such as the one run by Joslin. Instead, he was part of a medical team faced with managing public health issues on a scale he had never seen. Resources allocated for combat were instead directed to transporting and caring for the sick.

Thus, the influenza epidemic markedly hampered the war effort. It is part of the recorded history of America's participation in the First World War that influenza killed more servicemen than enemy fire.

Given the high incidence of influenza amongst the troops as well as the treating team of doctors, nurses and orderlies, it was only by good fortune that Joslin himself did not contract the serious, often fatal, illness.

Joslin's contemporary Harvey Cushing was not as fortunate.

Not only did Cushing contract a severe bout of influenza but he also developed a lingering complication which affected the nerves of his lower limbs causing severe pain in the legs. He was to be troubled by the discomfort in his legs for the rest of his life, not that it dampened his ardour for work.

Cushing went on to pursue an illustrious career pioneering the sub-speciality of neurosurgery. In his time he was regarded as the premier exponent of that demanding and high-risk speciality, and the world's outstanding neurosurgeon.

Diabetes was not a common condition encountered during Joslin's war service. Pneumonia, frequently a complication of influenza, was the most common and serious problem and as there were no antibiotics, the mortality rate was high.

Although Joslin and Cushing did not serve in the same area of France, the two men, who had both been at Yale around the same time, kept in touch and remained friends for the rest of their lives. Joslin practised in Boston throughout his life whereas Cushing started at Johns Hopkins in Baltimore, before being lured to Boston. The two acted as each other's medical advisers. Joslin had conducted an examination for life insurance on Cushing, who in turn had inoculated Joslin against smallpox.

Cushing's admiration of Joslin, which had begun during his student days at Yale, was undiminished throughout his life. Writing to his parents during preparation for an examination, Cushing had remarked, "I think that man Joslin will be at the top of the class." According to Michael Bliss, who wrote a biography of Cushing, "Keeping up with Joslin was to become one of Cushing's self-imposed goals".

On 1 March 1919 Lieutenant Colonel Elliott Joslin was discharged from the army of the United States of America and resumed life as Dr Elliott Proctor Joslin of Boston.

Joslin was always proud of his military service. He said, "The service in the army was one of the greatest pleasures I have had in life and has done more than anything else to broaden my point of view." His rank was an abiding source of immense pride. He made a point of including that in his annual report to the Class Secretary of Yale. He was equally proud of his son Allen's Army service and his rank of major which he mentioned when acknowledging the latter's assistance in producing the textbook by shouldering some of the clinical responsibilities of patient care.

In the second edition of Joslin's diabetic manual for patients, published in 1919, included in his credentials on the title page was "Formerly Lieutenant-Colonel, M.C., U. S. Army." He did not include it in his later manuals or in any editions of his textbooks. He was careful to avoid giving any impression of superiority amongst his colleagues. In fact he seemed much more at ease when in the company of patients, as he was in the manuals. Any public recognition of a physician is noticed by his patients and often is a source of pride for them.

Upon his return Joslin was a changed man. It was clear to all who knew him that the experience of war had a profound effect on him.

The experience, not only of the fighting but, from a medical viewpoint, for one accustomed to working in the comparatively genteel environment of the city of Boston, memories of the suffering and death visited upon the large numbers of young men and women, as much from influenza and its complications as from war wounds, left a lifelong impression on him.

Throughout his life he donated funds towards organisations supporting returned servicemen and their families. His memoirist, Anna Holt, describes an older Joslin taking produce from his farm in Oxford to a lady in the town when he heard that she was serving a meal for several young soldiers.

On another occasion when visiting Britain, upon hearing of an organisation established in one of the hospitals to help returned servicemen, Joslin left a sum of money with one of the professors to be donated anonymously. He had been invited to deliver a lecture on diabetes. Such invitations, especially from England, had become much more frequent since the publication of his book just before the war.

Joslin had turned 50 while serving. But war makes young men old beyond their years.

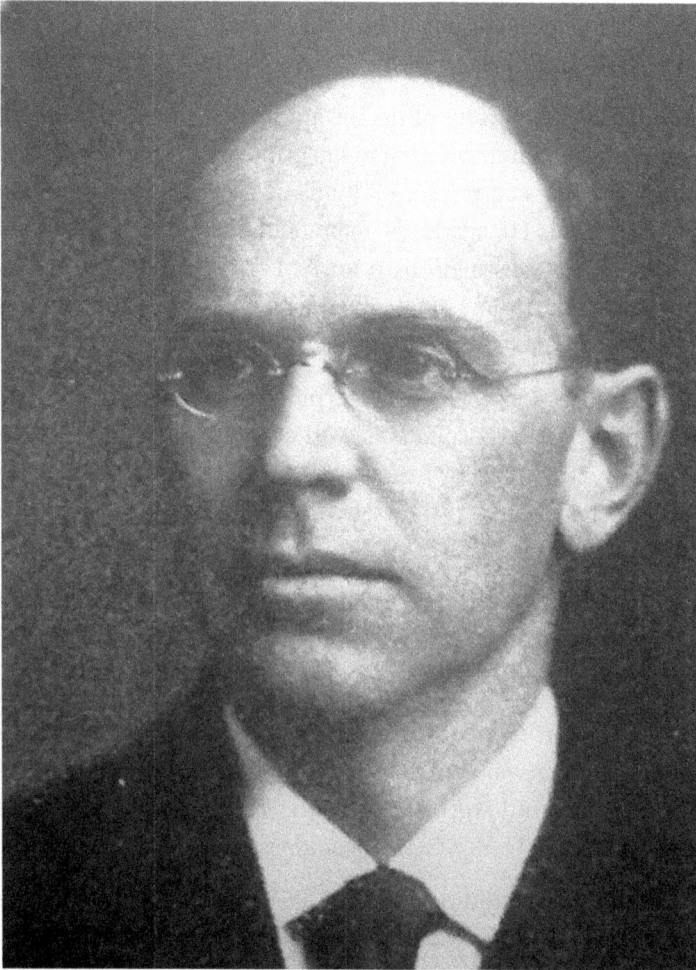

Joslin in 1920

Recollections of a Joslin Assistant

During the celebrations for the centenary of Joslin's birth held on 6 June 1969, one of his former assistants Dr Albert A Horner (later to become

Physician-in-Chief at the New England Baptist Hospital) was invited to describe this stage of Joslin's career and in particular, events pertinent to his callup for military service. Horner also made some interesting general comments on this stage of Joslin's professional life. I have included extracts of this speech from documents kindly provided by Cathleen Sullivan, Assistant Librarian at the Oxford Public Library.

"The hundredth anniversary of the birth of Elliott Proctor Joslin prompts me to remind you that in addition to his prime interest, diabetes mellitus, he spent many years caring for all kinds of illnesses in the speciality of Internal Medicine. He made as many publications on other medical subjects as on diabetes mellitus prior to 1914. His contributions to the knowledge of gastrointestinal diseases, of typhoid fever and of pulmonary tuberculosis were great.

"He developed a very busy private practice, seeing patients in their homes, and in private hospitals as well as in his office. To help in the care of the great number of patients, he needed, and easily acquired as assistants, men who had just finished their internship,– there were no hospital residencies in those days. I was his assistant from 1915 to 1920."

Horner also shared his own observations on Joslin's attitude to the 1914-18 war.

"Early in his career, Dr Joslin studied in Germany and wrote articles in German but after Germany entered Belgium in August 1914, he recognised the great dangers to the world of what the Kaiser was doing and trying to do. Until April 1917, when Pres. Wilson declared war, he kept hoping that the United States would not become involved.

"However after hearing three officers of the French Army speak at the Harvard club in 1917, he came away anxious to get overseas as quickly as possible.

"Of course his responsibilities here (that is towards patients in the various facilities in Boston) were great, and it took him some months to get relief. *[Horner, out of modesty, did not mention that much of the care of Joslin's patients had been left to him.]*

"Initially, when Joslin entered the United States Army Medical Corps, he spent six months as Head of the Medical Service at Fort Devens, Massachusetts.

"Finally he went overseas where he served for several months both before and after the Armistice, in November 1918, as a Consultant in the hospitals of the American Expeditionary Force in France. After his return from World War I Joslin resumed his practice of Internal Medicine with increased emphasis on Diabetes Mellitus."

(Horner's comment on the time when Joslin's special interest in diabetes may have begun, as indicated by his publications prior to 1914, is at odds with the information contained in "A History of Joslin's first 100 years through its Publications" published by the Joslin Diabetes Centre in 1998. Indeed, as early as 1910, Joslin and Francis Gano Benedict had co-authored the Carnegie Institute of Washington paper, "Metabolism in Diabetes Mellitus." There were also several publications on different aspects of diabetes to the end of 1913.

So, although it is true to say that Joslin had patients with other conditions, especially in the field of gastroenterology, his own interest in diabetes was clearly coming to the fore as early as 1910.)

Sunday 6 May 1917

The first American army units sent to war were essentially medical, base hospitals with doctors, nurses and support staff. The soldiers of the American Expeditionary Force (enlisted or conscripted) followed later.

It is interesting to note the difference between Joslin and his contemporary Harvey Cushing at the time of leaving for war service.

Joslin left (and returned) without fanfare.

Cushing reported for duty a few months later but, unlike Joslin, the well-known surgeon was not shy of publicity!

The departure of Base Hospitals Numbers 4 and 5 had occurred with much fanfare and a celebratory service held on Sunday, May the 6th, 1917, at St Pauls Episcopal Cathedral in the presence of many dignitaries, including the Governor of Massachusetts and Mayor Curley. The processional hymn played by the Harvard band was "The Son of God goes forth to War":

"The Son of God goes forth to war,
A kingly crown to gain:
His blood red banner streams afar:
Who follows in his train?"

The church service had been suggested by Harvey Cushing.

The Reverend Endicott Peabody, the respected headmaster of the exclusive Groton School, known for his oratory, had addressed the congregation. Endicott's rich baritone voice held the audience spellbound as he spoke of "the bleeding in France and this unit's mission of mercy."

Women wept during the singing of the Star Spangled Banner and the Battle Hymn of the Republic.

Although not a pacifist, Joslin did not display any great enthusiasm for the war effort. The only mention he made in any of his writings was a footnote in the second edition (p.24) of his manual for the use of diabetic patients, simply noting:

"February 6, 1918–March 1, 1919, absent on duty, Medical Corps US Army."

Resumed practice April 1, 1919."

Joslin was part of the medical units which have gone down in history as the first Americans officially to serve in the war zone in World War I. He never mentioned this in his writings.

Part 13.
1919

1 March 1919

Starting Medical Practice – Again!

By early 1918, prior to his call up for military service, Joslin had completed the manuscript for *A Diabetic Manual for the Mutual Use of Doctor and Patient*. He had already put in place the arrangements for the publication of the manual by Lea and Febiger, the publishers of his textbook. However, the task of handing over the patients to his assistant Horner took priority.

This meant that he had to leave the final proofreading to his secretary Helen Leonard, who duly delivered the material to the publishers after Joslin's departure. The unexpected assignment clearly made Leonard apprehensive. Holt mentioned this in her memoir of Joslin, noting the task had been left to "a faithful and fearful secretary Miss Helen Leonard [who] saw the book through the final throes of publication." The first edition of the manual was therefore released in 1918 while Joslin was serving in the Expeditionary Forces of the United States in France. Leonard's assistance was acknowledged in the preface to the work. Joslin wrote, "I am especially grateful to my publishers because of their continued courtesies, and to my secretary, Miss Helen Leonard, upon whom has devolved the final revision of the proof."

A reprint of the first edition was also issued during Joslin's absence on military service.

Holt went on to say, "The need for this primary text, so clearly written and so readable, was so great that it was accepted with great rejoicing. During the next 43 years it went through 10 editions in the United States and translations in several foreign countries. Its popularity has never waned. All 10 editions were completed under the guidance of Dr Joslin. In fact, the book so proved its worth from the very beginning that it became a worldwide guide for the treatment of diabetes."

Interruption to his work, as well as several projects which were delayed due to his military service, had to be attended to on his return. Publication of his studies with Benedict was delayed further by two factors. The main reason was that Joslin gave priority to restarting his medical practice, but this preoccupation was swiftly relegated to the background because of news of the isolation of insulin by two Canadian researchers, Frederick Banting and Charles Best, in 1921. For these reasons the Carnegie paper did not see publication till 1925.

Joslin was one of the few practising physicians to fully recognise the significance of this event and the extent of its impact on the lives of patients with diabetes and on the practice of medicine. He realised that treatment with insulin was going to markedly change the treatment needs of the patient – as it would Joslin's writings on the subject.

As was typical of the man known for setting himself goals to be reached in minimum time, he allowed exactly one month to get back into harness, regardless of the additional tasks!

It soon became clear that Joslin had underestimated the work needed to get his practice restarted.

He realised his need for more secretarial assistance. Helen Leonard, who had continued working for him after his call up, was retained, but Joslin needed someone to take charge of reorganising the broad range of his activities and responsibilities associated with his practice and academic duties Although his medical practice took precedence he was also keen to resume his writing, especially since he had a binding contractual agreement with the publishers for both his books. He promptly resumed his membership of the various committees in the hospitals where he had been admitting patients previously and expected to do so again.

The person who came to mind was a young woman he had known for many years. Her name was Anna Holt.

Anna Holt

Anna Holt was born in 1890 and had lived in Oxford where her family was well known. Her father had been associated with the A.L. Joslin Shoe Store since its establishment in 1871. At one time she had helped in the Joslin household as governess to the young physician's family.

Holt had been educated in local schools and academies but had later gone to Radcliffe College in Boston, Class of 1914.

In 1919 Holt was employed in the Department of War Risk Insurers in Washington, DC. Joslin wrote to her offering her a job as an assistant and promising to match the salary she was earning at that time. He told her about his plans for writing the second edition of the manual in the near future. Joslin expected that both the manual and the textbook, the latter in preparation for the third edition, were going to need extensive revision and editing. Up to that time both books had sold briskly.

Holt, clearly taken by the physician's energy and enthusiasm, also recognised the opportunity to participate in the production of the books. For her this was a unique opening. Being part of a smaller team so unlike the Washington bureaucracy; working with a respected physician; being back in Boston, a short train journey from Oxford, were all seen as a heaven-sent gift to the young woman.

She accepted the offer, secured her discharge from government employment, and joined Joslin's practice immediately.

The manual in its second edition was released later in the same year. In its preface Joslin acknowledged Holt together with his assistant Dr Albert Horner, stating that " [to] my assistant Dr Albert A Horner and to my secretary, Miss Anna Holt, I am most grateful."

Horner, who had continued as Joslin's assistant during the latter's absence, had cared for the patients who were in hospital at the time of Joslin's call up. However, the number of patients had dropped dramatically, proof of the dependence of the size, even the survival, of the practice on the presence of Joslin himself.

That patients, as well as doctors who referred patients, sought Joslin in particular is shown in a chart in the second edition (p.24) of Joslin's manual for patients published in 1919 and is partly reproduced below. The number of patients Joslin had treated in Corey Hill and New England Deaconess Hospitals starting in 1913 had seen a steady increase from 164 in 1916 to181 in 1917. However, after Joslin's call up in February 1918, that number fell to 23. By contrast, upon his return in 1919, even though he did not start till April of that year, the number jumped to 105.

Number of patients treated by Joslin at Corey Hill and New England Deaconess Hospitals, January 1913 to November 1919.

Year:	1913	1914	1915	1916	1917	1918	1919
Number of cases:	43	60	109	164	181	23	105

Joslin never described himself as a specialist let alone a sub– specialist. In fact he insisted that to be a good internist a doctor had to be a good general practitioner. It is clear, however, that even at this early stage Joslin's practice was heavily weighted in favour of caring for patients with diabetes.

Doctors not only from Boston but also from neighbouring states including New York were referring diabetics to him. This was as much from his reputation through word of mouth of patients and doctors as from his writings in medical journals. The publication of the textbook on diabetes, the first of its kind in the English language, also provided a spectacular increase in referrals. Joslin could not possibly have imagined that the popularity of this publication was to give him prominence in the English-speaking world as a pioneer in the management of diabetes.

Today, diabetology constitutes a sub-speciality which ranks with cardiology, respiratory medicine and infectious diseases as a branch of internal medicine, and deservedly occupies an important place in the clinical spectrum of medical practice and care.

At that time medical practice was divided into surgery and medicine, with the former being almost entirely concerned with surgical operations which had, during this period, received added impetus through the introduction of anaesthesia. The agent used for this purpose was ether. The procedure, which was to revolutionise surgery, had been pioneered at least in that part of the United States by the Massachusetts General Hospital surgical unit. It was here that on 16 October 1846 the highly respected Boston surgeon John Collins Warren had carried out the first surgical procedure. The administration of the ether anaesthetic, etherising, was carried out by a Boston dentist, William T G Morton. Indeed, the term anaesthesia was coined by Oliver Wendell Holmes, another medical luminary of that period.

Behind the Scenes

As planned, the Joslin practice at 81 Bay State Road, Boston was officially ready for business on 1 April 1919. But only officially! In reality, behind the scenes, there was frantic activity driven by the ambitious young physician. Given the sharp decline in the number of patients, could there even have been an element of panic?

Fortunately Joslin had retained his position as Principal Physician of the New England Deaconess Hospital. The smaller hospitals he had used previously were only too glad to provide beds for the patients of the popular doctor.

The various activities and strategies employed to re-energise the practice are better viewed from the recollection of some of his associates, particularly Holt.

While Horner continued to care for patients in hospitals, it was Holt who now took charge of the day-to-day activities designed to get the office practice off the ground. She described the various methods (tactics,) mostly thought up by Joslin, but also Holt and Helen Leonard, to get previous patients back to his practice. In her memoir of Joslin, Holt said,

"Upon return from military service in 1919, at the end of World War I, Dr Joslin faced the delicate task of putting together his practice and opening his office again. The first requisite was to discover how many of his former patients had survived during the war interlude. This necessitated extreme caution in the manner of approach. Letters were written to some patients who were good enough to include in the reply not only how they were themselves but also word about one or even several other patients whom they knew. It was felt more advisable to visit a few patients personally in their homes for some reason or another".

The Modern Age and its Newfangled Gadgets!

Joslin's first car.

According to Barnett, Joslin had bought a car in 1915 before joining the Expeditionary Forces, whereas Holt dates the acquisition at 1919. What is clear however is that, given the spectacular success of the T model Ford sedans, their price had come down after the end of the war. This may well have been a factor in persuading the thrifty physician to make the purchase at the later date.

Holt had quickly realised that having private transport was going to be of considerable help in facilitating transport to the various hospitals, clinics and medical school, not to mention visiting private patients at home.

A significant drawback, however, was that at that time these vehicles required considerable mechanical competence. Synchromesh gears, let alone automatic transmission, were unheard of. Engaging or disengaging the gears required coordinating the action with using the clutch. Neither was there power steering, which made parking or even taking sharp corners a challenge. Joslin, who was never mechanically inclined, was eventually persuaded to hire a driver, much to the relief of his assistants and family! One of the general practitioners who at that time was in a group being tutored by Joslin recalled many years later "a bumpy ride, especially going uphill" to Corey Hill Hospital for bedside tutorials by Joslin. The ride was probably bumpy because of the challenge of engaging the lower gears to negotiate the incline.

Resuming Holt's version:

"It was at this time that E.P.J. bought the first of a long succession of Ford cars. For this first one he hired a robust young man as chauffeur. Eventually, the Doctor learned to drive and continued to do so until the age of 80, when, to the great relief of family and friends, he decided to forego this never-too-perfect accomplishment." So, another robust young man gained employment with the now famous Dr Joslin!

Returning to the task of contacting former patients, the secretary set forth in the chauffeur-driven car to call upon many former patients who had not been traced otherwise. These quests took her to many parts of Boston and even into the suburbs where an automobile at that time had never ventured before. Sometimes the very person being sought would be among the charmed spectators around the little car, and all the information needed, and much more, would be forthcoming in torrential volume. This searching took time but gradually word got out about that the doctor was back and patients, both old ones and new, began coming to the office.

(Given the demands on Helen Leonard, the secretary in the office at this time, it is likely that the person who actually went searching was Anna Holt herself. Her comment on not having been to some of the less affluent suburbs would be consistent with her own upbringing in the genteel village environment of Oxford and later, at the other extreme, the bustling, metropolitan Washington, DC.)

It was not long before the full round of practice was underway and the workload became too heavy for the two assistants and the one secretary. The office force therefore grew to keep pace with the expanding demands.

A Machine Replaces a Secretary!

Soon added to the office equipment was a dictating machine which permitted Joslin to dictate letters at night when no secretary was on duty to take shorthand notes. The machine operated with wax cylinders that recorded in tiny grooves the sounds of the human voice spoken into the transmitter, and the next morning the typist, through the reverse process and using earphones to amplify the sound of the words uttered the night before, wrote the letters as recorded. The cylinders were reusable when shaved smooth again by a machine designed for the purpose–and which lived quietly in a corner of the doctor's bedroom!

Holt commented that "Mrs Joslin learned to live happily with strange roommates throughout her married life."

"The dictating machine and the Ford automobile were the first two members in a long sequence of time-saving equipment the doctor happily accommodated himself to using. In fact, in later years, the more modern and much smaller tape recorder dictating machine went with him on most occasions when he travelled, especially on trips to Oxford for the weekend."

To say that this machine improved Joslin's efficiency would be an understatement. He was now able to dictate letters to patients as well as write articles for medical journals and correspond with colleagues in the United States, Europe and England. What's more, instead of dictating to a secretary, he could dictate without being restricted to his office or office hours. Even though the machine was "most cumbersome", Joslin carried it everywhere, including to Buffalo Hill during weekends.

An example of Joslin's being in a relaxed mood can be seen in the final paragraph of the eighth edition of the manual dictated on a Saturday afternoon at Buffalo Hill. He says:

"As I send this final revision of the page proof to the publishers this Saturday afternoon, August 21, 1948, and bear in mind what I have written about uric acid diabetes and the new modified protamine zinc insulin, I can think of nothing more appropriate than the rubric on building D of the Harvard Medical School composed by Pres Charles W. Eliot and based upon the writing of Hippocrates:

> "Life is short
> and the Art long
> The Occasion instant
> Experiment perilous
> Decision difficult."

The modest and self-effacing Holt – she was a New Englander after all – does not say so, but it is likely that the introduction of the dictating machine, the tape recorder and perhaps even the car was her idea to get the very conservative Joslin into what was, for that time, the modern era.Her efficiency saw the second edition of the Joslin manual meet its publication deadline in early 1919, and its release later in the same year.

As was typical of Joslin the contributions of both, his assistant Dr Albert A Horner and his secretary Anna Holt, were acknowledged in the preface.

Holt was able to achieve all this in a little over one year. Judging by the number of patients seen in 1919, remembering that Joslin had only returned to work on 1 April it is clear that the word had spread quickly. Not counting any patients referred for conditions other than diabetes, in the seven months from 1 April to 1 November 1919 Joslin saw 105 diabetics in his practice, a marked increase from the 23 seen after his departure on 6 February 1918 until his return on 1 March 1919.

End of Anna Holt's Tenure

Whether or not Joslin, or for that matter Holt herself, had expected such a rapid recovery of Joslin's practice is unclear. However, given the punishing schedule he followed, it is not surprising that most, if not all, aspects of his work were resumed and he was again working at the hectic pace he had kept before his call up.

In today's labour market Holt would be recruited on a contract to get Joslin's practice off and running after it had essentially ground to a halt by the end of 1918, because, in retrospect, that description would befit the contribution she made.

However, as it would turn out, her several character traits including a remarkable capacity for organisation and sheer hard work – the latter being one of Joslin's strengths which he was quick to recognise in others–forged a relationship between the two which was to last a lifetime. But for now her association with Joslin was at an end.

Officially then, by late 1920, Holt was no longer employed by Joslin.

So what was the dynamic Miss Holt to do next?

If coming back to Boston was an attraction, as it possibly was, what else could she do? Given the alacrity with which she had left her job with the insurance company in Washington, there is no indication of her wanting to go back to that city or to that work.

On the other hand, I was not able to find any information on any effort on the part of either Joslin or Holt for her to remain in Boston. Not that there was any commitment or expectation on the part of the employer or employee for finding new employment for her.

However, given Joslin's commitments, influence, and popularity at Harvard Medical School and his extensive professional and social network, it is perhaps not surprising that late in 1920 Holt was offered a position as Assistant Librarian at Harvard Medical School. She had no previous experience in this field.

A clue to the possible role of Joslin in securing the position for Holt may lie in an article by Alexander Marble published in the *Transactions of the Association of American Physicians* in 1962. On the occasion of Joslin's death that year, Marble recalled that "Dr Joslin had a strong and abiding interest in medical education and research and had much to do with the early development of the Boston Medical Library."

His experience in this field and therefore his opinion on the suitability of Holt to work in the library may well have been a factor taken into account by the authorities looking to fill the position. Indeed, one could read more into this influence given that the position of Assistant Librarian was a new one. Was the position created at Joslin's suggestion?

Whatever the circumstances which led to her new employment, contact between Joslin and Holt continued, and was regular and consistent as much from his needs as from her willingness to give prompt attention to any requests by him for material from the library for purposes of research and scientific writing.

I found handwritten notes from Holt to Joslin when he was looking for biographical information on Dr Richard Minot, one of his patients (and the one he regarded as his most famous), in order to prepare his (Joslin's) submission to the Nobel Committee nominating Minot for the Nobel Prize. Minot received the award in 1934 as a co-discoverer of the treatment of pernicious anaemia. In another note, handwritten in pencil, the ever devoted Holt assured Joslin of her loyalty saying, "I will of course, respect the confidentiality in this matter as you have asked."

The Joslin archives contain several other handwritten notes from Holt to Joslin whom she continued to help in numerous ways. It is clear that Joslin had been an enduring influence in the young woman's life.

Joslin himself had been on several committees, including some associated with the library where Holt remained an assistant until July 1935 when she was made the Head Librarian of the Harvard Medical School, School of Dental Medicine and School of Public Health. She held this position until her retirement on 29 June 1957.

At a reception held in her honour at that time, Dr C Sidney Burwell, formerly Dean, and then Samuel Levine Professor of Medicine at Harvard Medical School, called attention to the high regard in which Holt was held among the leading medical librarians in the United States.

He remarked, "She knows more about the history of Harvard Medical School than anyone else. The library has been the repository for all the School's historical material and Miss Holt was the first to classify and organise this material."

During more than three decades of service, Holt was of "immeasurable assistance to more than 10,000 medical, dental and public health students at Harvard."

In her time she had supervised a remarkable expansion in the library's facilities.

Holt's personality was praised by Dr George P Berry who was the Dean at the time of her retirement, stating that Miss Holt had won "a warm place for herself in the hearts and minds of the Students and Faculty of the three Schools. She has contributed immeasurably to the growing intellectual life of the Harvard medical area."

After retirement Holt continued to live in Providence, where she established a connection with the local library, working on a part-time basis.

The affection and esteem in which Holt held Joslin was described in a statement she prepared in 1964 for the 50th year publication of the Class of 1914 of Radcliffe College which counted her as one of its distinguished alumni. It was quoted by Alexander Marble in the foreword he wrote for Holt's memoir of Joslin published in 1969. The language is typically restrained.

She said:

"My long and happy association with Dr Elliott P. Joslin lasted nearly 50 years. Working with him on many and varied undertakings was a liberal education, for Dr Joslin was a scholar as well as a true physician to his patients, who always came first in his life. Also, he was a wonderful teacher at all times and in any place where he saw a chance to impart a bit of knowledge. By just listening to him I absorbed much that has guided and helped me over the years."

The comment by Alexander Marble that the statement reflected her warm regard for Dr Joslin may be regarded by some as something of an understatement.

As is clear, Holt's original official appointment as secretary in Joslin's practice had in fact embodied a much broader role, and although her official appointment to Joslin's practice only lasted a little more than 12 months, the young woman had become deeply attached to the dynamic, albeit demanding, physician.

Theirs was a unique association which was to last till the end of Joslin's life.

The reader would therefore not be surprised to learn that nearly 40 years later Holt would return to the side of her mentor when he most needed her even though, especially in his senior years, he was disinclined to admit that he needed assistance with anything!

Joslin's many commitments which saw him spending long hours at work left room for little else. One new task he had given himself upon returning from war was to add to his teaching commitments by inviting primary care practitioners to his ward rounds, especially in the smaller hospitals like Cory Hill, and Faulkner. One of these doctors recalls accompanying Joslin to Corey Hill mentioning that "he packed everyone into the car. The ride was uphill, hectic, and hot". She stopped short of commenting on his driving skills which, according to Holt, were not one of his strengths. However, including general practitioners in his teaching fold would have spread his reputation even further.

Howard Root Joins Joslin

In 1920 Joslin employed a new assistant called Howard Root. According to Priscilla White it was the practice at that time to appoint assistants, not associates. That Root went on to become Joslin's first associate might well have been a conscious decision on the part of Joslin to change the nature of this practice. Whether or not he had realised that the delivery of medical services was going to require change, especially given the larger numbers of patients in his practice, is unclear. But he did appreciate the necessity for able assistants to provide the kind of meticulous attention required in the management of a diabetic as he himself had practised and, through his books, had also urged other physicians to do the same.

One of Joslin's strengths was to maintain contact with his colleagues not only in Boston but throughout the country. He did this by attending meetings all over the country, and further bolstered professional relationships through his letter writing. Recognising the importance of keeping in touch with physicians in Canada, England and Europe, he made regular trips to conferences held there. His attendance at medical meetings was appreciated, even sought, after the enthusiastic reception accorded his book. This was particularly so in Canada and England.

That the Canadians regarded Joslin as a peerless authority on diabetes was shown by their decision to award the first Banting Medal and the invitation to deliver the inaugural Banting Lecture to the Boston physician. Of course his close relationship with Banting's friend and associate Best may also have influenced this decision.

Although he never said so, Joslin also enjoyed his popularity in England. In many ways Joslin was more English than the English. His impeccable bearing, immaculate dress and faultless manners endeared him to medical colleagues and the lay public wherever he went. The English embraced their American cousin with an enthusiasm not usually associated with the reception they accord strangers.

Outside of the United States a Boston Brahmin would more likely be referred to as an English aristocrat (until his accent revealed his true origins!). In former English colonies and territories like India and the Indian population of ex-British colonies such as Fiji, he would be referred to as a "Pukkah Sahib" (a Hindi term for a "real" Englishman.) But that is a story for another day.

Of course the outstanding characteristic which left Joslin's audiences–medical and the lay public alike– almost speechless was his grasp of the practical as well as the scientific aspects of diabetes. Today Joslin would be regarded as a master communicator. This he certainly was–and some!

Remember that Joslin had seen literally hundreds of diabetics and written a book on the subject even before insulin had been discovered!

In retrospect, the appointment of Howard Root could be seen as the beginning of the Joslin Clinic. Not that this was regarded as anything momentous at the time, and even if it had, it was going to be overshadowed by one of the most momentous medical discoveries in history.

Part 14.
Insulin

The Dawn of a New Era

"It is natural to man to indulge in the illusion of hope."

Patrick Henry

The discovery of insulin and its successful application to the treatment of diabetes transformed the lives of diabetics. It averted death from diabetic coma. At the time of its discovery in 1921, for patients treated with insulin the experience was a miracle and insulin was a wonder drug.

According to Michael Bliss in his book *The Discovery of Insulin*, accounts of the event vary according to the teller. "Well into the 1950s the oral history of the discovery of insulin was more interesting than the written history. There was a kind of underground of gossip, centring in Toronto medical circles and usually becoming more interesting after each round of drinks."

Perhaps the main reason for the heated debates was disagreement about who was really responsible for the discovery and therefore deserving of the Nobel Prize, an award coveted by, amongst others, scientists involved in medical research. In late 1923, the Nobel Prize for the discovery of insulin had been awarded to Frederick Banting and John Macleod of the University of Toronto.

The controversy over who did what is not part of this work. What is not controversial about the roles of different claimants is that only after the Canadian discovery did the work on insulin proceed to large scale commercial production. It was the successful implementation of this essential step which made insulin available for treating the thousands of diabetics in America and around the world.

The important scientific and experimental steps in the discovery of insulin can be summarised fairly simply.

The role of the pancreas in diabetes, at least in dogs, had been demonstrated by Minkowski in Germany towards the end of the 1800s. Banting, a surgeon by profession, with little in the way of experience in laboratory research, managed to isolate an extract made from the *islets of Langerhans* which are small nests of cells situated in but different from the rest of the pancreas. These islets were named after Paul Langerhans (1847-1888), a German medical student who had first made the observation in 1869, the year of Joslin's birth. But at that time it was not known that the islets were the source of insulin.

Banting then injected this extract into dogs made diabetic by removal of the pancreas. The technique he used for removing the pancreas had been developed by Frederick Allen in animal experiments he had carried out in Boston between 1908 and 1911.The method had been described by Allen in his magnum opus *Studies Concerning Glycosuria and Diabetes* published in 1913.

As a gift to mark the end of my Fellowship in 1970, Leo Krall gave me a highly valued photograph. It was the page from the notebook of Banting and Best which recorded the dramatic results of their experiment on 7 August 1921. It detailed for the first time the falling levels of blood sugar in the experimental animal, a dog, which had developed diabetes after removal of its pancreas by the surgeon, Frederick Banting, assisted by a medical student, Charles Best. The experiment had proceeded throughout the night, and the blood sugar recordings were made at 1am, 2 am, 3 am and 4 am following injections of the extract. With each injection the blood sugar value had fallen. This was the critical experiment which showed that the extract made from the insulin-producing cells in the pancreas could control blood sugar in a diabetic animal.

Joslin Hears Whispers About Insulin

The first time Joslin heard of the work going on in Toronto was when he had gone to a meeting of the Southern Medical Association in Arkansas in late 1921. There he had talked with a Canadian called Dr Llewellyn Barker who at that time was working at the Johns Hopkins Hospital. Barker was a University of Toronto graduate who had recently been back there for a visit, and had learned about the Banting and Best experiments which were the number one topic of conversation in the medical circles in Toronto. He mentioned it to Joslin.

Always on the lookout for any promising advances in the treatment of diabetes, Joslin could not wait to get to his dictating machine! He wrote to John MacLeod, the head of the Department of Physiology where the work was being carried out.

Joslin wrote, "Naturally if there is a grain of hopefulness in these experiments, which I can give to patients or even can say to them that you are working on the subject, it would afford much comfort, not only to them, but to me as well, because I see so many pathetic cases."

MacLeod, an academic without any experience in, or exposure to, the treatment of diabetes, wrote back in a typically cautious tone counselling restraint in making any promises until the extract could be tried on human beings.

It is here that another man, who is perhaps given less prominence because of his commercial connections, also learnt of the work in Toronto from Barker. His name was Dr George Clowes, the research director of Eli Lilly & Company, a pharmaceutical manufacturing company located in Indianapolis, Indiana. Clowes had a background in medical research and was known to and respected by John Macleod.

Both Joslin and Clowes were told by Macleod that the Banting and Best findings were going to be reported at the next meeting of the Physiological Society in New Haven later in the year.

On Friday afternoon 30 December 1921 a paper with the title "The Beneficial Influences of a Certain Pancreatic Extract on Pancreatic Diabetes" was presented in New Haven by Banting and Best. MacLeod was also listed as an author. Banting and Best were not members of the Physiological Society and were listed as being there by invitation.

Most, if not all, doctors in North America who were prominent in diabetes research and interested in the treatment of diabetes were present. This included Joslin, Frederick Allen and George Clowes, of the Eli Lilly Company.

Afterwards, Joslin expressed reservations typical of a physician in clinical practice. "They might be onto something up there in Canada; we look forward to hearing more."

Frederick Allen was more generous towards the Toronto workers but also cautious. He said, "If you have solved the initial difficulties (preparing the extract), your method is better than mine could ever be..... *It is high time we had some treatment beyond mere diet*, though I recognise the difficulties in the way of a practical application of any extract."

Allen's comment on diet is in italics to emphasise the fact that both he and Joslin were conscious of the limitations of diet in the treatment of diabetes, but being practitioners in that field were all too aware that that was all they had to offer the patients. I believe this point needs to be made in view of the frequent criticisms of both these men for the parlous physical condition of patients subjected to a restricted diet. They used it because there was little else to offer their patients.

The actual announcement of the discovery of insulin was made by Macleod at the meeting of the Association of American Physicians in Washington on 3 May 1922. Banting and Best were not there. They had excused themselves, saying that the trip from Toronto to Washington was too expensive.

Joslin was present at that meeting and said that the standing vote of appreciation to Macleod and his associates was the first of its kind he had seen in the 20 years he had been involved in the society.

Frederick Allen described Banting's and Best's accomplishment as "one of the greatest achievements of modern medicine. It may justly be called epoch making."

Rollin T Woodyatt, another leading American physician, said, "I think that this work marks the beginning of a new phase in the study and treatment of diabetes. It would be difficult to overestimate the ultimate significance of such a step."

Once the work of Banting and Best had been developed to the extent that they were able to produce an effective extract containing insulin, the entire medical world, and indeed the whole world, was transfixed by the dramatic effect of the discovery, particularly on the children so afflicted.

As for the extract, every diabetic wanted the treatment immediately. So did their parents, wives, husbands – and doctors! Any strings available were there for the pulling.

The effect of the discovery of insulin on millions of patients suffering from diabetes all round the world is part of medical history.

What is less well known is the impact of this discovery on Joslin himself. Although he did not suffer from diabetes, his deep involvement and almost single-minded interest in caring for those who did placed him at the very centre of this dramatic discovery. That he was fully aware of the significance of this finding was very much in evidence from the outset. His mastery of diabetes was recognised and respected throughout the English-speaking world, including in Canada and especially by both Banting and Best. The archives of the Joslin Diabetes Centre house personal letters from both these men to Joslin on his 70th and 80th birthdays expressing their appreciation of his friendship and unreserved admiration for his experience and expertise in the treatment of diabetes.

6 August 1922. Joslin's Insomnia Rewarded

".....When I said she [the patient] was to have bread and potato, both patient and nurse thought that I was joking and breaking faith with the gods, Joslin and Allen".

*Frederick Banting 1922

"Banting was different. Having never treated any diabetics, he had no preconceptions about the relation between insulin and diet... "

Michael Bliss 1982

*Frederick Banting, the discoverer of insulin, was actually a surgeon by profession and had no experience of treating diabetes. Joslin on the other hand was a leader in the field, and at that time had treated in excess of some 3000 patients with the condition.

Joslin received his first supply of insulin from Toronto on 6 August 1922. Having already witnessed its effects on several diabetics during his visit to Toronto, Joslin was barely able to keep his emotions in check. "I remained awake all night," he wrote in his manuals and textbook. He never forgot that event which he knew would change the destiny of millions of people around the world.

Even nearly 40 years later in the last manual he edited in 1959 (the 10th edition), he recalled the sleepless night. He quoted Keats:

"Then felt I like some watcher of the skies
when a new planet swims into his ken..."

At the time of the introduction of insulin and its early dramatic effects on previously wasted patients Joslin had compared the transformation to that described in the Old Testament in the book of Ezekiel: "I will bring flesh upon you.... And ye shall live."

It is well known that the first injection of insulin in that part of the world, was given not by Joslin but by his assistant Howard Root. Whether it was because Joslin was nervous, given his oft admitted difficulty with things mechanical, has not been explained in his or anyone else's writings on that particular event.

The injection was given on 7 August 1922 in a cottage known as Broadbeck Cottage next to the New England Deaconess Hospital. The cottage was similar to houses which served as accommodation for patients not considered ill enough to need admission to a hospital.

The patient was a 42-year-old, ex-nurse, Miss Elizabeth Mudge, who in five years of diabetes treated with a restricted diet was down to 69 pounds in weight, "just about the weight of her bones and a human soul," said Joslin. Debilitated from diabetes, she had only once in the previous nine months managed to go for a walk. Six weeks after starting insulin she was walking four miles a day.

When I was in Boston, Broadbeck Cottage had been demolished for further expansion of the New England Deaconess Hospital. The hospital laundry had been built there, but to mark the actual spot where the injection had been given there was a brass plaque.

In later years Joslin still spoke of the life-changing impact of insulin. In the first manual published after the introduction of insulin (the third edition in 1924), he had said, "Insulin has wrought a revolution in the lives of severe and moderately severe diabetics."

The photographs of Banting and Best appeared in every one of his manuals from 1924 on.

It is interesting to look at the discovery of insulin from the point of view of a physician so steeped in the care of every aspect of diabetes for well over a decade prior to this discovery. Joslin had published several articles on diabetes in scientific journals, and had written a textbook for physicians as well as a manual for the use of patients. Both the textbook and the manual had gone through two editions. This was very different from physicians coming upon insulin without a background of treating patients with diabetes. This also applied to many physicians in Toronto.

The increased survival of diabetics with the use of insulin so dramatically shown in the diabetic children was carefully documented in the records kept by Joslin. He introduced the survivor medal for patients who through conscientious management avoided complications of the disease for 25 years. The quarter-century medal was not only for his patients, but for any patient who upon examination (including laboratory tests and specialist eye checks) fulfilled the criteria. This practice has continued, and was later extended to include 50-year survival. Today, one of the staff members is assigned the task of attending to the Joslin medal matters virtually full time. Following my last visit to the Joslin Centre in 2014, when I met Matthew Brown, the Joslin archivist told me that the medal task was assigned to him. Matthew said long survivors now numbered in the hundreds.

Stories of the dramatic rescue by the introduction of insulin in patients who were alive but in dire straits without insulin were also highlighted. One of the best remembered and oft-repeated stories of such a rescue was that of an English physician, Dr Robin Lawrence. After regaining his health Lawrence devoted his life to the care of diabetics. With the writer H G Wells, also a diabetic, he founded the British Diabetic Association. Lawrence was befriended by Joslin and in a tribute recounted an incident when Joslin sent him to his shoe store to be given a new pair of shoes when the Englishman had visited Boston, his own English variety proving unsuitable for the New England winter! Whether or not Joslin told him of his family connections in the shoe trade is not recorded.

Joslin and the Nobel Prize Controversy

"It is the molecule that has the glamour, not the scientists."

Francis Crick

Joslin did not take part in the controversy surrounding the Nobel Prize but made his personal view clear in a brief comment. His initial remarks in the third edition of the manual published in 1924 avoided any comment which could be regarded as indicating him taking sides. In fact, the third edition of the manual made only a brief mention of Banting and Best. He said, "Banting, a young orthopaedic surgeon with zeal for research undampened by four years of service at the front, discovered insulin, the hormone of the pancreas, which regulates carbohydrate metabolism. He received the assistance of his friend, C.H. Best who, although a second year medical student, was trained in physiological research."

The chapter is a concise summary of the discovery together with the development of insulin. The contribution of other workers in Toronto to isolate insulin from the pancreases of cattle and hogs was also mentioned.

It is clear that at this stage Joslin was not aware of the vehemence of Banting's protestations about what he considered was unfair attribution of the credit (and therefore the Nobel Prize) to MacLeod instead of to Charles Best. Five years later, when Joslin released the fourth edition in 1929, he added one further comment on the subject in a new paragraph:

"When "Charlie" Best, the medical student, helped Banting to discover insulin, he proved that a medical student was *ipso facto* an investigator and deserved to be regarded as such". However, he never omitted the fact of the research being carried out in Macleod's department.

(What is not widely appreciated as far as Best not receiving the award is

a straightforward yet irrefutable explanation provided by none other than the Nobel Committee which, when asked about it, simply responded that <u>Best had never been considered for the award because he was never nominated!</u>)

There were, and still are, many controversies within the profession in relation to diabetes, including but not restricted to its treatment with reduced diets. It is clear that Joslin tried to steer clear of controversies as much as possible. There is little in journal articles or other reports about him to indicate that he had an argumentative nature. Rather than getting involved with who should get what, he was keener to get back to his own work.

As with his approach to the efficacy of treating diabetes with reduced food intake in the pre-insulin era, Joslin was very conscious of the fact that what was needed as far as insulin was concerned was its production in commercial quantities. He had thousands of diabetics in his practice, and even if one accepts the incidence of 10% of an average diabetic population being young people including children, the need for supplies of insulin was obvious.

He was one of the first to write to the head of the Lilly Company. Copies of letters between the director of Eli Lilly and Joslin showed the obvious esteem in which the physician was held by Lilly.

Largely, if not entirely due to their production of insulin, Eli Lilly and Company became a leader in the American pharmaceutical industry. In the first year of its marketing insulin, the company earned more than$1,000,000. The insulin extract used on Banting's and Best's dog was from a dog's pancreas. but the large quantities needed for thousands of human diabetics were made from cattle and hogs.

Joslin did not get involved in the establishment of various committees and clinics in Toronto following the discovery of insulin in 1921, because his own practice as far as diabetes was concerned was years ahead of any counterparts in Canada. The Diabetic Clinic at Toronto General Hospital was started in June 1922.

Although a member of the Insulin Committee, established by Toronto

University to advise on matters relating to granting a license to manufacture insulin, he did not go to its initial meeting on 17 August 1922. However he did attend a roundtable conference some months later (25 November 1922) together with other clinicians from America, including Allen, when clinical issues and supplying insulin to different doctors were discussed.

Joslin and Allen, regarded as among the foremost authorities on the subject, were the first American recipients of the extract from Toronto–but only in limited amounts.

Joslin's overall mastery of the theoretical and practical aspects of treatment is clear in his writings in those early years of the use of insulin. He was quick to grasp the fundamentals of insulin usage, and given his facility for presenting scientific and technical information in simple language, his patients were able to embrace the new treatment and the challenges of managing the many practical problems comparatively easily, especially with the additional help provided by the Joslin- trained dieticians and nurses. He could see, and was able to explain clearly, the place insulin had in the day-to-day treatment of the condition.

His manuals for patients are exemplary in their clarity of instruction, supplemented by drawings, charts and photographs starting with the way insulin needs to be stored, followed by the method of drawing it up into the glass syringe, getting rid of gas bubbles drawn up in the syringe with insulin, before cleaning the area to be injected and then injecting the preparation–but not before describing, again with drawings to match, the parts of the body best suited for the injection. Years later, using his instructions made management of diabetes infinitely easier for all concerned.

The discovery of insulin and its successful application to the treatment of diabetes transformed the lives of diabetics by averting death from diabetic coma. For those afflicted with the condition at the time of its discovery in 1921, insulin was life-changing.

Given the dramatic improvement in the treatment of diabetes achieved, it is appropriate to reflect upon certain aspects of the lives of diabetic patients before insulin became readily available.

The Parlous State of Diabetics Before Insulin

It is thought-provoking that the treatment of diabetes when Joslin completed his medical training was restricted to chemicals including opioids and arsenic! Neither were there any specific dietary prescriptions being used by physicians in America at this stage.

In Europe, especially Germany and France, dietary restriction had been employed by some physicians, notably in Germany and France, for many years. Bouchardat, in France, also advocated exercise as part of the treatment, the first physician to do so.

Little emphasis was placed on any specific treatment used, or tried, on the series of diabetics compiled from the records of Massachusetts General Hospital and studied by Joslin during his internship in 1898.

Having visited European centres in the early years following his graduation, Joslin was clearly aware that the Europeans were ahead of American physicians in the treatment of diabetes. He used the diet and exercise prescription for his patients from the outset. Treatment strategies including both these elements were designed for children as well as his adult patients.

Joslin was quick to recognise the importance of establishing a partnership with adult diabetics and, where possible, also with children. This was very different from the traditional method of giving orders to patients and/or others involved in their care. He encouraged both parents of children to engage in the treatment program.

However, he was strict and insisted on dietary restrictions being followed at all times. Any lapses were regarded as cheating. With the difficult children he employed his kindly gentle manner to try and win them over, in order to cultivate a relationship where they wanted to please him. He believed that giving children responsibility helped the young as well as their parents.

"Give any child, diabetic or otherwise, an opportunity to manage something or somebody and the chances are that he or she will come out all right. They need to be given responsibility."

His staff noticed that, without exception, his admonition was gentle when it came to children. Gentle admonition, however, was not always used by other members of Joslin's team, especially, as some of the Fellows, myself included, discovered many years later!

I was told of one such instance in 1969. The patient, then in his late 50s, told me that he had been a patient of Dr Joslin's about 40 years earlier, and he and his mother had stayed in a hospital–he couldn't remember the name–near the Joslin practice to be taught insulin treatment and dietary restriction by one of the Joslin nurses. One night, he and another boy sneaked out of the hospital and went downtown because they were starving for ice cream. On their return they had the misfortune of running into the supervising nurse waiting for them at the entrance of the hospital. He said he remembered the nurse's name because it was a source of great amusement for both the boys.

He said, "Miss Winterbottom marched the two of us to the mortuary and showed us several dead bodies. If you break your diet, this is what will happen to you, she said."

The patient told me that his current visit was the first since what he called "the Winterbottom incident" 40 years earlier!

Clearly not all Joslin patients were compliant. This case was presented at the usual morning (8.00 am) conference, much to the amusement of the other Fellows as well as some – but perhaps not all – the staff members.

(Later that day I ran into Leo Krall and asked him if he had heard any more about the case presentation that morning. "I hope we didn't upset the senior members of the staff," I said. I was particularly concerned about stepping on the toes of one or more of the five surviving members of the "original seven." No", said Leo, "that was good – even Dr White laughed – and she was closer to Dr. Joslin than any of us.")

According to Holt, Joslin was not above using "a bit of sarcasm mildly administered or a few words of ridicule which made the individual appear a little foolish ......" when dealing with non-compliant adults. At other times he refrained from reacting to such patients, as he relates in one of his manuals (sixth edition, p.61):

"When a patient comes to my office with a single specimen of urine instead of a portion taken from the 24-hour quantity, without any record of the food eaten during the preceding day, and starts to recount that he had nothing but eggs, meat, and fish, then later remembers that he had a little cream and various vegetables, then with prompting recalls butter and an orange and a little oatmeal, potato or bread, I always pity him and on very exceptional occasions am able to recall with satisfaction after the interview, Solomon's soliloquy in Proverbs, chapter 16, verse 32."

(As noted above, more often than not Joslin spared the rod. When he did, the satisfaction he received was from a biblical verse in the Old Testament mentioned above – "he who is slow to anger is better than a warrior…"

All those associated with diabetics before the discovery of insulin were fully aware that the starvation diet treatment for many patients literally meant starvation. Unbearable hunger and craving for food, especially in children, was heartbreaking for them as well as their parents and the staff. Doctors, including Joslin, had the unenviable task of watching helplessly as their patients wasted before their eyes. Some, as Holt said, were able to hang on by a thread literally until the fortunate ones were rescued by the miracle of insulin. The waiting room for diabetics today is a far cry from the times before the discovery of insulin.

Supplies of insulin for the general diabetic population in America did not begin till 1923. In the 1920s, specialist care of diabetes was not readily available, especially in the more remote areas. Barnett relates the heartbreaking story of a woman from Nova Scotia. This 37- year-old mother of two had decided to make an appointment to consult Dr Joslin or his associates in May 1921. She had made a steamer trip to Boston. Barnett quoted her story as follows,

"We were awakened at 6 AM Sunday and were within a few miles of Boston with a heavy fog and rain coming down simply in torrents. We really had a very long, fussy morning, passing the quarantine and then the immigration officials…. Pitt (her cousin), appeared suddenly and rescued me from a very fussy medical officer who insisted on my

producing a doctor's certificate when I had explained to him 50 times that I had no doctor except the Joslin manual for over two years, and therefore had no doctor's certificate.

Dr Joslin came in for a few minutes Sunday night to the ward and I liked him so much from the very first. The next morning, he examined me himself. His hospital assistant Dr Root was with him and the two graduate nurses who made rounds every morning with the doctors. My weight, undressed, was 73 1/2 pounds when I came..... I have been measured standing and sitting. I have had to blow into different glass tubes with clock faces. I have had blood drawn from my arm twice a week for the blood sugar list. I didn't think there could be any more sensations left.... I do not know yet how long I may be able to stay, but I shall do whatever Dr Joslin advised now that I am here and it cost so much to come! My ticket was $50.50 and I had to pay the same for Marie. (The fee was for a three-week stay).

I can't understand why my strength does not come back quicker. Dr Joslin seems to think I am all right. In every single lecture he has given, he has explained to newcomers that I managed my diet alone for two years and always speaks of me as a "very remarkable" patient.

I shall much prefer being fattened up a little to be pointed to as a model."

The final sentence which I have underlined emphasises what mattered most to patients at that time. Although prepared to follow the advice of the doctor to stick to the restricted diet, the perpetual hunger and the attendant weakness was for most, if not all of them, almost unbearable.

Barnett related the tragedy of this patient's final years. She died in the early months of 1923, leaving children under the age of 10 years. Although she had been seen by Joslin in May 1921 when insulin had already been discovered, she did not receive the wonder drug. Supplies for the general public in America did not become available till late 1923.

I have quoted this letter nearly in its entirety because it illustrates several points of interest in the way Joslin conducted his day-to-day practice. It also allows the reader a glimpse into the way diabetics were managed in-house, being hospitalised as much for treatment as for education. It shows Joslin's practice of making a patient feel important by seeing her on a Sunday evening, even if he left the formal examination till the following morning. He expected his staff to be in attendance by eight o'clock, often earlier, when he came to examine patients. It also shows the involvement of nurses as noticed by the patient.

The story reveals the plight of those living in remote areas, a situation which persists in many parts of the world to this day including in the so-called developed (first world) countries. Not only do these patients suffer from inadequacies in the availability of specialist care, they also have to meet increased costs involved in travelling and accommodation – the tyranny of distance.

Joslin's Prize Patient

The good fortune that saved the lives of many patients who happened at that time to be hanging on and barely surviving on their starvation diets was to be treated with insulin. The dramatic rescue of such patients brought the phrase "saved by insulin" into common use.

One such patient in Joslin's practice was a man called George Minot, case number 2383 in the Joslin ledger. George Minot came from a well-known and distinguished Boston family. He was the son of James Jackson Minot, a physician. Minot's great-grandfather James Jackson (1777–1867) was a co-founder of Massachusetts General Hospital.

Minot, a medical graduate, was working as a haematologist in Boston. Nine years out of medical school, at the age of 36, he developed what is now known as Type 1 or childhood diabetes, presenting with 7% glucose in his urine. Measurement of glucose in his blood gave the result of 430 mg/dl, more than four times higher than in normal people. He recognised that he had diabetes. He had been a robust young man, nearly 6'2" in height weighing 147 pounds. The weight fell rapidly to 135 pounds, which on his tall frame gave him a haggard appearance.

Minot consulted Joslin who promptly put him on a reduction diet. Joslin's instruction was precise: "The record of food intake will be an essential guide to treatment, equal in importance to the record of sugar in the urine." The total caloric value of the diet was reduced to 525 calories per day, as opposed to some 1500 cal which would be the normal requirement for a man of Minot's age and build. Within two weeks the urine sugar was diminished and the blood sugar had fallen from the initial 475 to 190 mg/ml–"a marked improvement", said Joslin.

The diabetes was better but the patient was haggard and miserable!

To his credit, and Joslin's delight, George Minot turned out to be the ideal patient. When his diabetes was diagnosed in late 1921, early 1922 (the records are vague about the actual date of his first consultation with Joslin), after initial control of his high blood sugar the diet was increased. Joslin kept his carbohydrate around 2000 calories for most of 1922. On this, his original weight of nearly 150 pounds was reduced to 120. His blood sugars were in the range of 150 mg/ ml which, though not ideal, was acceptable. Minot's wife Marian was equally conscientious and very supportive, not only in making herself familiar with the diet but also in measuring/weighing each item of food even when they went to dine in a restaurant.

In January 1923 Joslin started treating Minot with small doses of 1, 2 and 3 units of insulin. Within a few months the dose was up to 14 units, and by 1924 the dose was 18 units before breakfast and 14 units at night. Minot's wife Marian said, "This is the first winter since marriage that he has not lost 7 to 14 days from his illness."

With his mastery of English and weakness for colourful phraseology, Barnett could not resist the temptation. He described Joslin's diet for the suffering Minot as "involving ordering, monitoring, titrating, and tinkering."

He provided a detailed account of Minot's early period of treatment of his diabetes, largely drawn from the 1956 biography of Minot called *The Inquisitive Physician* by Rackemann.

"The diabetes was severe. Both George and Marian [his wife] had courage – a much deeper courage than might have appeared... When George and Marian travelled anywhere – even up the street to dine out – they brought along a little black leather slouch bag which had seen

better days, but which was still all in one piece. It contained a Chatillon scales and a tin pie-plate, and, sometime later, it contained the bottle of insulin, with syringes, the alcohol and gauze sponges, not to mention the little block of blue paper and a couple of pencils. In helping himself to food, George put it first on the pie plate, to adjust its weight on the scales, before moving it to his dinner plate. The amount was noted on the blue paper... Often he would turn to Marian: "how much spinach, did you say?".... I have allowed for the cracker and cheese. I had with a cocktail – that's right, isn't it?" Marian could remember the values of food better than George and she knew what he should have."

Minot, in spite of the burden imposed on him by diabetes, pursued a brilliant medical career as Chief of Medicine in a Boston hospital and head of the Thorndike Laboratory, where his work contributed to the discovery of the treatment of pernicious anaemia and for which he won the Nobel Prize in 1934.

Joslin used the inspirational story of George Minot in his manuals and his textbook. In the last manual he wrote (the 10th edition in 1959), the frontispiece bears a full-page photograph of Minot. The caption reads,

Dr George Richards Minot, 1885–1950.

Saved by Insulin – Co-discoverer of the Treatment of Pernicious Anaemia. Nobel Laureate , 1934.

Joslin's treatment of Minot with the very small doses of insulin in the beginning shows how conservative he was in his clinical practice and that he certainly was not going to go overboard with the latest treatment. This is in sharp contrast to the liberal doses of insulin used by Frederick Banting in one of the first patients treated in Toronto shortly after the discovery of insulin. It must be remembered that Banting had not treated diabetes previously, while Joslin had been doing so for about 20 years. It also indicates that Joslin was initially reserved in his judgment, as indicated by his description of insulin and its discovery in the third edition of his manual published in early 1923, when adequate supplies of insulin for American patients had only just begun.

Insulin is now available in comparative abundance, especially in the developed countries, but many less-developed countries are still struggling with challenges imposed by the lack of, or inadequate, medical supplies, including insulin.

Joslin's New Friend and Admirer

Joslin was well known to the Canadian medical authorities largely through his writings, but particularly since the publication of his book *Treatment of Diabetes Mellitus* which had been reviewed in the *Canadian Medical Journal* as well as other medical publications. However, what many Canadians had not appreciated were some of his personal qualities.

Shortly after the development of the extract in Toronto and its use on patients in the university hospital there, Joslin was one of the American doctors invited to see these patients. Not only adults, but children also were taken by his warm, personable manner when meeting him for the first time. This was documented in detail in the book, *The Discovery of Insulin* by Michael Bliss.

That he had a presence dominated by his impressive carriage, impeccable manners, charm and immaculate attire was well known in Boston. He was also blessed with a winning approach, especially to patients including young people, because of his warmth, concern, and the gift of imparting the sincere impression that he understood their suffering.

It seems to have been more a case not so much of Joslin discovering Canada, but rather of Canada discovering Joslin.

As far as the medical fraternity was concerned, Joslin had been well known for many years. He was a frequent invited speaker at conferences and was much sought after, especially since the publication of his textbook and manuals for patients with diabetes. He was particularly supportive of younger physicians, especially those involved in medical research. This resulted in many friendships.

One such relationship was his friendship with Charles Best (although for much of his life he was called Charlie). The relationship between Best and Joslin had started from their first meeting in Toronto after the discovery of insulin.

Best, who considered himself partly American because his father had been a physician in Maine, became very fond of Joslin, who in turn, in spite of his New England reserve, showed great affection for the talented young Canadian.

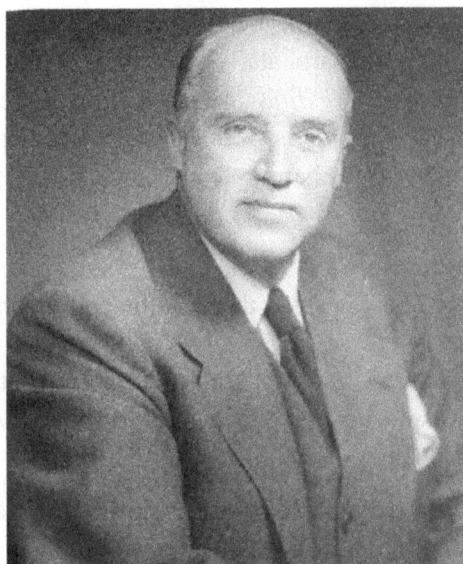

Charles Best

During a visit to Joslin's country retreat, Best, an accomplished horseman, decided to buy a pony. When he had selected one, Joslin approved of his choice, pointing out that transporting the animal by railroad to Canada was not going to pose any difficulty. For some reason Best thought that Joslin was giving him the pony as a gift. Some months later the postman delivered a bill for $125 with a note from Joslin, saying that he thought that was a fair price!

If there is a gene for trading (which, after all, is one of the oldest activities known even in ancient civilisations), Joslin had certainly inherited it from the merchants on both sides of his family. Although well known for his generosity, he was also a stickler for correct conduct, especially, it appears, when dealing with younger colleagues.

Best, who married his childhood sweetheart Linda Mahon a few years after his year of insulin fame, spent part of his honeymoon at Joslin's country retreat, Buffalo Hill. The bonds of friendship between Best and Joslin remained strong throughout their association and lasted to the end of Joslin's life. For his part, Best maintained an interest in Joslin's family and the Joslin Clinic for his entire life.

(My wife and I met Best at a reception in 1969. He was charming to my wife and asked me if I had read Joslin's textbook. He smiled when I said no, and told me that he had read every one of them. "Yes all ten editions, and the last one by Dr Joslin was the best," he said.)

Joslin's Practice After Insulin

"Insulin does not cure diabetes but it is a priceless gift to the severe diabetic provided he is intelligent and faithful." E P Joslin 1923

Joslin's personal rejoicing was best seen when he spoke to the thousands of patients and their relatives as well as medical and allied health professionals through his manuals. His public pronouncements were quoted by Michael Bliss when Joslin expressed wonderment that the limpid liquid injected under the skin could metamorphose a baby.

Although by nature a private person, Joslin could not contain his excitement upon first seeing the practical benefits of insulin and again, unusually for him, quoted the prophet Ezekiel's vision as described in the Old Testament. But as already noted, it was in his manuals that he gave full expression to his unbridled joy in the ninth edition of his manual published in 1953(pages 39–40):

"When I think what the diabetics were when I treated them in the days of undernutrition (1914–1922), and what they are now with insulin, I'm reminded of the words of the prophet Ezekiel about 2500 years ago. No truer description of the transformation which has taken place in the life of a diabetic patient can be found than in the account of his vision of the valley of dry bones."(Ezekiel 37, 1–10.)

Joslin then proceeded to quote the entire 10 verses. Perhaps he thought of the first two verses as describing the lot of the starving diabetics who had been treated with undernutrition:

1. "The hand of the Lord was upon me, and carried me up in the Spirit of the Lord, and set me down in the midst of the valley which was full of bones.

2. And caused me to pass by them round about; and, behold, there were very many in the open valley; and, lo, they were very dry."

To describe the transformation wrought by insulin, Joslin quoted verses 6, 8 and 10:

6. " And I will lay sinews upon you, and will bring up flesh upon you, and cover you with skin, and put breath in you, and ye shall live...

8. And when I beheld, lo, the sinews and the flesh came up upon them and the skin covered them above......

10....and they lived."

The conservative physician in him, however, was cautious in his approach to the actual use of insulin in his patients, warning that the new treatment was still in its infancy. If this indicates that Joslin may have underestimated the remarkable improvement made possible by insulin, the impression will be quickly dispelled by a glance at the third edition of Joslin's textbook published in 1923.

This edition was dedicated "To Banting and Best and the Toronto Group of Insulin Workers."

The beginning of the preface is almost a sentimental soliloquy as he remembers earlier workers in the field:

"In the early months of the century Naunyn taught me with [my] Case number 8 that his methods enabled a diabetic of 60 years to live out the full expectation of life. In 1914 Allen's development of Guelpa's crude theories of undernutrition, together with insistence upon the patient's use of the Benedict test [to estimate the amount of sugar being lost in the urine] and of food scales, increased the average diabetic's outlook by two years...."

He spoke of physicians and scientists involved in the study of diabetes whom he had known personally. The list reads like the "Who's Who" of diabetes over the previous 50 years or so. It also confirms just how effective Joslin was in his capacity for regular communication, mostly through his assiduous letter writing, with workers not only in America but in Europe as well. The list also includes what may be regarded as his understated tribute to those who had helped him, including the physiologists with whom his association and friendships went back to his college days in Yale some 30 years earlier.

"These contemporaries, and I omit the youngest, it has been my good fortune to know personally – the clinicians, Allen, Falta and Gayelin, Minkowski, Magnus Levy, Naunyn, Newburgh, von Noorden, Wilder, Williams and Woodyatt; the chemists, S. R Benedict, Bloor, Folin, Schaffer and Van Slyke; the physiologists and metabolists, FG. Benedict, Boothby, DuBois, Lusk and McLeod; the pathologist, Opie and to have had for teachers, R. H. Chittenden, and R. H. Fitz. All these are still alert with the exception of the last, and even he lives in his son. With such trained minds interested in diabetes the time was ripe for new discoveries."

Joslin then makes a statement which would strike a chord with any physician in practice coming upon a new treatment promising a significant advance in managing a condition which has had such adverse consequences, including death, for his patients over a period of some 20 years. He says:

"Yet, can the reader imagine the feelings of a doctor with a background of 1000 fatal cases, who has lived to see what the ages have longed for come true in the discovery of insulin by F.G. Banting with the help of his student friend, C. H. Best".

He then lapses into a wistful tribute to the physicians of the past, especially Bouchardat whose writings had influenced him greatly.

Unchallenged as a leading practitioner treating diabetes, the numbers in the Joslin practice rose steeply after the introduction of insulin. The huge publicity generated by the discovery and its production in commercial quantities had also publicised the names of physicians associated with various aspects of the introduction of insulin for the treatment of diabetes, especially in children where the effects of insulin were widely publicised, correctly, as literally life- changing.

However, the spectacular success of insulin in achieving dramatic results in treating diabetes did not blind Joslin to other as yet unresolved, even unrecognised, aspects of the condition.

Joslin was one of the first physicians to comment on a rise in the incidence of diabetes which had not been recognised at that time. In an article, "The Prevention of Diabetes," written in 1921, he described a group of inhabitants in Oxford, Massachusetts.

"Although six of the seven persons, or heads of families... living in (three) adjoining houses... on a peaceful, elm-lined street in a country town in New England, succumbed to diabetes, *no one spoke of an epidemic.* Consider the measures which would have been adopted to discover the source of the outbreak to prevent a recurrence... (as it would)...if these deaths had occurred from scarlet fever, typhoid fever or tuberculosis. Because the disease was diabetes, and because the deaths occurred over a considerable interval of time, the fatalities passed unnoticed." (Joslin's father's first wife, Lucretia, had died of scarlet fever.)

The global incidence of diabetes has now reached epidemic proportions in the developed countries in particular.

In 1948 Oxford, Joslin's birthplace, was chosen as the town where the incidence of diabetes was investigated by Wilkerson and Krall. Leo Krall was later recruited by Joslin to join his staff in 1953. He was the last member of the original seven. If Joslin was regarded as almost evangelical in his enthusiasm for spreading the word on the treatment of diabetes by strict adherence to the basic rules of dietary restriction and other tenets, history would show that Krall was the disciple to spread the word internationally.

Multilingual, affable and quick to establish friendships, Krall proved to be the internationalist Joslin would have wanted to publicise his teachings. Leo Krall also wrote several books on diabetes, including two successive Joslin manuals, the 11th and 12th editions following Joslin's last, the 10th. He was elected to the presidency of the International Diabetes Federation in 1982 and, through his writings in several languages, enjoyed international recognition and a faithful following in academic circles.

(Leo Krall remained a close friend even after we returned to Australia in 1971. He and his wife Lois stayed in our home in Sydney on several occasions. Our friendship had begun within weeks of our arrival in Boston, and at one stage they had invited us to stay in their home and look after their 12-year-old son Kenny. As they were leaving for their trip, Leo tossed me his car keys and said, "Don't drive the smaller car, drive the Mercedes!" The almost new, beautiful navy blue car with cream upholstery was a dream to drive, and for us quite a step up from our $120 early model Oldsmobile!)Watching TV at the Kralls, I developed a fondness for ice hockey. The Boston Bruins were one of the leading teams in the competition and their star Bobby Orr, was an exceptionally talented athlete. Leo's last letter to me was written a few months before he died in 2002 at the age of 87.)

Joslin also recognised the role of obesity in causing diabetes. He had noticed the presence of increased body weight in several of his patients when looking through his ledger. He repeatedly warned the patients of the risks of obesity. He also admitted in one of his manuals that he even gave his friends a hard time if he thought they were carrying excess bodyweight.

Quickly recognising the importance of the practical aspects of the use of insulin, Joslin devoted a great deal of time and effort to training his staff, especially the dieticians and nurses, in the day-to-day use of insulin including adjustment of the dose according to the blood sugar levels and the amount of sugar being lost in the urine. Joslin did not get involved in the establishment of facilities such as diabetic clinics in Toronto following the discovery of insulin in 1921. His own practice, begun more than a decade earlier was years ahead of any similar establishment in Canada. The Diabetic Clinic at Toronto General Hospital was started in

June 1922.

It is clear that he was one of the earliest physicians to see where insulin fitted into the treatment program of a diabetic. He saw its importance but also recognised that it was not the only measure to be used.

Joslin counselled that insulin was one, but only one, of the three basic requirements for successful treatment of diabetes, namely diet, exercise and insulin. He used various analogies, the most popular being a chariot drawn by three horses (a spiked team) to emphasise the challenges facing the patient in keeping all three horses in control.

Neither did Joslin allow the publicity surrounding insulin to divert him from his plans for his own practice. The first matter to be attended to was expansion of his facilities at 81 Bay State Road because of the influx of new patients.

Joslin Expands His Practice

In the years before insulin, according to the Joslin ledger, around 200 new patients came to his practice each year. After the introduction of insulin, during the first 10 years the number of new patients coming to the practice quadrupled.

The sheer weight of numbers dictated the need for increased space for secretaries, the laboratory and the reception area. Additional space and facilities for physicians to interview and conduct examination of patients necessitated substantial internal restructuring. An Otis elevator was installed to allow patients and staff access to the upper floors. Maids' quarters were largely taken over for collection of blood to be analysed in the laboratory. Radiology equipment and dressing rooms were now located in the renovated basement.

The maids were not the only ones to lose space in their quarters. The chief casualty of the expansion of the practice facilities was living space for the family. Even the master bedroom was not sacred! Wax cylinders used in the dictating machine, which was one of the innovations suggested by Anna Holt during the post-war restructuring, had to be stored in the bedroom. Whether the delicate negotiations for this particular encroachment into the couple's personal space was handled by Holt or the master himself was not revealed.

A further issue complicating plans for alterations to buildings in this area was the city ordinances. Fortunately these applied largely to external alterations so as to protect the classical features of the style of buildings. This included their facades, external windows and doors. The colour of any paint to be used externally also had to follow the strict guidelines specified by the authorities.

Education of the patient for the day-to-day care of his or her diabetes, always a central issue in Joslin's philosophy on the management of the condition, now incorporated instruction on the use of insulin together with practical and detailed information which the patients and their carers needed for management with insulin injections. For more than 10 years after the introduction of insulin the only type of insulin available was soluble insulin. The effects of this preparation only lasted for 3 to 4 hours, which meant that the patient had to have as many as four, sometimes six, injections a day.

Joslin shouldered the teaching duties in equal share with his staff, including attending the morning conferences starting at 8 am sharp!

An oft-quoted account of Joslin lecturing to patients described one of his methods to impress the audience. After he was assured that everyone was seated, he would enter the lecture hall struggling with two large buckets overflowing with water, one in each hand, and refuse assistance as he splashed some of the contents when negotiating the two steps up onto the stage. Gasping, (perhaps slightly exaggerated!), he would put the buckets down, then turn to the audience, withdraw his handkerchief to wipe his brow, and say, "This is what a person who is overweight has to struggle with 24 hours a day, seven days a week until he loses the excess."

Written instruction sheets in the form of slim bound files, cards listing the caloric value of common food articles, diagrams showing the correct areas of the body where insulin was to be injected, and drawings showing the way to hold the syringe when injecting insulin were clearly spelt out for the patient and his carers.

Such teaching aids have remained in use to the present day, and have been adopted in diabetic clinics and practices throughout the world.

In the course of collecting all editions of the Joslin manual for patients, I came across many such cards with patient notes and markings. Similarly, in the textbooks I saw notes in margins made by doctors.

Joslin did not dwell unduly on the discovery of insulin, even though he lavished fulsome praise on the Toronto workers and kept closely in touch with various developments in insulin throughout his life. Rather, he saw quite clearly the place insulin had in the treatment of diabetes, and devoted his own and his team's efforts to incorporate it into the overall treatment of the condition. He took pains to emphasise the correlation between the amount of food eaten by the patient with the energy spent in the course of a day, and the dose of insulin required.

One of the most important changes which had to be made once the patient was having insulin was to have measurements of the amount of glucose present in the blood. Insulin reduced the level of glucose as did fasting and exercise. Food intake increased it.

From the outset, Joslin set about clearly explaining this in his manuals for patients.

It was this necessity for a greater role of the laboratory in the day-to-day management of diabetes that dictated the next major change in Joslin's practice.

The timely appointment of a pathologist to the New England Deaconess Hospital was a boon for him. By this time Joslin had become the Chief Physician at the Deaconess. However, here also, the increased demands following the introduction of insulin meant that the resources were stretched from the outset. An added factor was the increasing number of other specialists, including surgeons and competing physicians like those attached to the neighbouring Lahey Clinic, now using the hospital and demanding increasing space for their patients as well as their needs for laboratory procedures.

Clearly, there was a pressing need for more space but which simply was not available at the Deaconess at that time.

Yet once again, the gods smiled on the ambitious physician.

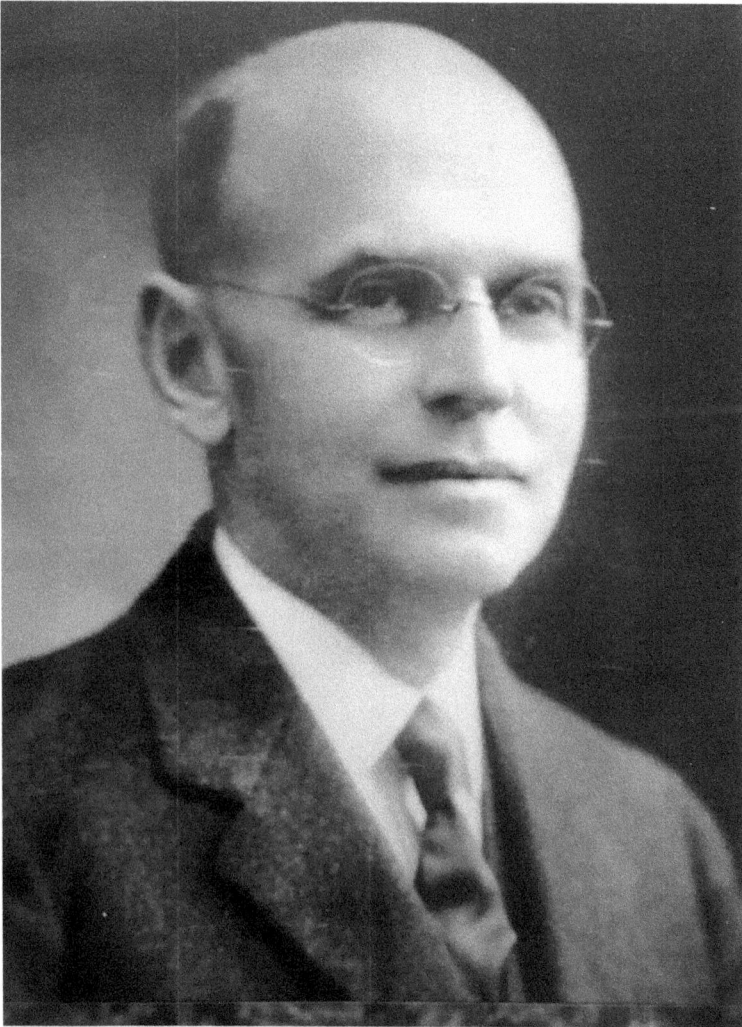

Joslin in his 50s. His signature in a careful cursive script.

307

Part 15.
The Banker

George Fisher Baker (1840–1931)

Given the prominence of the leather industry at that time, it is not surprising that Joslin would find himself in the company of sons from families which were associated with this enterprise. One such individual who became a good friend of Joslin was the chemist Otto Folin, whose family had been in the leather industry in Europe. Folin, a respected scientist, taught at Harvard University and helped Joslin with the chemistry of glucose assays in the urine of diabetics.

Another story, perhaps a more remarkable one, is about a man who was referred to Joslin for medical advice.

In 1925 a man called Baker travelled up from New York to Boston to see the distinguished Dr Joslin, as the latter had been referred to by Baker's Private Secretary.

Prominent in banking circles and often referred to as the "Dean of American Banking", Baker was regarded as the third richest man in the United States behind Henry Ford and John D Rockefeller.

Baker's father was a shoemaker in a small town called Troy, near Albany. This may well have been used by Joslin to put the 85-year-old at ease, as he was well known for remaining totally silent during interviews.

Joslin was proud of his own background, and not reluctant to share his childhood story of lacing 60 pairs of shoes at his father's shoe store in Oxford and banking his earnings of six cents at the local Webster Bank! Furthermore, Joslin's birthplace bore a similarity to Troy where Baker had spent his childhood. Both towns had been occupied by an indigenous tribe before, in Troy, the arrival of the Dutch and later the English. Such similarities in their backgrounds will no doubt have been used by Joslin to establish initial rapport.

Baker had not had much education, having gone to the Seaward Institute at the age of 14 and leaving two years later to work as a junior clerk at the New York State Banking Department. He had not gone to university. Instead he had joined the Massachusetts Volunteers at the age of 16, and fought in the Civil War.

Perhaps this was a reason for his making generous donations to Cornell and Harvard University libraries.

Joslin's approach to patients, dominated by humility and kindly concern, obviously struck a chord with the taciturn banker known for having the hardest shell and softest heart. He was also referred to as the Sphinx of Wall Street for his extensive share portfolio which he never discussed with anyone, on one occasion mentioning that he had not spoken to any journalist for thirty years!

Baker's association with Joslin also attracted the interest of Joslin's younger associate Donald M Barnett, the writer of Joslin's *Centennial Portrait*. When compared with most of Joslin's other patients, Barnett's book contains much more than the usual amount of information on the relationship between the physician and the banker.

It is clear that despite their difference in age – Baker was nearly 30 years older – the patient was very impressed with the physician. Joslin, for his part, knew that in 1924 Baker had donated $5 million to help establish the library at the Harvard Business School.

Barnett refers to correspondence between Joslin and Baker showing the high regard the latter had for the physician. That Joslin's geniality and charm had won Baker's admiration is clear. When Harvard conferred an honorary degree on Baker for his generous donation, the nervous recipient, perhaps daunted by the rarefied atmosphere of academia, asked Joslin to act as his escort at the presentation ceremony.

As was Joslin's custom, there was always a follow-up letter from him to the patient after a visit to the Joslin practice. Putatively, this was to inform the patient of the results of any laboratory investigations which had been carried out during his visit, but Joslin also used this as a way to reinforce the doctor-patient relationship. Another of Joslin's methods of persuasion in such matters was to enclose a stamped, self-addressed envelope in his letter to encourage a reply. One wonders if he did this in his letter to Baker!

However, Baker did respond to Joslin, and in one of the letters preserved in the archives asked if he could do anything for him. Joslin suggested that he establish a foundation at Harvard Medical School for the study of chronic disease. Baker donated $500,000.

Sometime after Baker's visit to Boston, Joslin's secretary was intrigued to receive a letter, which on the envelope bore the insignia of the Cadillac Car Company. In those times unsolicited advertising was unusual and in sharp contrast to the practices of e-mailing, texting and tweeting rampant in today's society.

If the envelope's cover had piqued her interest, its content left her speechless. The letter from the Director of the Cadillac Company informed Joslin that Mr Baker had sent a written request for them to deliver to Dr Joslin the car of his choice.

According to Barnett, Joslin declined this because he did not want the car to "force me to change my standard of living and I would have no time to enjoy it." Ever the fundraiser, however, he was quick with a counter-proposal!

He told the generous donor that he had just completed the fourth edition of his textbook on diabetes. (He had already given Baker a copy of the third edition of the manual for patients). Joslin suggested that if an equivalent amount of money could be donated to his practice, he would put it towards meeting the expenses for secretarial services for the forthcoming publication. Baker, who needed no convincing of Joslin's dedication to his work, readily agreed.

(After his earlier cars, which were from the Ford Motor Co., Joslin in later years drove Buicks. He was not a good driver, and was eventually persuaded to hire a young man to help in this regard, much to the relief of his staff and his family! He was always careful to avoid giving any impression of showing off, especially any signs of being wealthy. This carried over to his dealings with members of his staff. Although he was generous to them – he underwrote Priscilla White's Fellowship to study paediatric diabetes in Vienna – he impressed on them the importance of being seen to be careful with their money. As late as the mid-1950s holidays were, in many sections of the community, regarded as a privilege of the wealthy. So when members of his staff went on vacation, Joslin encouraged the use of the German term *arbeit* which actually means work!)

There is little information on the actual health of the banker, but it is reasonable to assume that he had what is now termed maturity- onset diabetes. Clearly Joslin did not discover any signs of serious complications of the disorder and reassured the patient. Hence his comment in the preface to the 4th edition of the textbook, praising the 85-year-old Baker for his habits in the management of diabetes and holding him up as an example and "a stimulus to the middle aged." To say that the patient was buoyed by the comments of the physician would be an understatement.

The Baker Clinic

A major expansion of Joslin's practice in the 1930s was the building of the Baker Clinic. It had been his long-term plan to establish in Boston a facility similar to that built by the German professor Carl von Noorden of Hamburg.

Demonstrating once again his habits of careful planning, Joslin did in Boston what he had done in Oxford. There his ambition of being a gentleman farmer had been accomplished by starting with the acquisition of a comparatively small block of land on which his country home was built. Then, over a period, he bought small parcels until he reached his goal of Buffalo Hill becoming a 300-acre holding.

He followed a similar plan for the Baker Clinic. In the early 1930s Joslin bought land near the Deaconess Hospital. Two boarding houses called Leatherbee and Lewis cottages at 160 and 170 Pilgrim Road respectively were acquired to be used as accommodation for ambulatory patients. In addition there was land near the Palmer Building of the Deaconess Hospital which Joslin bought so as to build the Baker Clinic in a central position within the Deaconess Hospital complex. Baker's donation provided the funds needed to finance the construction.

Joslin approached the authorities at the Deaconess to begin building as soon as he had received funds from the banker. A major stumbling block was that at that time America was in the depths of economic depression, and understandably there was great reluctance to embark on such a project. Furthermore, the value of Baker's stocks had fallen. However, Joslin argued that the loss in value of the stock could well worsen further. Whether it was his knowledge of the stock market or his dogged persistence which won the day is unclear, but the authorities were eventually persuaded to accede to Joslin's request.

The Baker Clinic was completed in 1933–1934 and its expanded facilities allowed Joslin to improve the delivery of care to the diabetic patients. The five-floor building included offices for Joslin and his staff. Joslin was the first Director of the Baker Clinic. Foot care was a priority given the large number of elderly patients with diabetes who had ulcers on their feet. The first floor also included a dental clinic and a classroom. The second floor contained research and clinical laboratories .The third and fourth floors were devoted to childhood and adult diabetics respectively. Surgical facilities on the fifth floor were for obstetrics and surgery on eyes. The sixth floor, also called the Baker Roof, was for exercises which were emphasised by Joslin as an adjunct to diet, and other measures for treatment of diabetes.

Joslin's Dreams, Fulfilled and Unfulfilled

"No man is an island entire of itself......"
John Donne

Joslin saw the Baker facility as the fulfilment of his long-held dream of replicating in Boston the European model for the treatment of patients with diabetes.

That the dream would turn out to be short lived had not occurred to him. There was one important difference between his plans for a single composite facility like the one housed in the new Baker Building and the establishments in Europe. Joslin devoted the multipurpose centre to the treatment of a single condition, diabetes, as opposed to the broader range of diseases seen in a more general hospital. The European masters like Joslin's hero, Naunyn, although knowledgeable in diabetes and writers of comprehensive books on the subject, were not single- disease specialists like Joslin. Neither were their facilities. This difference would play a critical role in a challenge to his best-laid plans.

The first few years after the completion of the facility were trouble free.

Baker's other donation, which Joslin had committed to cover secretarial expenses for the next edition of his textbook, was put to good use. The fourth edition, released in 1928, is one of the best. It was the last to list Joslin as the sole author.

The preface to the fourth edition is an excellent summary of the knowledge of diabetes and its treatment at that time.

The first two sentences are revealing. "Diabetics and especially diabetic children are here to stay," he began. The solace provided by this concise but emphatic declaration, especially for the parents of diabetic children, would be inestimable.

Then, what was unusual for the normally reserved and formal New Englander, Joslin lets his colleagues into his personal realms of introspection. "Years ago I longed to buy them an island or a continent where they could grow up without realising what they missed, but they would resent such an habitat today, because modern medicine has made them superior to their disease. Furthermore, we should miss them dreadfully, and scientifically we cannot spare them, until we learn how to prevent those complications which their one-sided diet develops both in them and even more subtly in ourselves.

Diabetic Utopia, therefore, we want in our midst and I cannot help being happy that one of the islands of that blessed archipelago will be at the New England Deaconess Hospital and near the Harvard Medical School."

Unfortunately he did not elaborate on his thoughts of isolating the children for the reader to determine if he, like all those associated with their care, was desperate for a way to relieve their suffering before the discovery of insulin. Or, was he wanting them to be away from the general population which may not understand the burden imposed on children being given painful injections several times each day?

Insulin more than fulfilled Joslin's dream of a better life for children with diabetes. And the Baker facility, complete with a research laboratory, replicated the European model of which he had dreamt.

Baker died in 1931.

Joslin kept an autographed photograph of his generous patient in his office to the end of his life.

He also kept his promise to the banker in the fourth edition of his textbook.

Treatment of Diabetes Mellitus Fourth Edition 1928

This volume, at 998 pages, is one of the longest of the 10 editions of Joslin's book. The details of the different sections are listed in the contents and reveal the broad extent of the coverage. Joslin penned a comprehensive description of diabetes in children, but his description of insulin and the practical aspects of its use in the diabetic patient is a matchless primer and a detailed scientific essay of surpassing excellence. The chapter is written with a facility of expression which would encourage doctors with far less expertise and knowledge of metabolism to study the subject, thereby gaining the knowledge needed to underpin the practical use of insulin in the treatment of their diabetic patients.

Just as diabetes received barely a mention in my medical course in the 1960s, it is worth noting that in the 1920s and 30s knowledge of the basic aspects of the condition, let alone the finer details of the physiologic aberrations, was even more limited, and for that reason often left out of the medical course altogether.

As always, Joslin drew heavily on his own practice, mentioning in the preface that 895 cases had received individual citation.

This volume included a short but excellent chapter on experimental diabetes in dogs at the beginning of the book.

Starting with the Strasbourg dog of von Mering and Minkowski in 1889, Joslin went on to describe the experiments on the New York dogs of Allen in the early 1900s. He then wrote about the Toronto dogs and the discovery of insulin in the 1920s before launching into a detailed ten-page description of the Montpellier dogs especially 440, the Montpellier dog without a pancreas, complete with several black-and-white photographs supplied by Hedon, author of the original article in a French journal of physiology (which Joslin translated but at the same time counselled that every student should translate himself.)

If, as he claimed, this was to "inveigle the doctor into a search for details", the succinct presentation complete with photographs and charts would be hard to fault–or resist.

Joslin's conclusions drawn from the experiments are worth quoting.

"The power of insulin to maintain the totally depancreatised [sic] dog for an indefinite survival in good condition is thus proved, provided it is associated with the administration of pancreatic ferments by mouth....

If dogs in Montpellier and Toronto can recover from such a state, is it strange after what I have lived through these 29 years that I should lay emphasis in this book upon the needlessness of deaths from diabetic coma, and record here my indebtedness to the dogs who have helped to save my patients' lives?"

Two more areas of study which today dominate treatment of diabetes, as well as the attention of healthcare providers, were discussed in detail by Joslin. These were the increasing frequency (incidence) of the disease and the awareness of complications through damage to arteries especially in the brain and the legs.

Emphasis was placed on the importance of statistics which allow the physician to gain a broader perspective on the different aspects of the condition, including its mortality rate. Joslin never directly discussed the many benefits of his diabetic ledger, and it is possible that he may not have realised the long-term benefits of recording the basic details of each patient.

It is a matter of record that life insurance companies were always receptive to any information from the Boston physician.

I was interested in an addition made by Joslin in the introductory chapter in this edition of his textbook. When discussing the increased lifespan of the general population as well as those with diabetes, he said:

"The danger of growing old, whether diabetic or non-diabetic, is now double what it was in 1860 and hence it is the part of wisdom that all prepare for a long life. Mr Harold Vanderbilt recognised this and made provision for it in the new dormitory of the Harvard Medical School which bears his name and was opened last fall. In this building he placed a gymnasium to promote the health of doctors-in-the-making."

What Joslin did not say was that he was the leader of the committee of students who raised the funds for the project and had approached the philanthropist. Joslin was also the unanimously chosen spokesman, and there is a record in the Harvard Medical Archives of him speaking on public radio urging members of the public to make donations to this cause. Another member of the committee was Harvey Cushing.

In the accompanying fourth edition of the manual for patients three themes were developed. Joslin stated that the patient could "master his disease if he so wills; second, that his own length of days after his diabetes begins, is in some degree, a measure of the success he achieves; and third, that he has an excellent chance by living long and well to be an explorer of regions of diabetes, hitherto unknown, and thus to open up trails toward health and cure of diabetes which others can more easily follow."

Then, waxing lyrical, he quoted John Bunyan's "Author's Apology" from the classic Christian allegory *The Pilgrims Progress,* published in 1678:

"Art thou forgetful? Wouldst thou remember?
From New Year's Day to the last of December?
Then read my fancies, they will stick like Burrs,
And maybe to the Helpless, Comforters."

One could argue that, given his reference to "explorer of regions…" and "open up trails" in the preface to the manual, some of the earlier lines of the poem would have been more appropriate as an introduction to all of Joslin's manuals for patients:

"This book will make a traveller of thee,
 If by its counsel thou wilt ruled be;

It will direct thee to the Holy Land,
If thou wilt its directions understand."

One explanation for his choice may be that, although a devout Christian and a regular churchgoer, Joslin rarely, if ever, referred directly to his religious beliefs in his writings or in his medical practice. Perhaps the third line of the above verse accounts for his preference for the lines used.

Part 16.
Leadership

Joslin's Organisational Capabilities

In the 1920s Joslin recruited several individuals with a range of expertise he felt would be needed in the care of diabetics in the future. Their progress under his guidance repeatedly demonstrated the founder's organisational capabilities.

After Howard Root, Joslin recruited Priscilla White, the only woman in the original seven. The daughter of an otolaryngologist, White had been an outstanding student at Radcliffe College before attending Tufts Medical School. Joslin was quick to recognise in her the qualities he sought in his staff: early rising, energy and curiosity, hard work and stamina. Years later, he described these in his first impression of the young medical student.

White had called upon him to write a preface to her 1932 monograph *Diabetes in Childhood and Adolescence.*

"…in 1922…. the writer of this monograph came to my attention. I could not help noting that when this early rising, young medical student had finished at 7 AM her two hours of metabolisms for my friend, Dr Frank H. Lahey, she emerged with enough energy and curiosity to take time to entertain and observe (and eventually, it has proved, capture) my diabetische Wurmschen before she started her classes at the Tufts College Medical School….in sickness and in health…. through childhood and adolescence to manhood and womanhood, they [patients with type I diabetes] have come to depend upon her as physician and friend."

Once employed, White was encouraged by Joslin to pursue her own goals even though he provided guidance and support. In addition, he used incentives which would put many of today's employers to shame. Thus, in 1928 he financed White's studies in Vienna to add to her knowledge and experience in treating children with diabetes. To inclusiveness and incentive he added the third "I" of independence by putting her in charge of the treatment of children in his practice. This culminated in White's becoming a world authority on children with diabetes.

In a career spanning fifty years, White wrote extensively on paediatric diabetes and pioneered the management of diabetes during pregnancy in diabetics.

Unlike some current researchers, Joslin never sought to attach his name to scientific articles written by his colleagues unless he had actually done some of the work on the project including the writing. This was evident in several single-author articles written by his assistants.

Joslin's organisational expertise as the head of his enterprise may also have lessons for some of today's CEOs. His generosity towards his employees/colleagues manifested itself in ways which delivered lasting, even lifelong, benefits.

And he did so without fanfare.

It was his idea that all physicians attached to his practice, as well as their secretaries, be offered full time employment to the age of 75.

He did not give bonuses, entry or exit packages.

The fifth edition of the textbook, issued in 1935, saw the inclusion of his three associates, Howard Root, Priscilla White and Alexander Marble as co-authors (although the title page lists them–in smaller print–as providing "cooperation"!). Although unfailing in his generous acknowledgment of their efforts, Joslin never left any doubt as to who was in charge.

Donna Younger told me that even when he was 90 years old, and much of the work as far as the medical care of hospitalised —patients was concerned was carried out by his younger associates, Joslin insisted on his name being on every Joslin patient's file as the attending physician"!

There is little doubt, however, that the 66-year-old Joslin had an unmatched grasp of the nature of diabetes, including findings from the latest research on its causes as well as the most recent advances in treatment. Neither did he feel that he had to wait for new findings to be reported in scientific journals to pursue any information which could be used to improve the lot of the diabetic. Thus in the "Baker edition" (the fourth) of his textbook he had written:

"In fact, during the last five years wherever I have read, heard or seen

anything which I thought would be of value in the treatment of my diabetic patients, I have recorded it and later, if on second and third perusal it has seemed worthwhile, inserted it into this book."

Ever the conservative clinician, he was quick to notice, but careful to avoid, jumping on the bandwagon of "the latest "when it came to treating his patients. Even with insulin he had tempered his own excitement and counselled caution before full acceptance.

The most dramatic illustration of Joslin's organisational capabilities, however, is to be found in his professional networking, which included not only the doctors on his staff but extended back to associations formed during his college years. For example, Harry Fowler, who had been his roommate for three out of the four years at Yale, kept in touch throughout his life. Many years later a notice in a Yale newsletter mentioned that Joslin had been a pallbearer at Fowler's funeral.

His capacity for maintaining contact was largely due to an extraordinary capacity for letter writing. The Harvard Medical Archives I visited in 2014 preserve handwritten letters by Naunyn and Minkowski to Joslin. Yet he was also able to write to his young patients, often only eight or nine years, in simple language without a hint of condescension. Neither did he forget the third part of his rule for writing letters – report, affirm, solicit–even when writing to his young patients. In Barnett's book there is a photograph of a letter dated 31 August 1931 from a 15-year-old shoeshine boy, enclosing one dollar which was the total earned for shining shoes on a Saturday in his father's shoe shop.

Joslin's foundation membership of the Interurban Club from the early years of his medical practice established an association with the elite of the medical profession of that country for his entire working life.

He travelled extensively in America, Canada, Britain and Europe, usually to take part in medical conferences. In the last decade of his life, the formation of the International Diabetes Federation in 1955 provided an added attraction to travel overseas.

He was generous and willing to extend his hospitality to visitors who were usually entertained at his country home in Oxford.

If one were to engage in a network analysis of Joslin's contacts it would include medical students, doctors, nurses, dieticians, patients, insurance executives, journal editors, international friendships and associates, book publishers, librarians, College (Yale) associates, church associations and farmers as well as his powerful family members, especially the wealthy and influential Proctors. The list, in all probability incomplete, leaves one almost breathless.

The Confident Author

An avid correspondent, as is evident from his numerous letters in the archives, (and as mentioned above), Joslin did not necessarily wait for documentation in scientific journals of any new information on diabetes, preferring to write to the researcher, especially if he knew him. Even if he didn't know the person in question, as was the case with the Toronto workers, as soon as he heard of the possibility of insulin being isolated he had written to McLeod. Given his reputation in the wider medical community, largely through the publicity generated by his textbook, an enquiry from him did not go unheeded.

An added advantage was his persuasive writing style, which was exercised almost daily if one counts his letters to patients. Correspondence was probably the main reason for Joslin's habit of being at his desk at midnight and beyond.

He knew how to deliver a punch line. His use of the short sentence at times resembles Hemingway's prose. For example, in the preface to the fifth edition of his textbook Joslin said:

"Diabetes is a disease for young doctors. It is the young doctor who has explored it."

Once he had the attention of the reader he followed up with examples from history, in this case, including Minkowski, Banting, and Best amongst others.

Neither did he shy away from controversy.

It is said that over the sixty years in medical practice Joslin had seen more than 52,000 patients with diabetes. With the practical and theoretical knowledge of his subject at his fingertips, he could, and did, speak with authority on diabetes.

By this stage in his life and career he was less guarded about expressing his personal views. He cautioned against the use of unproven remedies. In encouraging the young doctor he advised, "To retain his patient for 20 years he must shun proprietary remedies as the devil does Holy water... (and) ever sift wheat from the chaff, remembering that faithful treatment in season and out of season is rewarded."

In a prescient comment on the current practice of specialisation, Joslin reminded doctors that "to practise diabetes today one must be, first of all, a general practitioner, although one longs, in addition, to have training in a dozen specialities."

He did, however, recognise the benefit of specialised knowledge of different manifestations of diabetes, citing the work of William R Jordan who had been an assistant in his practice. Jordan had published a detailed review of nerve complications of diabetes. Joslin admitted that Jordan's work "revealed much that we have overlooked."

I devoted part of my Fellowship to a study of one of the complications of nerve damage in the feet of patients with diabetes, and had used some of Jordan's findings as background for my paper. By chance, I had the good fortune to meet Dr William Riley Jordan at a medical conference in 1969. A typical Southerner, Jordan was friendly, correct and courteous. He told me, "A good article can bring you new patients. The one you mention brought me about 30. When you stop publishing you are quickly forgotten." He was also candid!

My copy of the fifth edition of Joslin's textbook was acquired in 2011 from a bookseller in Maine. Just inside the front cover, in neat handwriting, is the name of its previous owner, Deborah Cushing Leary, who was a highly regarded physician and is fondly remembered by many, especially those receiving the award named in her honour in the medical school in North Carolina where she worked. I was unable to determine if she was related to Harvey Cushing. Needless to say, that copy has a special place on my bookshelf. Such are the joys of collecting old medical books!

Joslin's Son Dr Allen Proctor Joslin

The fifth edition of the textbook, records for the first time Joslin's professional association with his son Allen. Allen Joslin had joined his father's practice in 1934 at the age of 28. He had attended college at Yale (Class of 1927), and from there had gone to Tufts Medical School. He had trained at the New England Deaconess Hospital. At the clinic, he was on call for unscheduled walk-in patients and phoned-in requests for consultations at short notice.

Doubtless Joslin would have preferred his son to follow in his footsteps and go to the Harvard Medical School. Presumably Allen Joslin did not satisfy its academic criteria for admission. However, as A W Stearns, the Dean of Tufts had come to realise, some students rejected by the more academic medical schools, as Allen Joslin had been, possessed other qualities which fitted them for useful and successful careers in medicine.

Even Harvey Cushing, known for being a stickler for tradition, protocol and exclusivity verging on elitism, had come to realise the folly of this narrowness. "Perhaps we had better be courageous rather than proud and take selected individuals whose personal qualifications are more important than their scholastic deficiencies," he conceded in his senior years.

Barnett comments on "a general tension" between father and son. He attributes this to Joslin's "lifelong demand that his son should practise medicine with the same intensity as he himself did." In a conversation with me in 2014, Barnett also mentioned Joslin's visiting a grandson (Allen's son) at Yale and being unhappy upon hearing that the young man was not preparing for a career in medicine.

Dr. Allen Joslin was still in full-time practice during my time at the Joslin Clinic. Then in his 60s, I found him to be a gentle and courteous physician with a kindly manner. Unlike many (if not most) of the staff members, he was not a driven practitioner. Neither was he slim or of erect posture as his father had been and was described as such repeatedly in the writings of both Barnett and Holt. Allen Joslin was portly and slightly stooped and looked older than his years. In a phone conversation with me one of his grandchildren spoke of him as "a very loving grandfather." (Any grandfather would trade his appearance for that compliment any day of the week!).

In Joslin's defence of expecting high standards not only of scholarship in medical practice but also in his personal life, it was clear to all associated with him, including patients and colleagues, that he practised what he preached. One can only speculate on conversations around the family dinner table during the early years of his children's upbringing. There is little if any information on his eldest child and only daughter, Mary, or the youngest, the son who carried his father's name. The one photograph of Elizabeth Joslin during the early years of their marriage, in Holt's memoir, shows an attractive young woman with a round face and perhaps a fuller figure than seen in photographs taken with grandchildren during her senior years. Was she able to temper Joslin's wishes (even demands?) on his diet and exercise mantra for their children? Joslin admitted that he gave his overweight friends a hard time. And what of his paternal grandfather Abel Proctor who tipped the scales at 300, yes, 300 pounds? Fortunately, or unfortunately, Joslin was only 10 when Abel Proctor died. It is part of Joslin's family history that his mother also had a history of obesity and developed diabetes. But she bore the full brunt of her son's dietary prescription with, as far as is known, uncomplaining fortitude and grace! Holt described attending a Sunday dinner at the Joslin's and watching the family enjoying a rich dessert while his mother had an apple!

Joslin's leadership in the profession in America and indeed in the English-speaking world is unquestioned, and attested to by countless awards, medals, honorary degrees, visiting professorships, invited lectures and elected positions in different medical societies, associations and committees. None would argue that he was highly respected and admired.

But was he loved? Certainly there was deep affection between him and the men and women who worked for him. Holt's memoir, actually a hagiography, can be placed alongside the obvious affection in which Priscilla White held Joslin. Barnett called it a father-daughter

328

relationship. In my conversations with Dr White when I worked with her at the Clara Barton Camp in Oxford, she expressed great affection for Joslin. Neither can there be any doubt of the admiration and affection which his patients had for him.

One other comment on the dedication of Joslin's textbook edited by others following his death is that not a single edition has been dedicated solely to him. Neither is there a photograph of Joslin in any of them. Leo Krall, the last of the "original seven," wrote two Joslin manuals for patients. The 11th edition, published in 1978, was nineteen years after Joslin's last manual. It was the longest interval between successive editions. Its frontispiece was a full-page photograph of Joslin. The 12th edition was published in 1989 and showed Joslin in a group photograph taken on the 25th anniversary of the discovery of insulin.

It was Krall who had said to me, "I'm not into hero worship, but Dr Joslin was the greatest man I ever met." Krall was not known to lavish praise or engage in exaggeration. He had been Joslin's personal physician before passing that responsibility to Donna Younger.

So, the question of love, respect, admiration and other feelings and emotions evoked by this man in those who were closely associated with him, especially his family, remains an enigma for a distant watcher like this writer. I believe that it is best left in the private domains of the hearts and minds of all whose lives he touched personally, or indirectly through his contributions in countless ways.

Joslin Looks Ahead

In addition to the need for education brought about by the introduction of insulin, Joslin quickly realised that the lifespan of the child with diabetes would be markedly increased. The survival into adulthood of the millions of diabetic children all round the world, (20-40 million according to one estimate in 2014), shows that he was right, although it is doubtful that even he could have foreseen just how successful the modern treatment of diabetes would prove in terms of increasing the lifespan of the children contracting the disorder.

The recognition of complications of arteriosclerosis affecting especially the feet and legs of adult diabetics who had had the condition for more than a few years led to the inclusion of a surgeon, Leyland McKittrick to the Joslin team in 1926. Although McKittrick was accomplished in abdominal surgery, Joslin referred patients with foot problems to him. The speciality of foot care in diabetes, later to become an established surgical subspeciality, as well as vascular surgery of the lower limbs, owe at least part of their beginnings to Joslin's vision.

William Beetham was an ophthalmologist who had been seeing patients from the Joslin practice for many years. His location at 109 Bay State Road, the same street as Joslin, facilitated the cooperation between the two men due to the ease with which patients could go from one to the other. The City of Boston, out of respect for Joslin had instructed the parking police not to issue tickets to patients attending Joslin's practice at 81 Bay State Road.

Starting in 1932, Beetham extended the study of diabetic complications in the retina by pioneering the use of laser treatment for the disorder.

William Beetham was still in practice in my time at the Joslin Clinic in the late 60s. His son-in-law Dr Lloyd Aiello had joined him and later took over as a senior ophthalmologist associated with the Joslin clinic.

Joslin also expanded the group of physicians working as his assistants to cope with the increased number of diabetic patients. As mentioned previously, the number of patients coming into the Joslin practice had increased fourfold within 1 to 2 years of the introduction of insulin.

By the second half of the 1920s, Howard Root had taken much of the burden of the day-to-day management of hospitalised diabetics from Joslin. Priscilla White was involved in office practice as well as inpatient care of the pregnant diabetics and the children. Alexander Marble, the man Joslin had hoped would be involved in research because of his studies in Europe, actually turned out to be of more help in editing parts of Joslin's textbook and manuals. Robert F Bradley proved to be a superb internist, and made seminal contributions to cardiac abnormalities in diabetics. Leo P Krall, the last to join the original seven, was especially useful in dealing with patients from South America and Mexico because he was fluent in several languages, including Spanish.

In 1928 Shields Warren was appointed to the Deaconess Hospital clinical laboratory as a pathologist. He respected Joslin and agreed with the latter's views on the need for frequent measurement of blood glucose as a necessary adjunct to the treatment of diabetes in hospital. With his cooperation, Joslin was able to persuade the hospital authorities to agree to the increased workload on the nursing staff.

Warren's work was the seed for the later self-monitoring of blood glucose by patients which is now the mainstay of the treatment of insulin-requiring diabetes.

Warren's monograph *Pathology of Diabetes Mellitus* became a standard reference, and remained in publication through many editions until it was incorporated into the Joslin textbook.

In summary: Joslin's medical accomplishments included, but were not restricted to, developing a comprehensive medical facility for the treatment of and research on diabetes; issuing at regular intervals over 40 years a textbook on diabetes and an instruction manual for patients; as well as active participation in national and international organisations devoted to the care of patients with diabetes.

To manage all these aspects of the "Joslin Complex" would require exceptional organisational capability.

The shoemaker's son from a small town in Massachusetts had become a consummate manager of men. Clearly Priscilla White had seen this, which explains her comment to me that "he could have been anything."

Part 17.
Arizona

The Statistician

Even in his 70s, with unflagging zeal, Joslin made further inroads into several aspects of diabetes. In 1948 he made representations to the Surgeon General of the United States to embark on a study of the incidence of diabetes in the entire population of one town. The town chosen was Oxford, Joslin's birthplace. The study involving the entire population of a single town was another first. Headed by HLC Wilkerson, the study conducted interviews and laboratory tests on the entire population numbering 3516 individuals. It was during this time that Joslin had first noticed the capabilities of LP Krall who was an associate of and assistant to Wilkerson.

(Shortly after employing Krall in 1953, Joslin asked him to be his personal physician. Later, with Krall's increasing popularity overseas requiring frequent trips abroad, the task of being "the old man's" personal physician was passed on to Donna Younger, who took care of Joslin to the end of his life. Leo Krall told me many stories about Joslin. On one occasion he commented on Joslin's generous tipping of a taxi driver. "The tip was more than the fare," said Krall. "Yes", replied Joslin. "Have you ever seen me waiting for a taxi when it's raining?"

The confidentiality of Younger's doctor-patient relationship with Joslin proved to be an inconvenience from my point of view because of the constraints which had to be respected when it came to seeking personal details, especially of Joslin's health, including his mental state towards the end of his life. In spite of this Dr Younger always tried to be helpful with her recollections of other details of her patient's life. I avoided asking her about personal incidents of Joslin's health, relying instead on the Barnett and Holt books.

For example, I had to be satisfied with the description in Holt's book of the amusing episode which related to Joslin's hospitalisation for emergency appendectomy. Having correctly diagnosed the condition, he booked a bed at the New England Deaconess Hospital – remember he was the hospital's Chief Physician so there would have been no argument about providing an emergency bed! He then organised a consultation with a surgeon, but completed his medical consultations before admitting himself for surgery. Within 24 hours of his operation, contrary to nursing protocol, he was sitting up in bed dictating letters. It was only when the surgeon read the riot act that there was grudging compliance!

Later, Matt Brown from the Joslin Diabetes Centre Archives sent me a letter relating to this incident showing the date of Joslin's appendicitis being late 1953 when he was 84. The letter was from Percival Proctor Baxter, a cousin of Joslin and the son of James Baxter whose poem ("..plows, but never sows ") was used as an epigram by Joslin. Like Joslin, Percival Baxter was not inclined to draw attention to himself. At that time he was the Governor of Maine!).

As early as 1921 Joslin had made an important observation on the frequency of diabetes in his own home town. Although he did not mention Oxford by name it is clear that that is where the subjects of his comments lived.

"Although six of the seven persons, or head of families ...living in (three), adjoining houses... on a peaceful elm-lined...street... in a country town in New England.... succumbed to diabetes.....no one spoke of an epidemic.... Consider the measure which would have been adopted to discover the source of the outbreak to prevent a recurrence... (as it would)... if these deaths had occurred from scarlet fever, typhoid fever or tuberculosis... Because the disease was diabetes, and because the deaths occurred over a considerable interval of time, the fatalities passed unnoticed."

These observations quoted by Barnett were supported by an important addition in Holt's memoir. She said, "the recollection of his mother and several other overly stout near- relatives, all living near one another when he was a boy, *all well- to- do and who almost surely over-ate,* and who all developed diabetes had made a lasting impression on him. In addition to his mother, an aunt Ellen Osborn Proctor was also a diabetic. Continually he warned everyone against becoming overweight, especially those who had relatives with diabetes."

Obesity in affluent communities is now widely recognised as an important cause of the epidemic of diabetes, especially in the developed countries. Joslin's observation on obesity was confirmed when he recognised its frequency in the information recorded in his diabetic ledger. Most adults presenting with diabetes, when asked about the history of their weight, recalled that at some stage they had been obese. Joslin never tired of reminding his patients, colleagues, and readers of his manuals and textbooks (and his friends!) to avoid obesity.

Joslin Does His Own Survey

One detail in the United States Census Reports and Mortality Rates published in 1937 caught the attention of the eagle-eyed Joslin. As he himself had said, he was always on the lookout for anything which might have a bearing on diabetes. Recording his 1921 observation of the incidence of diabetes in his home town, he noticed that two states, namely Rhode Island, and Arizona, had markedly different death rates from diabetes. His own ledger had been used by the Metropolitan Life Insurance Company to make its actuarial calculations in relation to deaths caused by diabetes. The government document revealed that the smallest state in the union, namely Rhode Island, had a higher death rate from diabetes as compared with Arizona, which was much larger – three times the size of New Jersey –but had the lowest reported death rates in the United States. Rhode Island, being much closer, was conveniently located for its reports to be checked, but Arizona was closer to the West Coast. Unable to contain himself at discovering this, to him, "astonishing discrepancy", Joslin asked his secretary to make arrangements to travel by aeroplane to Arizona on 12 February 1940.

Well known throughout the United States, largely because of his manuals and textbook, Joslin was not only afforded access to any information he wanted but was feted everywhere he went. Conferences in hospitals with medical and nursing staff were liberally sprinkled with lunches, dinners and sightseeing! He visited a number of Indian reservations as well as the State Penitentiary. Typical of his thoroughness and planning was Joslin's approach to every doctor by mail and being forthright in his reason for doing so. He asked each doctor if he was a diabetic himself! Being the person he was, very few of his colleagues showed any hesitation in sharing personal information with him. He did the same with the clergy, not forgetting to remind them that he was a Deacon of the Old South Church in Boston! The incidence of diabetes between the clergy and the doctors was the same.

Although as recounted by Holt, Joslin enjoyed himself in the mountains and delighted in the beautiful sunsets in Arizona, he was perhaps being diplomatic when writing to his wife, saying, "You would not like the scenery here." Neither Joslin nor his faithful Anna Holt provided any explanation for Joslin's opinion on his wife's likes and dislikes. On the other hand, Anna Holt said that Joslin "wrote repeatedly how good everyone was to him, never seeming to realise that his enthusiasm, charm of manner, consideration for others and his ever present graciousness endeared him to all he met along the way. His friendliness was contagious."

And the gentle Elizabeth Joslin was not going to like any of this? Hmm. It gets better, or worse, depending on your point of view, dear reader.

To quote Holt further, "Usually, somewhere in his daily letter, he tucked in a request or two asking Mrs. Joslin to tell the secretaries to send a book, some dietetic cards, history sheets used to record information about each patient, a small cheque to help with a fund for a new gymnasium for the Indian School or just to write a note of appreciation to a doctor's wife for opening her home so hospitably to the busy, inquisitive doctor from Boston. Always mindful of how much the little things often please people, on one occasion he even remembered to have her mention the family's dog Skip, a beloved member of the household where he had been entertained. It was his concern for the smaller, less important things of life as well as the larger ones that made him so beloved by all manner of people."

Yes, there are repeated instances of Joslin being "mindful of how much the little things often please people." So it is difficult not to notice his seeming indifference to his wife's likes and dislikes versus his own enjoyable experiences in Arizona. There is no mention of her having difficulty travelling or having any aversion to mountain scenery or enjoying the hospitality of doctors!

Although not an active sportsman himself, Joslin took an interest in the

Boston baseball and football teams. The Boston Red Sox were a favourite. He is said to have had a brain for the statistics of their win/ loss records. Whether or not he actually attended any games or took Elizabeth with him to Fenway Park (home of the Red Sox) to watch any games is not known.

References to his wife are mostly in the context of her as the hostess entertaining guests including last-minute additions and/or unexpected ones.

I recall a retired Presbyterian minister commenting on men who were street angels and house devils! One would hesitate to append this label to the venerable physician even though other prominent men have had similar observations made on their private/domestic "selves", Winston Churchill being an oft-quoted example.

I could not find any further reference to the survey in Rhode Island and Arizona in Joslin's writings for many years after this trip*, but I have enclosed the information above, fairly or unfairly, because it does provide an insight into Joslin's social interactions and Elizabeth's role in his work as observed and described by Holt.

(*In fact, it was in the last edition of his textbook, in Chapter 2 titled "Incidence of Diabetes," that Joslin spoke about the study he had done more than twenty years earlier. He gave no reason for the delay, but I can almost hear Leo Krall the co-author known for his diplomacy, persuading Joslin to describe his findings as a suitable opening for the chapter. The comprehensive 30-page dissertation has the unmistakable imprint of Krall's writing except for Joslin's typically lucid contribution at the beginning.)

Joslin Medals

"When one of my own patients earns a medal I feel I am in the presence of a Spartan soul.."

(From a handwritten letter by Joslin to Reginald Fitz (Junior), January 1950).

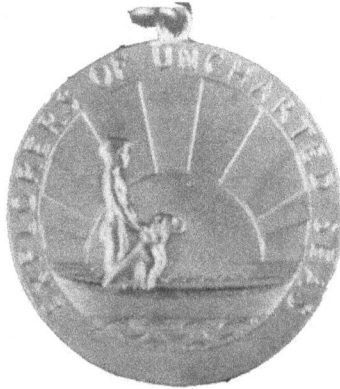

Joslin Medal

The idea of a tangible recognition of the patients who were able to exercise the self- restraint and discipline needed to control their condition had been stated by Joslin in a lecture he had given at Harvard Medical School and which was published in 1930. Acting as a champion for those who suffered from diabetes he said:

"How can we measure the success or failure of a diabetic career? Any standard has its deficiencies, but if a diabetic with his disease can live longer than his neighbour of the same age without it, I consider that he has attained distinction, and should be recognised as outstanding."

The Quarter-Century Victory Medal instituted in 1947 was for people who after 25 years of diabetes were free of complications.

The complications for which they were examined included damage to the eyes (retinopathy), to the kidneys (nephropathy), and to the nerves in the legs and feet (neuropathy). Joslin's first associate, Howard Root, coined a new term to cover all three conditions, triopathy.

Joslin had designed the motif which was used in this medal – and, (in 1953), in the Diabetes Foundation Inc. seal. It showed three horses representing diet, insulin and exercise. In order to manage his diabetes satisfactorily, a diabetic had to control all three.

"So far as I'm aware, this was the first time in medicine that a medal has ever been given to a patient in recognition of his personal share in the management and control of his disease," declared Joslin. Aware of the need to provide proof of his claim, Joslin documented details of the patient he used as the model. The medal called "Expectation of Life Medal" struck in 1961 was for those whose duration of diabetes exceeded the life expectation of a non-diabetic of the same age. The imprint on it read "For prolonging life's span after the onset of diabetes. A scientific and moral victory."

Later, a third medal was struck to acknowledge those surviving the condition for 50 years. The 50-year medal reflected the remarkable improvement in the survival of the diabetic, attributed largely to insulin but also to many other advances and innovations in medicine, including new antibiotics, improved surgical techniques and better nursing care. Before the discovery of insulin, in Joslin's practice only 10 patients had survived for 50 years. The first 50-year medal was awarded on 12 May 1970.All three medals were the work of the well-known sculptress Amelia Peabody. Peabody (1890–1984) was more than a patient to Joslin. She was an admirer, a friend, as well as a generous supporter. The sole heiress to a considerable family fortune from her father and stepfather, Peabody also had a farm in Dover, Massachusetts. She shared Joslin's love of horse riding, and there was between them a feeling of being fellow gentlemen farmers.

(According to Barnett, Peabody was part of a group of women who were second only to Joslin's wife Elizabeth in their support, loyalty and affection for him. The group also included his mother, Sarah, and his daughter Mary, daughter-in-law Barbara Joslin, the Deaconess School of Nursing students and their faculty, and last but certainly not the least, Priscilla White. Barnett also made special mention of Holt because of her several roles in Joslin's professional and personal life, starting with being a governess for his children when she was 20. She then helped with editing his research papers during his Carnegie laboratory period. Joslin assigned to her the task of checking the references in his textbook as well as completing various tasks for him when she was employed in the library of the Harvard Medical School, firstly when she was Assistant and then Head Librarian. It is clear that Holt was never too busy to accede to any requests from Joslin). These were important factors in Joslin's ability to maintain his effectiveness on so many fronts for some 60 years.

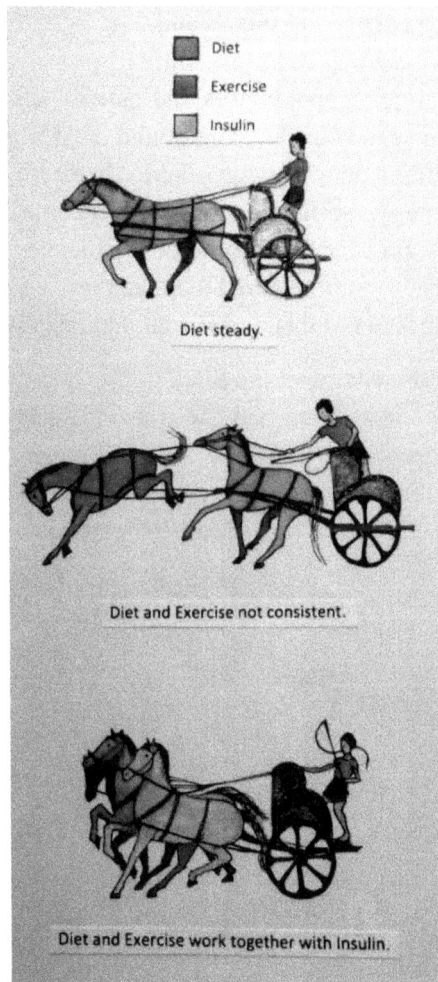

Diet and Exercise

Joslin's use of horses to illustrate the different aspects of treating diabetes, particularly to help patients, was beautifully described by Barnett, and the following (Joslin) quote is taken from his book.

"Three horses draw the diabetic chariot and their names are diet, exercise and insulin. In fact, all of us in our life's journey depend upon the three, but seldom recognise the third although we often realise that we are poor charioteers. Yet we fortunate ones have instinct to help us hold their reins, but the diabetic cannot trust his instinct as a guide, and in place of it must depend upon dieticians, nurses and doctors unless he understands his disease. To drive a pair requires skill, but to manage a spiked team [three horses] is no joke, and doctors and patients alike remember that ponies are more mischievous than horses and must be expected to upset the diabetic children's pony now and then. Therefore, the education of the diabetic charioteer is serious business. It sometimes needs a woman's hand to tame the team because her intuition, patience, mastery of detail, sympathy and even love are required to make these crude drivers, young and old, become masters of their steed, and incidentally, of their fate."

(The imprint of the medal with the three horses and the charioteer with the word "victory" over them and the triad of "insulin exercise diet" below has since been adopted by the Joslin Foundation in many of its documents and publications. It also adorns my certificate of graduation at the end of my Fellowship from the Joslin Clinic in 1970).

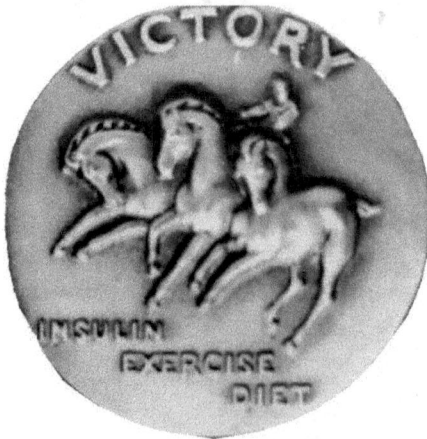

Joslin Medal
Camp for Diabetic Children "Islands of safety."

In 1932 Joslin and the Women's National Missionary Association of the Universalist Church joined to create the Clara Barton Birthplace Camp. As much a place for diabetic girls to enjoy outdoor activities, the camp was also established because Joslin was all too aware of the burden imposed on parents caring for children with diabetes,. The camp also provided an opportunity for the patients to be instructed in the care of their diabetes when occupied in outdoor physical activities.

The Universalist women provided property and funding and Joslin became the first medical director. The camp was used by eight girls in the first summer. The numbers soon increased and more than one camp was established in the grounds of the homestead. Its establishment was hailed as the first "hospital in the woods" and many programs were to follow its model in later years.

Joslin termed the camps "islands of safety". In the fifth edition of his manual, published in 1934, he said, "Summer camps for diabetic children are splendid."

In 1948 Joslin bought a property in Charlton, Massachusetts. Additional resources provided by Dr and Mrs George G Averill and Dr Classen Mowry contributed towards the cost of the construction of the additional facilities needed to fit out the property as a camp for boys with diabetes.

George Averill, the same age as Joslin, had graduated from Tufts Medical School in 1896 and had a practice in Cambridge, Massachusetts. Although he left medical practice in 1910 to manage a fibre company, he never forgot Joslin's support and help with the management of his diabetic patients. Averill kept in touch with Joslin throughout his life. He also donated funds for the Joslin Auditorium at the Deaconess Hospital.

Built on the shore of Putnam Pond in Charlton, the camp was away from any main road. The rolling fields and wide open spaces on the 115-acre site provided an idyllic setting for the summer holidays for the boys. The camp was named in Joslin's honour, but only after the Averills and Classen threatened to withdraw their support unless he agreed!

The property is owned by the Diabetes Camp, Home and Hospital Fund, Boston Safe Deposit and Trust Co, Trustee. What was known only to his closest associates was that, especially in the early years, Joslin and his wife provided monetary assistance to help the camp over its many financial challenges.

Even though the Universalist women were officially in charge of running the camps, Joslin's hand was clearly evident in the whole operation. No child was ever refused admission to the camp even if the parents were in financial difficulties. Joslin never forgot, and always acknowledged, the important role played by the Association of Universalist Women in establishing the original camp for girls at the Clara Barton birthplace in North Oxford. Here also Joslin and his wife, who visited both camps frequently, provided financial assistance whenever needed.

The two camps are 3 miles apart, a distance easily conquered by the enthusiasm of the boys from the Joslin Camp wanting to visit the girls. When I was in charge of supervising medical management as the resident physician, Dr White who visited each week, told me that Dr Joslin never approved of the practice (of boys visiting the girls' camp), but pretended not to notice! Perhaps he was a kindly curmudgeon after all. Whenever he was in Oxford, Joslin made a point of visiting one or both camps. He was good with names, frequently remembering first names from previous camp visits.

To encourage the girls to engage in exercise, the girls' camp frequently received invitations to visit Buffalo Hill on Sunday afternoons. Camp counsellors, nurse and the resident doctor joined in with helping children ride on the backs of docile horses. In the early years Joslin's children, especially his daughter Mary and son Allen, would lead the horses ridden by the smaller children. In later years Joslin's grandchildren performed the same duty. The young and more timid girls were taken on a ride in a circle on the lawn in front of the house. The bigger ones went down the long driveway. The more adventurous children could get in the hayrick which was drawn by the sturdy draft horses and be taken across the fields. In later years the draft horses were replaced by a tractor and the hayrick by a platform truck which held some 30 or more happy passengers!

The treat after these activities was a generous slice of watermelon or a peach. The children were expected to put the paper napkins and stones from the fruit into the appropriate receptacle provided by the very correct host and hostess. Joslin always joined in, frequently being in the centre of the circle, surrounded by children. Nor did he ever let the occasion end without a short talk – always with a moral. Perhaps the Sunday School teacher (and Assistant Superintendent of the Sunday School in Bethany) had remained alive and well in him after all.

The Elliott P Joslin Diabetic Camp for Boys was one of his proudest achievements and remains in operation to this day.

The experience in the camps showed that diabetic boys with careful supervision could be managed effectively while still able to take part in all the usual activities of non-diabetic boys' camps. Each year facilities continued to be increased and improved with new buildings and other equipment, much of the money coming from gifts from parents of diabetic boys and friends and supporters of the Joslin practice. As with the girls' camp, Joslin persuaded the Universalist women to provide administrative support with Joslin and his associates managing the medical side.

Miss Winterbottom, the chief Wandering Nurse at the New England Deaconess Hospital and the first nurse in charge of the camp, described in simple terms the relationship between physical exercise and food intake on the one hand, and blood glucose on the other.

"One appreciates the sensitiveness of diabetic children after studying them under the strict regime of camp life for two months," she said. "They are sugar free when the sun shines and spirits are high: sugar is present when it rains and spirits are low.

Sugar vanishes with exercise, but returns with its lack.

A long interval between insulin and sugar makes for sugar freedom, but a short interval between insulin and food causes its appearance. When the dessert is orange, grapefruit or watermelon, the Benedict test is blue, but when the dessert is banana, prunes or ice cream, the test is green, yellow or brown.

When the child is happy and gay, contented or excited, he is more apt to be sugar free than when upset emotionally, homesick or worried."

Joslin commented that "of all Miss Winterbottom's comments, I am sure that [the comment] relating to exercise is the most valuable and that all else is closely dependent upon it." His emphasis on exercise in the management of diabetes was second only to insulin.

Photographs taken during the haying season in the early years of Buffalo Hill showed Joslin with the farmers employed on his property. Joslin is wearing a coat and tie and an alpine hat. The hat is indistinguishable from the Tyrolean and German versions, but there is no information on whether it was acquired locally or during one of his European trips. It may even have been a favourite gift he chose to keep as a souvenir. Given his interest in his attire, which is almost an inconsistency given his otherwise ascetic nature, he may well have made an exception, especially since he was on his farm and not in public view. Both Barnett and Holt commented on Joslin's careful attention to his appearance, Holt noting that "he was one of those fortunate people to whom dirt did not stick." Barnett said that Joslin wore Brooks Bros. suits, a fob watch on a chain in his waistcoat, and polished lace-up boots.

After he turned 60, Joslin's medical commitments became such that he was not able to spend the amount of time on his farming as in the earlier years. In the mid-1930s he leased the farm to professional farmers. However, the stables and horses as well as the grooms were retained to the end of his life.

Part 18.
Triumph

Joslin in His 80s Birth of The Joslin Diabetes Centre

"The ultimate measure of a man is not where he stands in moments of comfort and convenience, but where he stands at times of challenge and controversy."

Martin Luther King Jr.

National and international recognition and honours had been heaped on Joslin from the mid-1940s on. One he especially cherished was the first Banting Medal and the invitation to deliver the first Banting Lecture in 1941. He was introduced by Charles Best, who had almost hero-worshipped the accomplished Bostonian since their first meeting twenty years earlier.

In my meeting with Best in 1969, he had said, "Dr Joslin helps people but never talks about it. He helped me from the first time I met him, and that's more than 40 years ago, you know."

An added interest for Joslin in the last decade of his life was the International Diabetes Federation. Formed in 1950, its congresses, held every three years, were an opportunity for him to meet up with his European contacts and colleagues in the one visit. At the first congress in Leiden, the Netherlands in 1952, 15 countries are represented. The second congress was held in Cambridge in 1955 and the third in Dusseldorf, West Germany in 1958. The number of countries joining the federation had risen rapidly and by the time of the third Congress, 42 countries were represented.

Joslin was present at every IDF Congress, the last in 1961 when he was 92 years old. It was held in Geneva. Albert Renold, the brilliant Swiss researcher whom Joslin had chosen to succeed him as director of the Baker Research Laboratory was there to welcome him. Joslin was elated with the election of his first associate, Howard Root, as the president. He himself had been elected honorary president of the IDF at its inception. It was during this visit that he was honoured by the Swiss Academy of Medical Sciences in the ceremony described later (Part 19). This was Joslin's last visit to Europe and indeed his last visit to a major medical conference.

A Challenge Emerges from Fading Light

"Authority forgets a dying king." Tennyson.

Perhaps Joslin's greatest challenge was to be visited upon him in the evening of his life. Although he was respected and honoured overseas, the situation back in Boston, as far as his medical practice was concerned, was not as rosy.

Joslin's various involvements and duties, particularly in relation to his position in his beloved institution, the New England Deaconess Hospital, were showing signs of change. Joslin had been its principal physician from the very beginning of its establishment near the Harvard Medical School. In the early halcyon days of his practice, he admitted as many patients as most surgeons. He was also one of the hospital's most effective fundraisers, using skills which had been honed over the years starting from his medical student days. He had been the director of its original clinical laboratory and adviser to the Deaconess School of Nursing. The hospital had been started by a group of Methodist deaconesses who valued the assistance and support of the courteous, popular physician known for his strict adherence to puritanical religious principles.

Joslin had taken an active role in helping with the expansion of the hospital's services, the most dramatic example of which was the George F. Baker Building which had opened in 1934 and had been funded entirely by the donation from the banker who was one of Joslin's patients. It had been built on land purchased by Joslin. The donation and, as already indicated, the design of the building, were entirely the result of Joslin's efforts.

One of the first things I noticed during my initial period of the Joslin Fellowship in 1969 was a small brass plaque in the elevator of the Baker Building. The inscription named the donor, but what struck me and what I still remember was the phrase "because of his regard for Dr Joslin." It was the first time I had seen or been in a building which had been built with funds donated because of a person's regard for an individual.

To say that Joslin had enjoyed privileges as a result of his position of power and influence would be an understatement. At least that is how his situation was viewed by some of the younger doctors who had arrived on the medical scene in Boston in the post-war period.

The period after the Second World War (1939–1945) saw a distinct shift in the politics of medical, especially hospital, management. Barnett called it the "age of hospital medicine". There were increased demands for resources ranging from hospital beds and operating theatre facilities to emergency services. There were calls for streamlined financial management. In addition to doctors, laboratory staff and nurses, new forces came into play with business executives given a higher position on the totem pole. In many hospitals, business managers came to occupy the position at the top which had, in Joslin's time, been occupied by doctors. And at the Deaconess, it was Joslin who had been at the top of the totem pole for much of his professional life.

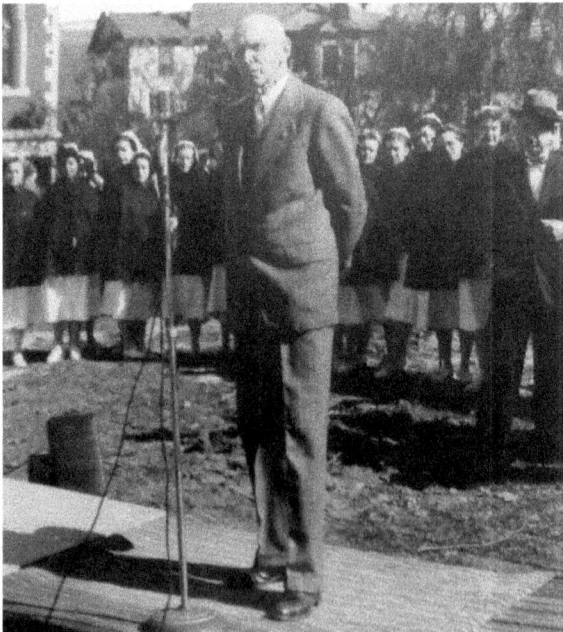

Joslin aged 81 in 1950

Some may see an irony in Joslin's being asked to speak at the dedication of the Central Building of the New England Deaconess Hospital in 1950, because this, in effect, spelt the end of his favoured status in this photograph taken on, and perhaps for, the occasion shows an impressive looking Joslin, at the age of 81, almost reduced to being the front man. In the background of the photograph was a young administrator whose expertise was in the area of hospital finances. This was the beginning of the use of a new range of non-medical personnel in hospital administration, and indeed the forerunner of many hospitals being run as part of corporations. It was the beginning of the era of the hospital CEO.

These changes had not escaped Joslin's notice. Perhaps he had a premonition of the shift in the balance of power in the delivery of medical care more than a decade earlier when he had established his own fund for supporting different aspects of diabetes care in his practice. As was his nature however, there is no record of his voicing any thoughts about, let alone objections to, these changes. But the changing loyalties of organisations he had helped, even nurtured, had a profound effect on the highly principled physician. According to Barnett, "perhaps the stress of these years was having its effect on EPJ's disposition despite his Yankee civility. Photographs of EPJ with his trainees in the years 1948 - 1953 show him appearing very stern, even angry. He was known to dismiss office personnel for a breach of manners to patients. One story that was repeated frequently and probably exaggerated, came during these years and relates to EPJ's attitude towards liquor. Apparently when EPJ was given whiskey as a Christmas gift by patients, he would lecture to his secretarial and nursing staff about the "evils of drink" and then proceed to pour the entire quantity available down the drain before the presenter had reached the first-floor door of Bay State Road."

A concession – at last?

Donna Younger, in a recent conversation, told me that a few years before he died Joslin, then in his late 80s, had invited some members of the staff to his apartment in the Longwood Towers for supper. They were speechless when he appeared with a tray carrying glasses of sherry!

"Yes, sherry," she said.

(I did not ask if the host himself drank the sherry or whether it was for staff members only!)

The Final and the Finest Ornament of the Joslin Legacy: The Joslin Diabetes Centre

Joslin realised that the Baker facility dream was over. In retrospect, the inadequacies of the facilities had become apparent towards the end of the first decade after its completion. To an observer, especially one with the benefit of hindsight, it is clear that Joslin had not foreseen the extent of the escalation in the number of patients, and therefore the demands on medical facilities and resources which occurred in the aftermath of the war. It is doubtful if anyone had.

Joslin had noted the increase in his own practice and made plans to move it closer to the Deaconess. However, it is clear that he was wrong-footed by the shift in the dynamics of power in hospital administration in general and the Deaconess in particular.

Given his age, he could have retired gracefully. He was in good health. He was known and respected throughout the English-speaking medical world after a glittering career. He was independently wealthy, with a flourishing private practice.

Yet what he did next is second only to his legacy as a physician, writer and teacher. Whatever the thinking behind the project, Joslin decided to go it alone. That he demonstrated the capacity for changing direction at this late stage in his life is a testament to his tenacity and a quiet and understated but fierce independence.

So Joslin, in his 81st year decided, and immediately embarked upon, building his own facility.

It was this decision which resulted in the Joslin Diabetes Centre.

Revisiting an Early Lesson

Joslin had never forgotten the hours spent with the distinguished architect Olmstead when, as a young man, he was planning Buffalo Hill. In 1946 he engaged the services of Henry Shepley of Coolidge, Shepley and Bulfinch, Architects. With him as co-author, Joslin wrote a paper,

"The Ideal Diabetic Unit – Of the Hospital, But not In It ".

The building was modelled along the lines of the Baker Clinic and situated on Joslin Road, separated by Joslin Park but still in close proximity to the Deaconess. This was to facilitate a continuing albeit modified association with the hospital necessitated by the nursing needs of short-stay patients in Joslin's Diabetic Teaching Unit (DTU).

His article included detailed drawings for patient accommodation, kitchens equipped for providing special meals, children's units, obstetrical areas, and accommodation for the parents or relatives visiting the patient. Dental and podiatry clinics were equipped with the appropriate instrumentation and furniture.

Emphasising the importance of education was a lecture hall for 60 patients. The inconvenience visited upon the patients having to travel from his Bay State Road practice to the Deaconess had not been forgotten. In his opinion, to be able to treat hospitalised patients and office patients in the one area together with facilities for teaching, research and accommodation for office and administration staff was the ideal, and had been his aim all along.

Joslin's suggestion that in addition to the treatment, teaching and research facilities there be a diabetic store in the new facility with the profits going to the needy was almost an overkill. (He was a merchant's son after all!).The architect and builders nodded their approval but relegated that suggestion to be followed up later and, as it would turn out, much later.

The approval of the plans by the city authorities was no hurdle, given Joslin's reputation and popularity in the city, and his friendly relations with John B Hynes, the Mayor of Boston. As soon as the first clod of earth was turned, Joslin inspected progress of the construction with daily visits.

Upon completion of the building, Joslin was honoured by the City of Boston, which named the street facing the building Joslin Road and the park across from the clinic building The Doctor Elliott Joslin Park. These joined the Joslin Auditorium built in the Deaconess Hospital with funds donated by Dr George Averill, a long-time friend and admirer of Joslin.

The high regard in which Joslin was held, not only by the civic authorities in Boston but internationally, is seen by the many awards and honours conferred on him by foreign governments and dignitaries. In 1950 he had been presented with The Cross of the Order of Leopold by the Belgian Consul in Boston, and in 1956 Le Croix de Commandeur de la Legion d'Honneur France at the French Consulate in Boston. His particular favourite was the Beloved Physician Award from the Massachusetts and Boston Council of Churches (possibly because he valued his role as a deacon in his church, a position he held to the end of his life). He was honoured by Pope Pius XII at the Pope's summer residence outside Rome when attending the Nutrition and Dietetic Congress there in the summer of 1955.

26 December 1956 A Red Letter Day

This was moving day from the old quarters in the Joslin home at 81 Bay State Road to the new address on the street which Mayor John Hynes had named after the popular physician. 15 Joslin Road became a mecca for patients and doctors not only from Boston but from around the United States and from countries as far away as Australia.

Joslin's office was located just inside the Pilgrim Road door of the Foundation building. He had brought his equipment from his home and office at Bay State Road: the old roll-top desk, bookcases with glass doors, an Osler-style examining couch with leather upholstery, the same pictures on the walls and the well-worn comfortable desk chair.

Joslin's practice had been legally converted to a group practice in 1952. The previously appointed assistants and associates officially became partners in the newly named Joslin Clinic. Joslin's practice however, had been known as the Joslin Clinic for many years before this and, according to Barnett, even the taxi drivers called it by that name. The respect and privileges accorded to Joslin by the mayor also included instruction to the parking police not to give infringement notices to patients visiting 81 Bay State Road!

At the time of the move in 1956 there were facilities for teaching in the basement, which also accommodated secretarial staff and some offices for the partners. The ground level floor which was entered from the street, was largely devoted to offices and consulting rooms for the doctors. The floor above was Joslin's pride and joy. This was the Hospital Teaching Unit, which opened in March 1957. It provided overnight accommodation for 40 patients who required minimum nursing care, the purpose of their admission being intensive instruction in managing their diabetes. The use the Deaconess nursing staff was the only significant area of association with the hospital. Eventually when fully developed, the Hospital Teaching Unit, later called Diabetic Teaching Unit, provided 70 beds.

Joslin and his associates boasted that within one week they could convert a diabetic with minimal knowledge of his or her condition to an individual capable of carrying out finger pricks to obtain blood for glucose determination, determining the correct insulin dose and injecting themselves.

Joslin's early recognition of teaching as the solution to easing the burden on diabetic patients of managing their condition had become stronger with the passing years. His emphasis on training nurses as teachers of patients with diabetes proved to be of lasting success and a major influence in the care of diabetics throughout the world. Today, nurse practitioners play a central role along with dieticians and several sub-specialists as part of the team in charge of diabetic care.

His earliest attempts at teaching had been in the small Broadbeck cottage. This was in the early 1900s before insulin had been discovered. Even then he was emphasising the importance of knowing about food portions in detail to avoid the development of acid accumulation in the blood, which almost invariably led to death. He never forgot the sense of desperation he experienced in those years. At that time, he used to say, "Education was all I had to give to the patients." Little wonder that he never forgot the importance of education.

After the demolition of the cottage the ambulatory patients had to live in boarding houses, and their education required attending classes either in the boarding houses or in other parts of the Deaconess. The logistics of combining education more than a mile away from his office practice near Kenmore Square had always been a challenge, especially for the elderly patients.

Even before the completion of the first part of the Joslin Clinic it had become clear to Joslin and his partners that additional finances were needed for future developments as well as diabetic programs. Barnett provides accurate details regarding the transition which took place for this process. He says that "Joslin wrote about his General Endowment Funds and a Home, Hospital and Camp Fund" which had been created in the 1940s.

Joslin said, "Although the three Funds, [Home, Hospital and Camp] were serving a useful purpose, it was felt an organisation of broader scope was desirable to protect the younger diabetics and the research [laboratory]. The conduct of such an undertaking would be much facilitated if the controlling body was incorporated and therefore the Diabetes Foundation was organised as a charitable corporation under the laws of Massachusetts. The charter states that corporation's purpose is the advancement of medical science and the promotion of the health of the community… with special emphasis upon research of all kinds in the field of diabetes and related diseases… and the establishment of one or more camps… clinics or hospitals (or units thereof)… the title of the hospital teaching unit is vested in the corporation…."

Joslin's fund-raising capabilities were well known, but the other members of the clinic were still astounded by his organisational prowess and also by the actual amount of money he had accumulated. His persuasive powers were seen in the substantial sums contributed by his patients even during the economic depression which gripped America during the early years of the 20th century. His younger associates could now understand Joslin's insistence upon conscientious contact best expressed in letters to patients, for which he preached another rule of three: "report, affirm, solicit".

A tragic personal detail emerged during the move from Bay State Road. Hitherto unknown to Joslin's associates was the change in Joslin's wife, Elizabeth, known for her gentle ways and faultless attention to detail. It was the astute Robert Bradley who had noticed a vagueness about her for some time, but during working hours Elizabeth Joslin was careful to keep out of the way of all activities relating to her husband's work. However, during the moving Bradley had noticed further deterioration which he only mentioned many years later. Elizabeth Joslin's disability progressed to a crippling loss of memory confining her to bed in the late 1950s. Joslin shared his heartache with his close and faithful associate and helper Anna Holt. He visited Elizabeth daily and spoke to her, even though he never knew how much of what he said penetrated his wife's wall of incomprehension.

Finish Line in Sight

Even though the facilities for research in the new centre were not in evidence at the time of the opening, Joslin clearly felt that his primary objective had been achieved. To him this was the fulfilment of a dream and, as is common with many who are rewarded with such success, Joslin felt that he was undeserving. "I have always been spoiled and gotten everything I want," he had said to Holt. Holt, being Holt, disagreed of course.

The completion of the Foundation building was still pending at the time of his death in 1962. Once completed and furnished and equipped as laboratories for experimental work, the Elliott P Joslin Research Laboratory of the Joslin Diabetes Foundation was officially launched on the 95th anniversary of Joslin's birth on 6 June 1964. Joslin's goal, indeed his dream, was given a concise yet succinct expression by Howard Root, his first associate, who said:

"In the Elliott P. Joslin Research Laboratory of the Diabetes Foundation, the largest known in the United States, exclusively devoted to research into the causes and eventual cure of diabetes, we work with one overriding consideration in mind: the well-being of diabetic patients."

Joslin Clinic, or to use its current name, the Joslin Diabetes Centre, is known and respected throughout the world for its excellence in the management of diabetes. The research laboratory, also founded by

357

Joslin, is at the forefront of research into the condition, and those who have worked there, including, perhaps especially, its directors, are counted amongst the most illustrious of research scholars in the world. The early history of the research laboratory boasted men like the late Albert Renold and George F Cahill being at its helm. The Swiss-German Renold, known for his infectious enthusiasm coupled with his brilliance and popularity, was followed by the tall, charismatic Cahill, whose impressive presence at the lectern, enhanced by magnetic oratory, made him one of the most sought-after speakers at scientific congresses throughout the United States and beyond. His opening address at the 1973 International Diabetes Federation Congress in Brussels in the presence of the Queen of Belgium held the audience spellbound, and is still talked about by those of us who were fortunate enough to be there.

Included in the plans for the Foundation building was a space on the facade facing Joslin Road left for the express purpose of erecting a set of panels telling the history of diabetes through the ages. The panels made out of stones were to have the artwork and texts carved by a sculptor. Not wanting to do anything by halves, Joslin wanted to know the cost of the project before embarking on it. Perhaps he had become more cautious, having underestimated the cost of the Foundation building which had necessitated deferring building the space for research.

So he had discussed the idea of the history panels with his wife and met some of the costs from their private funds. The texts were selected and written by Joslin.

The well-known New York sculptor Malvina Hoffman was approached and agreed to undertake the commission. Joslin provided the details as well as the legend for each of the 25 panels. The title carved in the first panel was:

"The evolution of Medicine is in reality the History of Man and his Religion. Those who have contributed to its advancement are legion. Progressive steps in the art of healing, especially as related to diabetes are here recorded."

The story begins with Egypt's Imhotep, about 2980 BC and continues through India, China, Babylon, Greece and so on up to the present, where panels 22 and 23 describe the history of insulin and its use.

The last panel declares: "This building given by thousands of patients and their friends provides the opportunity for many to control their diabetes by methods of teaching hitherto unavailable except to a privileged few."

Little wonder that when Dr Eugene Dubois of the Rockefeller Institute in New York, an old friend of Joslin, sent him a birthday greeting in July 1955 he told Joslin that he had been asked to outline the most important characteristics to be found in "a good piece of work." His answer was, "many hours of good, hard labour; infusion of a generous amount of Christianity; an impression of one's own personality."

Clearly the writer felt that this description was an appropriate description of Joslin's accomplishments.

It is said that Joslin never went home from his office without a quick visit upstairs to see that all was well with the patients' overnight stay. Till the very end of his life, Joslin familiarised himself with even minor details of his patients. His insistence on a complete physical examination regardless of the main reason for a patient's admission was a source of annoyance, especially for his junior staff. Donna Younger, the youngest member of the team when I was there, told me of an example of this during a recent visit to Boston. She said that she was called around midnight by Joslin and asked to come to the Hospital Teaching Unit to feel and record in the patient's chart the state of the arterial pulse on the patient's feet. Even all these years later, the gentle and ever-tolerant Younger rolled her eyes. "The patient had been admitted to check on a swelling on her thyroid!" she said.

Clearly, this was during the years when, according to Barnett, the stress of the changes affecting his position and status in the modern era of medicine around 1948 to 1953, "was having its effect on E.P.J's disposition despite his Yankee civility."(EPJ was the term frequently used by his staff when referring to Joslin.)

Increasingly he had left the day-to-day management of patients to his associates. This had begun with his plans for building his own facility when he had just turned 80.

Joslin also involved his senior associates, particularly Root, Marble and White, in contributing to the textbook. However, he remained very much at the helm, assigning to each of his associates a specific task. Recognising that the increased lifespan of diabetics following the introduction of insulin had led to the more frequent occurrence of complications involving the arteries in the eyes, the kidneys and the lower limbs as well as the nerves in the feet, Joslin tasked Root to study the records of the patients in their practice as well as in the literature .The findings were presented in the fifth edition of his text. The contributions of these three associates, particularly in the early texts, made their writings standard references on the respective subjects.

Joslin held Howard Root, his first permanent associate, in high regard. I found a copy of a handwritten letter by him to Root at the end of four years after the latter had joined him. At that time most assistants left the senior physician/mentor employing them after periods ranging from 2 to 4 years. Joslin expressed his wish that the association would continue. Root remained with Joslin, and succeeded him as head of the organisation until his sudden death at the age of 77 on 17 November 1967. A mere five years after Joslin's death, the loss of Root in some ways affected the organisation more than was appreciated at the time.

In retrospect, Joslin's practice was never able to recapture its glory days after the death of its founder and the first associate. Certainly none of the followers was able to replicate Joslin's feats of writing with the regular output of his textbook or the manuals for patients.

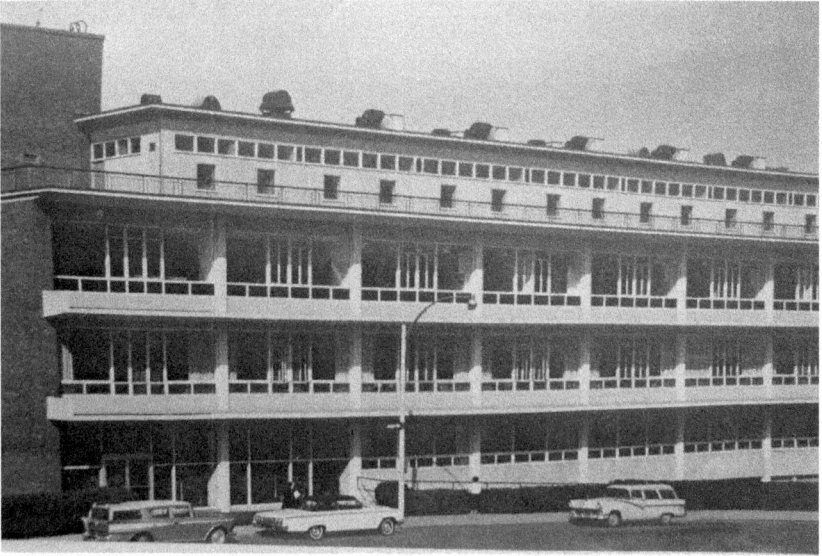

The Joslin Diabetes Foundation, Inc. Boston, Massachusetts

Part 19.
1959

Joslin at 90

"...I shall confine myself to a trot and eschew a canter."

EPJoslin.1959

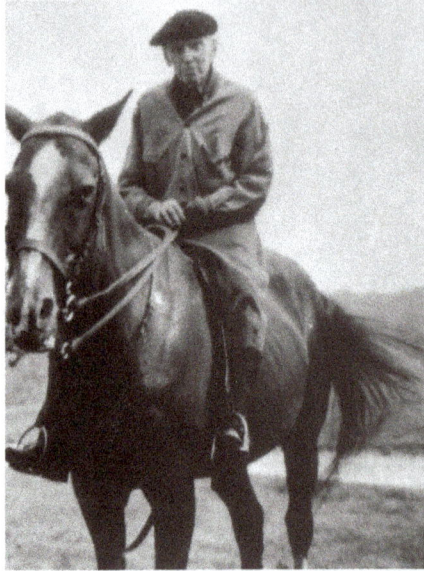

Joslin at 90 in 1959

In 1991 Mrs Carolyn J Donovan, the daughter of Joslin's son Allen sent Don Barnett a beautifully composed essay titled "Sunday Dinner." It provides some interesting and intimate glimpses of Joslin's life at home during his final years. In part it said:

"When we arrived for Sunday dinner, my parents, my brother and I, there was a routine, an order, a sense of ceremony at my grandparents, not a grand one, but one that suited the large oak table we would soon sit around. We came to the house in Boston at 81 Bay State Road which Elliott Proctor Joslin and his wife Elizabeth Denny Joslin built shortly after their marriage in 1902. Now it was the late 40s and early 50s. The one-room-wide five-storey building, with its graciously curving stairways, creaky Otis elevator and medicinal smells housed my grandparents, the Joslin Clinic <u>and</u> the fledgling Joslin Diabetes Foundation. The couple's three children Mary, my father Allen, and

Elliott Jr., had long since moved out. Over the years my grandmother's living quarters had been slowly squeezed onto two floors. Now, even the fourth floor front bedroom, lighted at night by the huge flashing White Fuel and Cities Service signs, was no longer available for guests. Would my grandmother end up in a closet, we wondered?

On these many Sundays we always arrived at a few minutes of one. My grandfather, having heard Dr. Meek preach at the Old South Church and having spent some time reading in his study was now on the second floor entrance hall or waiting room (what you called it depended on the day of the week), winding the stately grandfather's clock. We were followed by other guests, perhaps two or three practitioners, researchers or professors and their wives from Maine, England, Belgium or even sometimes from as far away as India. When everyone was assembled we would move towards the dining room. Ever the modest hostess, my gentle grandmother led the way. While she is strained to understand the heavily accented English of the most honoured guest, she was distracted by her concern that the black bean soup would be correctly diluted and the lamb, raised in Oxford would be neither too garlicky nor bloody red.

The dining room at the rear of the narrow house overlooked the Charles River, the Esplanade and, by the time I knew it, Storrow Drive. A metal fire escape crisscrossed the narrow French doors and the bowed window. This made the room appear rather dark when seen from the cream-coloured entrance hall.....

One of the bookcases flanking the fireplace held the 1920s edition of the Encyclopaedia Britannica, which would undoubtedly be consulted during the meal...

The oval oak table, extended to accommodate the guests and ringed with tall chairs, dominated but did not overwhelm. The style was solid, not ornate; grand, but not opulent.

After a grace, which thanked for mercies then begged for peace in whatever parts of the world were currently embroiled in conflicts, guests unfolded their linen napkins into their laps, the maid appeared with the soup, and we all waited for my grandfather to open the conversation. Invariably his first topic derived from the morning's sermon or scripture reading. St Paul and The Acts were favourite themes, and of course the Beatitudes. After that there would be comments on his favourite literature, a current non-fiction book, domestic or foreign politics (according to the origin of the visitor), the history of France (especially the woes of the Protestants after the revocation of the edict of Nantes, as depicted by Rodin's The Burghers of Calais), the history of medicine, the Clara Barton Camp for diabetic girls, a new camp for boys that my grandfather grudgingly allowed to be named in his honour, and of course the status of the new Joslin Diabetes Foundation and his efforts to raise money to build a teaching unit for ambulatory diabetics, which would be associated with the Deaconess Hospital.

During these dinners my grandfather often referred to the current treatment of diabetes, but he also expressed his theories through analogy and recounted stories of successful patients who were to receive medals for outliving their life expectancy. Great figures from history were his role models and he told their stories often. He was fascinated by Joan of Arc, Bernard Naunyn, William Osler, Harvey Cushing, John Hunter, Gen. Pershing, Teddy Roosevelt, Gandhi. During the meal the discussion might zigzag through history, but my grandfather had order and progress in mind. In the years I remember, he was choosing the greats in the treatment of diabetes who would be shown on the facade of the new Joslin Clinic building. He planned each scene carefully and made sure the panels were placed low on the building where passers-by would be able to see them.

The main course drew to a close. The Yale plates which had held the lamb, roast potatoes, green beans canned in Oxford, and of course, mint jelly, were cleared away and replaced by the dessert service. This more elegant setting posed a serious threat to followers of Emily Post. The maid set a painted yellow fruit plate with cream-coloured raised border in front of each guest. On the plate were a brass finger bowl with water, a lace doily, a dessert spoon and a fork. Now everyone, even the most sophisticated European, turned from my grandfather to my grandmother and waited for her silent instructions. Up until this point food had been simple, but this was Sunday and the day required a special dessert. I knew what it would probably be and mused about which fruit shaped ice cream

I would choose – a peach, a banana or a bunch of grapes. Once I'd made my choice I turned to wondering whether anyone would make the mistake of reaching out to pick a piece of fruit in his fingers. The convincingly coloured glaze of the ice cream delicacies had been known to fool serious newcomers engrossed in conversation.

I can't remember my brother and me saying much at all on these Sundays except when the immediate family were the only guests. Certainly I was not trained to ask questions, other people did that….

During these Sunday dinners my grandfather did not pontificate or lecture; he was a humble and truly mild-mannered gentleman who learned as much through conversation with others as from books. Even as I knew him in his 80s and into his 90s he was extremely vigorous. He still had so many dreams, so many people to teach, so much to do on the newest edition of The Treatment of Diabetes Mellitus, so many patient records to review and mark with the characteristic red "DM". I remember he spoke on these many Sundays of the greatest people in history, the greatest cities of the world, the greatest literature, and most importantly, of the greatest goals of mankind: love, peace, and learning."

The writing, though restrained, is evocative.

We can see Joslin winding the clock. We can hear the creak of the Otis elevator and sense the respectful, expectant silence as the guests head for the dining room. And at last–yes, at last–we see Elizabeth Joslin not in the background but leading everyone to lunch.

One senses the affection in which she is held by her granddaughter – "my gentle grandmother" and "ever the modest hostess."

Clearly this was before the practice had moved from 81 Bay State Road, and the crowding within the premises was clear even to a child.

Accolades

Feted overseas as well as at home, two events were representative of the high regard in which Joslin was held.

The New England Journal of Medicine designated its 27 August 1959 issue as the "Elliott P Joslin's 90th Birthday Issue." Joslin had been associated with this prestigious medical publication since its inception, as well as its predecessor *Boston Medical and Surgical Journal*. His first single-author article had been published in the latter in 1894.

As was typical of the man, he wrote to the editor of the journal expressing profound appreciation of the gesture. Clearly the contributions from his various younger associates and colleagues had given him much joy. He had gone horse riding after reading some of the articles and enclosed a black and white photograph of himself on one of his beloved steeds. The editor had written back to acknowledge Joslin's letter, gently suggesting that the nonagenarian (though he was careful not to refer to his age!) avoid being unduly vigorous. Joslin's compliant response, using equestrian terms quoted as an epigram earlier was typical of his respect for the norms and mores of such a discourse but not necessarily representative of his reaction to advice generally, as had been seen repeatedly by friends and colleagues, especially the latter, throughout his working life.

The articles from associates, students and colleagues related many personal and professional experiences. There was deep appreciation and unfettered admiration, not only of his academic and scholastic accomplishments but also of the many acts of kindness and generosity by him and his wife Elizabeth towards countless visitors and houseguests over a period of some 50 years. It was clear that he enjoyed the association and friendship of younger colleagues. Robin Lawrence never tired of repeating his own experience of Joslin's generosity when gifted a pair of shoes as his were very old and not suitable for the New England weather. Charles (Charley) Best spoke of his many visits to the Joslin's country home Buffalo Hill, as well as the academic activities he shared with the man he said had shown greater interest in his research work than any other individual.

The journal also included a special communication from the Queen of Belgium:

"Her Majesty Queen Elisabeth of Belgium has instructed me to convey to Dr Elliott Joslin her warmest congratulations on the occasion of his 90th birthday and wishes to join the scientific world in their appreciation of the outstanding services rendered by a great benefactor of humanity.

The private secretary."

The second event took place one month before his 92nd birthday, on 10 July 1961.While attending the fourth conference of the International Diabetes Federation in Geneva, Switzerland, Joslin was presented with a diploma from the Swiss Academy of Medical Sciences, a rare honour for an outsider.

The ceremony took place with much pomp and circumstance in the grand and impressive Great Hall of the Academy decorated with gold in the carved woodwork and flags of many nations on the stage. The honoured guest was seated centre stage on a huge chair resembling a throne. Joslin, still erect but frail (his weight had fallen to around 120 pounds from the usual 140 of his earlier years) was typically composed and alert.

There was nothing unsteady about his gait when, following the presentation, he walked unaided to the rostrum to acknowledge the honour. His short acceptance speech delivered in a clear, firm, and well-modulated voice with the unmistakable accent of a Boston Brahmin brought forth a burst of prolonged applause which almost drowned out the music of the brass orchestra. Remaining his usual calm self, Joslin acknowledged the gestures of goodwill before returning to his seat.

The Writer Who Sowed Till the End

In several of his manuals for the use of patients, Joslin had used the English translation of a Persian poem as an epigram:

Who learns and learns,
Yet does not what he knows,
Is one who plows and plows
Yet never sows.

Joslin's textbooks and manuals published regularly over a period of more than 40 years represent a remarkable, even unique, contribution to medical literature by a practising physician. The release of the manuals within one year of the publication of the texts – only the eighth edition was published two years after the release of the textbook in 1946–was another example of the writer's self-discipline.

Most of the textbooks were written to describe significant advances in the understanding or treatment of diabetes. Although Joslin did not say so, his writings did as much to publicise progress in the understanding of the condition as they did to report changes in treatment. The most outstanding example of this was his textbook written after the discovery of insulin. Although discovered in 1921, insulin did not become generally available for the diabetic population in the United States till 1923. Joslin released the third edition of his textbook in the same year, including on the title page, "third edition, enlarged, revised and rewritten." It was dedicated to "Banting and Best and the Toronto group of Insulin workers."

The fact that the longest interval between the release of textbooks over a 40-year period was usually no more than 5 to 6 years indicates Joslin's conscientiousness in keeping up with research into the condition throughout his working life.

The ninth edition of the text was released in 1953. The manual was released the same year. Joslin was 84 years old at the time. It is thought-provoking that over 50 years ago he devoted much of this textbook to the complications of diabetes. Today, that same problem besets millions of sufferers and is a major challenge for the service providers.

Many would have thought that he had done enough. They may well have suggested that he leave it at that.

But not Joslin!

In 1959, at the age of 90, Joslin wrote the 10th edition of *Treatment of Diabetes Mellitus,* and in the same year released the accompanying manual for patients. The differences in both works provide some interesting information on the writer. Known for his tact and diplomacy, Joslin was careful never to offend anyone. Thus, although he had firm views on the different aspects of the treatment of diabetes, he was usually measured in his suggestions and pronouncements on the subject. Not so in his 10th offering to patients and their treating physicians!

In the introduction to the manual, Joslin stated his conviction in what was then and even today a question asked by patients and doctors. And it is this. Does diabetes need to be treated that strictly? Joslin answered this in the first paragraph of the preface.

"60 years of experience with diabetes convinces me that aggressive and continuous treatment with strict control of the disease pays."

He also spoke of the effectiveness of the template of treatment he had introduced, and again spoke of his practice of teaching the diabetic in a 24-hour facility, meaning providing medical instruction and supervision in measuring and monitoring blood glucose and learning to alter (adjust) the dose of insulin needed. Joslin achieved this through establishing his teaching unit – H. T. U. (Hospital Teaching Unit) which he had established in March 1957 in his new facility, the Joslin Clinic which had opened on December 26, 1956.

In the 10th edition of the manual Joslin was more forthright about stating his opinions and beliefs in the best methods diabetics should use to treat their condition. It is at times forgotten that the manuals were also designed by Joslin to assist the doctor treating diabetics. Often manuals were as much to influence physicians as a way to persuade patients. For example, Joslin described the results of his method of treating mild or borderline diabetes. This is a controversial topic because it is often thought – by patient and doctor – that mild diabetes (at times referred to as having "just a touch of sugar"), need not be subjected to the strict diet and other measures recommended for the full-blown case of diabetes. Joslin produces results from his studies on 2000 patients studied over 20 years to show that if treated vigorously, 90% remained free of diabetes. Quoting the Bible as was his habit, he used the popular verse 22 from Psalms 118 in the Old Testament (King James Bible):

"The stone which the builders refused is become the head stone of the corner."

Joslin Loosens the Reins. The Return of Anna Holt

"I hope you will regard my insistence as a sign of tenacity, which is a virtue and not stubbornness, which is a vice".
Simeon Lock. (Neurologist, Boston.1970).

At this stage Joslin's health had begun to show certain signs of deterioration, nearly all due to his advanced years. He had developed congestive heart failure and was also troubled by the discomfort in his hip ascribed to age-related changes (*Pagetoid,* according to Barnett), requiring him to use a walking stick for steadiness and support. He had cut his patient load down to around 15 office consultations per week. A lifetime of the strict discipline he had imposed on himself appeared to defy any significant modification. He was already revising parts of his textbook in preparation for the 11th edition.

Joslin used his last manual to reinforce his conviction in the success of the methods of treatment he had used throughout his career, acknowledging always the teachers as well as the colleagues who had preceded him. What he never said, was how often he had helped some of these same colleagues he was praising. The most obvious example of this was Francis Allen.

Joslin maintained that heredity, which could not be controlled, and obesity were the commonest features associated with those who developed diabetes. Hence his lifelong campaign against excess body weight, even amongst those who did not have diabetes. He admitted more than once that he gave his overweight friends a hard time.

In my opinion the most important feature of Joslin's last manual was his open declaration of the details of his mother's diabetes and her influence on him and his career. Given that he had mentioned his mother's condition many years earlier, why he chose to reveal the identity of case eight now remains an enigma. What's more, it was stated, emphatically, almost at the beginning of the manual.

Chapter 2 carries the title "Control of Diabetes and why I believe it Worthwhile". It begins with a brief yet moving tribute to his mother:

"My mother's diabetes was recognised in 1900. She was my Case No.8.

Naturally, I went to Strasbourg to learn from Naunyn, the Nestor of diabetes, how to treat her. Following his methods and with a relatively low-carbohydrate, high-fat diet, which I can truthfully say I never knew her to break, the 6% sugar soon disappeared and she lived healthily and cheerfully for 13 years with diabetes which was as long as she was expected to live without it."

Joslin ascribed to Naunyn the profound influence based on the German professor's long years of experience in treating diabetes and emphasising the benefit of strict control of the blood sugar level. To Francis Gano Benedict, the brilliant chemist Joslin worked with when carrying out the metabolic studies on his own patients, he gave credit for demonstrating the importance of physical exercise in the treatment of the condition.

At the time his mother was diagnosed with the condition in 1900, Joslin had not branched out into specialising in diabetes. He himself never, at least in writing, gave any reason for specialising in the condition. The suggestion by White that his mother's diabetes may have been the reason for him doing so was contradicted by Barnett. However, Barnett did not provide any explanation for his opinion.

Joslin went further in ascribing to his mother credit for the benefit gained by his patients. His memorable tribute to her was stated openly for the first time.

"My mother's case was the first to teach me that control of the disease pays. Think of the effect of that one life upon the 52,000 which have come under my observation during 60 years of practice."

Then, disclosing another personal detail, he spoke of her love for a poem written by Ralph Waldo Emerson (who was distantly related to Joslin's Proctor ancestors). From the poem "Each and All" are reproduced the following:

"Little thinks, in the field, yon red-cloaked clown
Of thee from the hill-top looking down;
The heifer that lows in the upland farm,
Far-heard, lows not thy ear to charm;
The sextant, tolling his bell at noon,

Deems not that great Napoleon
Stops his horse, and lists with delight,
whilst his files sweep round yon Alpine height;
Nor knowest thou what argument
Thy life to thy neighbour's creed has lent".

"Emerson's lines which she loved are certainly appropriate," he said.

His acknowledgement also reflected his lifelong adherence to puritanical beliefs and codes of behaviour inculcated in him by the very religious Sarah Proctor Joslin and reinforced during childhood through his attending Sunday School and later, the churches at Oxford and Boston.

The freedom with which Joslin spoke in this chapter is quite unlike his tone and style in any of the previous manuals.

Could it have been Anna Holt who persuaded Joslin to put aside his New England reserve for once and openly declare his mother's influence in his life's work in this way? As Joslin had acknowledged in the preface, Holt had assisted with the rewriting. In the fourth edition of the textbook she had certified the references, a time-consuming exercise. In the tenth edition of both the manual and the text, Joslin stated in the preface, "Many secretaries have helped us but had we not had the benefit of the painstaking supervisory assistance of Miss Anna C. Holt, for 35 years at the library of the Harvard Medical School, the book would not have been completed this year."

In the manual, he said,"... And especially in the rewriting of the 10th edition to Miss Anna C. Holt, I am indebted..." I believe, Joslin used the words "rewriting of the 10th edition" to acknowledge just that, rewriting. It must be remembered that there had been frequent, even close, contact between Holt and Joslin, even while the former was employed in the library of the Harvard Medical School. Moreover, help with the final editions of his textbook and his manual was after she had retired and moved to Rhode Island.

Charles Best in his tribute to Joslin reported in the *New England Journal of Medicine* in honour of Joslin's 90th birthday had said that he had read all of Joslin's books. He did not specify whether he had read the manuals as well as the textbooks.

I did not read all the textbooks but I did read every manual and in my opinion the 10th is not only the best, but distinctly different from the first nine. It is for this reason that I have speculated on the contribution by Anna Holt, at least in its arrangement if not its contents. Holt had assisted with the writing of the second edition of the manual in 1919. At that time, however, Joslin was very much the writer and the role of his assistants was mostly confined to secretarial work. Clearly he had mellowed over the years and now gave his younger friend and helper a much freer hand.

It is interesting that there was one further publication by Joslin after his last textbook and manual. In 1960 the (Joslin) Diabetes Foundation Inc. published a book called "*Evolution of Medicine, Especially as Related to Diabetes.*" That it listed Holt as first author and Joslin second may have been his way of acknowledging her contributions to many areas of his life and work over the years.

It was to her during his last years that he confided his heartbreaking experience of the tragedy of his wife's illness. "If I could only do something to help her!" he said. However, as mentioned earlier, signs of Elizabeth Joslin's memory loss had been noticed in 1956 by at least one of Joslin's younger associates, namely Robert F Bradley.

He repeatedly recalled the wonderful day of celebration of their 50th wedding anniversary on 16 September 1952 when friends and relatives crowded Buffalo Hill. His children, grandchildren, great-grandchildren, and old and young relatives, were joined by friends and colleagues on the broad porches and grounds of "the Hill." "That's what I will remember," he had said to Holt. The sensitivity of Holt's record of Joslin's final days is memorable. It is recorded in part on page 382.

Anna Holt remained closely associated with Joslin to the end of his life and attended functions at the Joslin Centre even after his death. She was prominent in the list of guests invited to the celebrations of the centenary of Joslin's birth in 1969. In fact her book, *Elliott Proctor Joslin. A Memoir 1869–1962,* which was written for the occasion, had to be reprinted as the initial batch had run out within weeks of its release.

Holt died in 1977 at the age of 87. She never married.

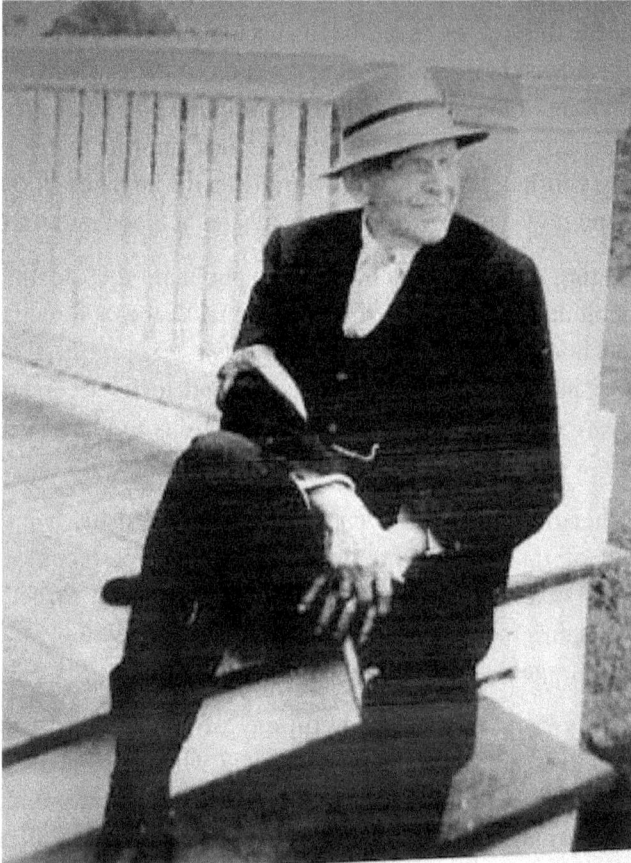

Mission accomplished – a smile at last

Part 20.
1962

The Death of Elliott Proctor Joslin

"I believe that it is quite possible that we shall never again in America see on the same scale, this combination of such widespread personal devotion by so many patients and such professional respect and achievement, concentrated in one person as we have seen in Dr Joslin."

F R Meek. 1962

"He still had so many dreams........he spoke on these many Sundays of the greatest people in history, the greatest cities in the world, the greatest literature, and most importantly, of the greatest goals of mankind: love, peace, and learning."

C J Donovan. 1991

"Dr Joslin dead at 92" (The Boston Globe 30 January 1962)

Joslin died on the night of Sunday 28 January 1962. His wife was unaware of his death.

He left three children, nine grandchildren and nine great-grandchildren.

Elizabeth Joslin died in 1964, a few months short of 97 years.

(A record of Joslin's funeral service was obtained from the Oxford Public Library through the kindness of Mrs Cathleen Sullivan.)

We May Not See His Like Again

The funeral was held on 1 February 1962 in the Old South Church in Boston where he had been a deacon for much of his adult life. The church was filled to overflowing with more than 1200 people. Doctors, nurses and patients, many from interstate and from Boston's major hospitals, medical centres and universities attended. The Governor of the Commonwealth of Massachusetts joined the mourners to pay his respects.

Except for Priscilla White and Allen Joslin, the other four members of

378

the original seven–Howard Root, Alexander Marble, Robert Bradley and Leo Krall–together with William B Hadley and B Dan Ferguson, who had been the first two physicians appointed to the original team on Joslin's staff, acted as ushers.

The eulogy was delivered by Dr Frederick M Meek, rector of the Old South Church in Boston's Copley Square. Meek, who with his wife and two children had been a frequent guest in the Joslin home, was known for his eloquence. His glowing tribute included reflections on Joslin as a physician and as a man.

Knowledge for him was something to be used as a tool for the benefit of people. In his work there was a thoroughness as if he were never to have the opportunity to review what he had done......

Always he was selfless, unassuming, with a humility that at times would lead him to apologise for taking another person's time – as if any of us did not covet the chance to do for him what we could.

He had a kind of questioning curiosity that in my experience was unique. It seemed to probe every unknown and unrecognised fact which he encountered in any field. Add to this, a meticulous attention to detail, and the load of work that he carried, becomes in part, understandable.

Dr Joslin dreamed his dreams – and he never ceased to dream – and then he built foundations under them. This was the pattern of his living."

I believe that it is quite possible that we shall never again in America see on the same scale, this combination of such widespread personal devotion by so many patients and such professional respect and achievement, concentrated in one person as we have seen in Dr Joslin.

Joslin's body was taken to the town of his birth for burial following a graveside ceremony. He lies in the company of his father and his mother in the same cemetery, not far distant from his childhood home in Main Street Oxford.

A simple headstone identifies his grave in North Cemetery, Oxford.

Joslin's Final Days As Recalled by His Colleagues

I discussed with both Barnett and Younger the actual circumstances preceding Joslin's death. Interestingly, neither agreed with the other! Barnett felt that Joslin had had a cold and should not have gone to church in Copley Square from his apartment in the Longwood Towers across the road from the Joslin Clinic by MTA. His opinion was that the cold had affected his lungs (pneumonia), causing his death.

What I found interesting was the vehemence with which each of these senior physicians stated his and her case. "He should not have caught the tram," said Barnett, shaking his head. It was one of the few times I had seen this very dignified individual becoming emotional, almost angry.

Joslin's personal physician Younger, however, was politely but firmly dismissive of that diagnosis. "He had aortic stenosis," she said." Aortic stenosis is a condition when there is a narrowing of one of the main valves inside the heart and which can cause sudden death.

I had hardly finished telling Donna Younger of Barnett's suggestion when she almost cut me off with "you don't develop pneumonia overnight." Then, perhaps realising that she had spoken almost sharply, which was contrary to her nature, she said, almost in an undertone, something like "guess it doesn't matter now" and looked away. With my own experience in internal medicine, I couldn't help noticing that in spite of being in her mid-80s, Younger's intellect was as sharp as ever.

Once again, I found myself reflecting, as I had done many times throughout this project, on the profound effect Joslin had on those who knew him, even more than 50 years after his death. I wondered if I was beginning to sense the dynamics in his relationship with his various associates and contacts. Then again, perhaps it was something that had to be experienced first-hand.

During my visit in 2014 I had asked Younger why, at her age, she was still working. She answered without hesitation: "Because I don't want to lose contact with Joslin."

At the time I assumed she meant the Clinic but later realised that the times and experiences with him were cherished memories.

Barnett, in his book, *A Centennial Portrait,* emphasised one of the motivating forces in Joslin's attitude to his work and his life. He said:

"Elliott Joslin never gave up. He seemed to be forever pursuing his mission. In his last textbook he had said:

"With a missionary zeal, one must convert not only the patient's mind and soul, but also his doctor to the realisation that it is worth the effort to control the disease as shown by the sugar-free urine, normal blood sugar and cholesterol."

Barnett was basing his opinions on the discovery of a portrait of John Wesley, the 17th century English Methodist evangelist, amongst the Joslin memorabilia in the home of his son Allen. Pointing to similarities between Wesley and Joslin he said:

"Wesley and Joslin were both missionaries. By train, ship and later by plane, Joslin and his disciples travelled with a set of "Scriptures." – Joslin's revised Manuals and textbooks. They preached Dr. Joslin's gospel: "Right living with attention to daily detail of exercise and a sparse diet control the threat of many diabetic complications."

John Wesley's rule could also apply to Joslin's way of life:

Do all the good you can, by all the means you can,
In all the ways you can, in all the places you can,
At all the times you can, to all the people you can,
As long as ever you can.

Barnett, like most Bostonians is not given to sentimentality. Yet his final remarks are wistful.

"Perhaps the next century would have as effective an educator as Dr Joslin....

... And perhaps that person will expand Dr Joslin's dream, and find a cure."

The only detailed account I found when searching for information on Joslin's final days was in Holt's memoir. The final chapter in her book is profoundly moving in its tenderness and devotion to her friend and mentor.

I have selected passages from that description. (The emphasis on the penultimate sentence is mine.)

On Saturday, January 27, 1962, he took part at the Joslin clinic in the making of a silent film, "Diabetes and Youth", to be used primarily for teaching. In spite of his struggle with a heavy cold over the preceding few days he was able to carry on to the end of the hour or more of the recording session. Throughout this period his voice was strong and clear as usual and his interest and enthusiasm for what was being said around him was as keen as ever. He seemed to love every minute of the proceedings...

On Sunday, January 28, 1962 he followed his customary schedule- church in the morning, dinner with some of the family, dictating a few letters to patients and "thank you" notes to friends for he was ever most punctilious in these matters...

Shortly after he had retired death came as he slept, just as he would have wished it to. Invalidism in any degree would have been unthinkable for a man of such great physical and mental activity.

A long, full life of infinite goodness and service to hundreds of people whom he had helped in so many ways, vastly productive in the results obtained toward the alleviation of suffering among diabetics everywhere, had come to an end as simply as it had begun nearly 93 years before.

On February 1, his beloved Old South Church in Boston was filled with mourners from all walks of life...who had come to pay their respects to the memory of this great and humane man so beloved by all who had known his gentle, kindly ways.

When news of his death spread abroad, letters, cards, telegrams and cables of condolence came pouring in by the hundreds from around the world to the family and the Clinic. Each one was carefully documented to be acknowledged–just as Dr Joslin would have wished.

Truly, Dr Joslin belonged to the whole world.

Looking back through his long and fruitful life one can honestly say with fervour and conviction the old Latin prayer- "Pax vobiscum."

A Personal Note

"Quite a guy."

About a week before I was due to leave Boston at the end of my Fellowship, I was sitting in the Deaconess coffee shop with Dr William Hadley, one of the most accomplished clinicians with whom I had worked. He was a golfing enthusiast and had brought a golf ball on a Monday morning to show me because "I got an eagle with it," he had boasted.

He said he wanted to tell me a story to give me an insight into Dr Joslin's effect on people.

The minister who had conducted Joslin's funeral service had spoken to Bill, who had been an usher, about an incident which, for some reason, interested the Rev. Meek. "As I stood up and was about to begin," he said, "I couldn't help noticing a man pushing past the attendant at the door to get in. He seemed quite agitated and I couldn't help thinking that the look on his face said that nothing was going to stop him coming in." Hadley had asked him to describe the latecomer and told me that he had no doubt about his identity.

"It was Dr Allen of New York. Dr Joslin provided unwavering support for him and his research work when many in the medical community mounted sustained attacks on his methods of treating diabetes. Allen never forgot that."

I detected that, just for a moment, the normally phlegmatic Hadley was lost in his own thoughts. It was only a moment, and when he caught me looking at him, and possibly feeling he had to say something, raised his eyebrows, shrugged his shoulders and said, "He was quite a guy." He then looked away, and after a few moments I had the distinct impression that he was once again revisiting earlier times. I felt it best to leave him to what were clearly very personal treasured memories. That was my last meeting with Bill Hadley.

Bill was keen on playing the stock market. He also liked cars and drove a Cadillac. "I always buy them second-hand," he confided.

383

Tragically, Bill died in a motor vehicle accident in 1979, aged 55.

That Which Endures

It has been said that every life is but a story. Yet some stories can be held up as mirrors for the world to see that life. Joslin's life was such a story.

The three tangible legacies of Joslin's work were the Joslin Clinic, the Joslin Research Laboratory, and his two publications–the textbook and the manual for patients.

Patient care and education continued at the Joslin Clinic after his death and remain active to the present day. There are many other facilities for the treatment of diabetes, as there are for research into the condition. Yet both these arms of Joslin's lifelong effort are not only active but have expanded their scope of activities and influence in their respective fields. The educational and patient care facilities now also operate out of satellite centres established by the Joslin Diabetes Centre. The Joslin Research Laboratory, respected throughout the world, has made numerous contributions of academic and practical significance in the study of diabetes and its complications.

As noted earlier, in Joslin's lifetime the publication of the manuals in most instances closely followed the publication of each of his textbooks over the period between 1916 and 1959. This ceased after his death.

The table below lists the dates of publication of the textbook and manuals.

Edition	Textbook	Manuals
First	1916	1918
Second	1917	1919
Third	1923	1924
Fourth	1928	1929
Fifth	1935	1934
Six	1937	1937
Seven	1940	1941
Eight	1946	1948
Nine	1953	1953
Tenth	1959	1959
Eleventh	1971	1978
Twelfth	1985	1989
Thirteenth	1994	
Fourteenth	2005	

The 11th edition of Joslin's manual for the use of patients published nearly 20 years later, was written by Leo Krall. He was the last to join the original seven. A full-page black-and-white portrait of Joslin in the frontispiece was Krall's dedication of the manual to his leader and exemplar.

As already mentioned, Howard Root had died by the time I started my Fellowship in 1969.The remaining five were fully active. Alexander Marble was the President and Robert F Bradley the Medical Director when I was there. Dr Priscilla White headed the Obstetric and Paediatric Divisions, with Leo Krall in charge of the Education Division.

Marble, White, Bradley and Krall edited the next (eleventh) edition of the textbook. They changed its title to *Joslin's Diabetes Mellitus* and dedicated it to Joslin and Root as follows:

"To our mentors: Elliott P. Joslin, and Howard F. Root.

Physicians devoted to the service of mankind whose extraordinary contributions to the knowledge and treatment of diabetes have benefited countless persons with diabetes throughout the world, this book is gratefully dedicated".

In addition to the contributions from several other members of the expanded physician team caring for patients of the Joslin Clinic, the book reflected the modern multidisciplinary approach to management, with collaboration from subspecialists including vascular surgeons, cardiologists, nephrologists and ophthalmologists. Also included were articles written by physicians engaged in full-time research in the Joslin research laboratory. Even though several of the contributors had left the Joslin facility, they were still more than willing to be included as authors. Over the years I met several of these men either during my visits to Boston or at medical conferences. Without exception these men held the staff members at the Joslin in high regard. Naturally there were many friendships with the members at the Joslin who had supervised them.

The 11th edition was issued in 1971.

Following the death of Priscilla White in 1989, Marble, Krall and Bradley, together with Richard Christlieb and Stuart Soeldner from the clinic staff and research laboratory respectively, edited the 12th edition released in 1985. It was dedicated to White. This was the last textbook edited by Joslin's original team.

Alexander Marble died in 1992. The 13th edition of *Joslin's Diabetes Mellitus,* released in 1994, was dedicated to him.

The quietly spoken Robert Bradley, who had retired in 1987, died in 2003 aged 83 years. He was the first member of the Joslin Clinic whom I met on arrival in Boston in 1969. He was the Medical Director of the Clinic at that time. The advice he gave me at the time of my leaving the Clinic stood me in good stead for my entire career as a specialist in internal medicine (with emphasis on diabetes and cardiology). Those two fields were his forte.

Leo Krall died in 2002 at the age of 87. He worked to the end of his life because, he told me, "Dr Joslin did that." Adjusting to changes in the method of delivery of medical care, services towards the end of his working life were a challenge for him, as they had been for Joslin. In one of his last letters to me Krall said that clinics for treating diabetes had become more like diabetes factories. He always had a way with words.

The 13th edition of *Joslin's Diabetes Mellitus,* released in 1994, was, for the first time, edited by two research scientists, C Ronald Kahn and Gordon C Weir. This no doubt would have pleased Joslin given his appreciation of the importance of this aspect of the study of any disease, especially diabetes. Having read much of his writings in his text and manuals as well as his contributions to the literature, I have little doubt that he not only valued research but had profound respect and admiration for those engaged in it. The lengths to which he went to engage in carrying out the metabolic studies on diabetics with Benedict made me wonder if Joslin's admiration for the research scientist was almost tinged with envy. (Perhaps this goes more to the mind of this writer, who was married to clinical medicine, and I hasten to add, happily, but like many clinicians, remains nevertheless a long-time admirer of those engaged in research).

Two other aspects of the 13th edition of the textbook deserve mention.

Firstly, the opening paragraph in the preface is an excellent summary of Joslin's capabilities:

"The 13th edition of *Joslin's Diabetes Mellitus* represents a fascinating point in the evolution of a book devoted to a single disease. The first edition was published in 1916, a single-handed contribution by a man of extraordinary dedication, vision, and energy – Dr Elliott P Joslin. Dr Joslin began his practice in 1898, in the pre-insulin era, and in this setting developed a unique understanding of the natural history of diabetes, as is evident in the first edition. The editions published shortly after the discovery of insulin show how quickly and clearly he grasped the principles of insulin therapy, adopting approaches that would be considered modern even by today's standards. He was unwavering in his conviction that blood glucose levels should be kept as close to normal as possible, even though the importance and even the existence of chronic complications of diabetes were not appreciated at that point. He clearly understood the critical role of education for people with diabetes and made it the cornerstone of all treatment programs. He quickly found that diet and exercise were a fundamental part of any regimen. His descriptions of the symptoms of hypoglycaemia are as well defined. This can be found anywhere today, and he rapidly determined the small quantity of carbohydrate required to treat insulin reactions. Any serious student of diabetes should spend time with these early editions."

The second matter which attracted my attention was the mention of a donor, the late Albert Y Samuelian, a businessman who had been a supporter of the Joslin Centre. His family had made donations towards the expenses incurred in producing the 13th edition of the Joslin text.

This brought to mind the generosity of an earlier Joslin supporter, the redoubtable taciturn New York banker, George Baker whose donations were put towards the production of the fourth edition of Joslin's text. I assume that the editors of the 13th edition did not have to request that the funds be spent on the textbook in place of a different gift offered by the owner as had occurred with Baker's unsolicited gift.

This was also the last text published by Lea & Febiger. It brought to an end an association begun by Joslin as documented in the publisher's archives more than a hundred years ago:

".... The memorandum of agreement made this 18th day of January, 1916 by and between Elliott P. Joslin, M.D. of Boston Mass and Lea and Febiger, publishers, for themselves and their assigns.

That Dr E.P. Joslin shall write and prepare for the press work on the Treatment of Diabetes Mellitus...."

The last Joslin textbook, the 14th edition, published by Lippincott, Williams and Wilkins, was issued in 2005. It's dedication honoured Robert F Bradley.

Joslin's textbook and manuals remain unique in the annals of medical history as the writings of a single individual whose medical practice lasted 60 years and who was witness to remarkable changes in the treatment of diabetes dominated by the discovery of insulin. His unique accomplishment was an ability to articulate in simple, everyday language the lessons learned over a long period, through the study of more than 50,000 men, women and children afflicted with what for many in the pre-insulin era was a fatal disease. This in itself would accord him a unique position in the pantheon of the greats of modern medical history.

Part 21.

1970

Postscript

In December 1970 my wife and I returned to Sydney. We left Boston with mixed feelings. We had made wonderful friends. Raj Saksena and his lovely wife Cindy had been our closest friends. Raj was a practising architect, and later the founding Dean of the School of Architecture at the Roger Williams University in Rhode Island. Their generosity towards us and love for our two girls was a bond that we found hard to break. The close ties I had formed with the physicians at the Joslin, I knew, were irreplaceable.

What we were relieved to leave behind were the Boston winters!

Joslin's final journey, on that last Sunday in January 1962, left those whose lives he had touched with their own private thoughts and recollections.

During the last few years, the time I have spent on reading, asking, and thinking about this remarkable man has been a different journey and its end has left me with a very different experience from my first departure from the Joslin Clinic in 1970. I do not feel that I am exaggerating the benefits of this exercise when I say that it has been a privilege to see his many virtues manifested in acts of service towards those whose lives he touched.

Of the many images of Joslin from his childhood through to the ninety plus years which come to mind, there is one which keeps recurring. I see the 90-year old Joslin as a lone horseman, riding in the forested area of Buffalo Hill, and in the distance I hear the sounds of a bubbling brook flowing to the French River as it wends its way southward through Oxford.

When Joslin mentioned Australia, which he did on several occasions, he called it "far away Australia."

That image of Joslin the horseman, still erect in the saddle at the age of ninety, reminded me of the words of a well-known Australian poet. A B Paterson, better known as "Banjo" Paterson, wrote "Clancy of the Overflow" about a drover called Clancy.

"And the bush hath friends to meet him, and their kindly voices greet him
In the murmur of the breezes, and the river on its bars.
And he sees the vision splendid of the sunlit plains extended,
And at night the wondrous glory of the everlasting stars."

The drover was herding his charges into the vast unknown of the Australian bush. Joslin, as a pioneer physician/educator, devoted his life to guiding children and adults afflicted with diabetes, into their uncertain future through simple and compassionate care.

Perhaps that is why the poem came to mind.

Or was it the memory of Joslin, a man of deep faith and unshakeable convictions, surveying the night sky and contemplating "the vision splendid" of his own final journey?

I don't know. I know only that I wanted someone from "far away Australia" to make a small contribution to the Joslin story.

September 2019
Sydney, Australia

Part 22.
Timeline

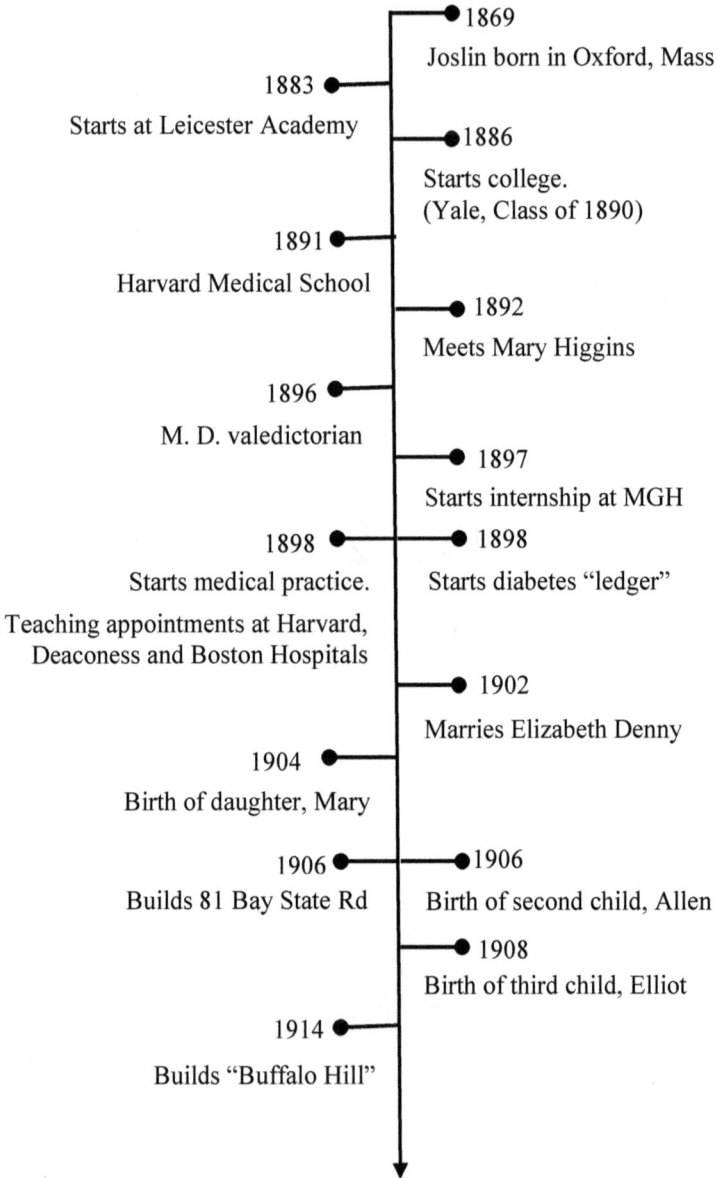

1869
Joslin born in Oxford, Mass

1883
Starts at Leicester Academy

1886
Starts college.
(Yale, Class of 1890)

1891
Harvard Medical School

1892
Meets Mary Higgins

1896
M. D. valedictorian

1897
Starts internship at MGH

1898
Starts medical practice.
Teaching appointments at Harvard,
Deaconess and Boston Hospitals

1898
Starts diabetes "ledger"

1902
Marries Elizabeth Denny

1904
Birth of daughter, Mary

1906
Builds 81 Bay State Rd

1906
Birth of second child, Allen

1908
Birth of third child, Elliot

1914
Builds "Buffalo Hill"

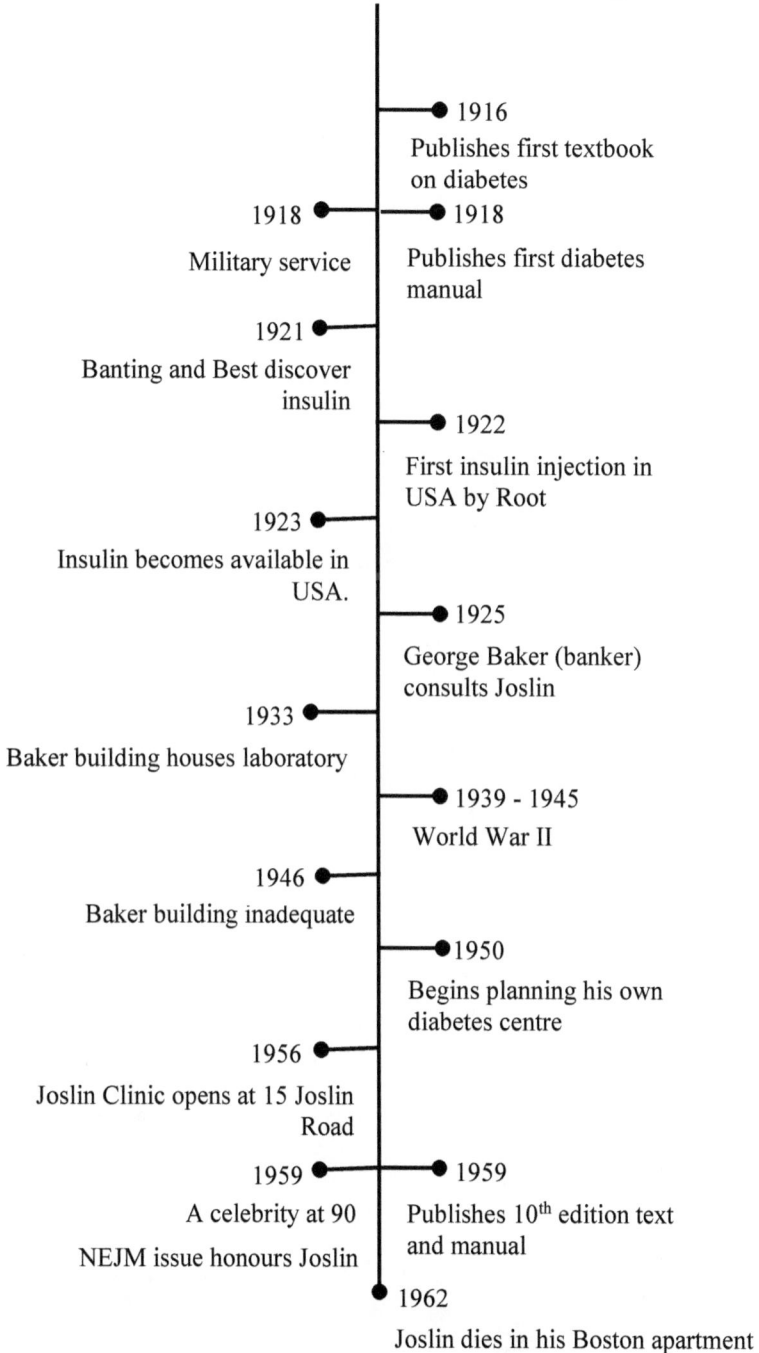

● 1916
Publishes first textbook
on diabetes

1918 ● ● 1918

Military service Publishes first diabetes
manual

1921 ●

Banting and Best discover
insulin

● 1922

First insulin injection in
USA by Root

1923 ●

Insulin becomes available in
USA.

● 1925

George Baker (banker)
consults Joslin

1933 ●

Baker building houses laboratory

● 1939 - 1945

World War II

1946 ●

Baker building inadequate

●1950

Begins planning his own
diabetes centre

1956 ●

Joslin Clinic opens at 15 Joslin
Road

1959 ● ● 1959

A celebrity at 90 Publishes 10th edition text
and manual
NEJM issue honours Joslin

● 1962

Joslin dies in his Boston apartment

Part 23.

Acknowledgements and Sources

My first and foremost debt is to the Joslin Diabetes Centre. Without its assistance and generosity this work would have been virtually impossible. Dr Donald M Barnett, who came out of retirement voluntarily to assist in establishing the Joslin archives, was of great assistance. All the photographs were obtained from the Joslin archives. Therefore, I would like to record my deep gratitude to the President of the Foundation, Dr Barnett and Matthew Brown, the archivist. Matt remained in touch by e-mail after my visit to Boston in 2014 and made my task not only an easier, but also a pleasant pursuit.

Dr Donna Younger, who with Don Barnett remains the only member of the Joslin staff who were there during my Fellowship in 1969 and 1970, was also of great assistance during my visit to Boston in 2014. She made several phone calls to the different centres, particularly the Countway Library at Harvard, to help with access to materials kept there. Since my return, Dr Younger has remained in touch answering my e-mails within 24 hours, which reminded me of the efficiency demonstrated by staff members – and expected of the Fellows – all those years ago!

Jeff Mifflin, archivist at Massachusetts General Hospital was the first archivist I met on my trip to Boston in 2014. I was captivated by Jeff's efficiency and quiet humility, and realised the potential of archives (and archivists) as potential stores of the kind of material I had been seeking.

Cara Marcus, librarian at Faulkner Hospital, Jack Eckert at Harvard's Countway Library, Cathleen Sullivan at Oxford Public Library, librarians and archivists at Yale, and Weckea Lilly at the Historical Society of Pennsylvania were all extremely generous with their time, sending material by post and internet with such promptness that I felt guilty being away from my task. Prof Milton Roxanas, a colleague and fellow bibliophile, has assisted with obtaining material from local libraries as well as from the Yale archives. Isabelle Redden provided much helpful advice on presentation and other matters in the completed manuscript. Mr Henry F Scannell sent a large number of extremely informative material from Boston newspapers (1909-1958) stored in the Research Services Department of the Boston Public Library. Richard Croall provided invaluable assistance with information on the history of the leather industry and shoe manufacture. Cheryl Fleming, my secretary for over 30 years, provided willing and prompt assistance with answers to my numerous queries. Philip Lentz, my grandson, was my go-to person for computer and word processing challenges, which were many! My son Tilak helped in many ways, including sourcing material from libraries in Paris on French physicians, and locating Apollinaire Bouchardat's grave in Pere Lachaise Cemetery – what a project that turned out to be!

Vijendra Kumar, was my friend in boarding school in a small village in Fiji when we were 13 years old and tracked me down some 50 years later, during which time he had pursued a distinguished career in journalism culminating in becoming the editor of the national newspaper, *The Fiji Times*. Vijendra is a remarkable man, held in high regard by all who know him, especially in the country of our birth. I am indebted to him for his advice and enthusiasm for this project and for reading the manuscript. Through Vijendra I met the generous and accomplished Praveen Chandra who made the task of turning the manuscript into a printable work look simple. My heartfelt thanks Praveen Bhaiya.

I regard everyone mentioned on this page, including those I have not had the pleasure of meeting, as a friend. To each one of you, including those I have inadvertently left out, I say Thank You. Without you I would not have achieved anything.

As mentioned in the preface, I have drawn much material from the books on Joslin by Dr Donald M Barnett and the late Miss Anna C Holt.

The substantial body of information available online from various sources, including the Joslin Diabetes Centre and various other libraries, filled many gaps in my knowledge of the overall conditions prevailing in New England, especially Boston, during the latter part of the 19th and the first part of the 20th century, the time of Joslin's childhood through to his late teens.

The account of Joslin meeting Mary Higgins is my construction of a tutorial for medical students by senior physicians, and is drawn from historical accounts and my own experience as a student and later as a tutor.

Lee Sinha's drawing of horses on page 341 is based on an illustration in the sixth edition of the manual, 1937.

Any errors and omissions are entirely mine and I apologise for them.

Finally, I say thank you to Lee for reading the manuscript and for listening to my endless stories about Dr Joslin.

Sources and Bibliography:

Barnett DM: Elliott P. Joslin, MD: A Centennial Portrait. Joslin Diabetes Centre.1998.

Bliss M: Harvey Cushing. A Life in Surgery. University of Toronto Press. Toronto 2005.

Bliss M: The Discovery of Insulin. University of Chicago Press.1982.

Daniels GF: History of the Town of Oxford, Massachusetts. Published by the author with the cooperation of the town.1892.

Holt AC: Elliott Proctor Joslin. A Memoir 1869-1962. Joslin Diabetes Centre 1969.

Joslin EP: Treatment of Diabetes Mellitus. Lee and Febiger. Editions 1(1916) to 10(1959) inclusive.

Joslin EP: A Diabetic Manual For The Mutual Use Of Doctor And Patient. Lee and Febiger. Editions 1 to 10 inclusive.

Kahn CR et al: A History of Joslin's First 100 years Through Its Publications. Joslin Diabetes Center 1998.

Krall LP: Joslin Diabetes Manual. Lee & Febiger. 1978.

Medical journals from archives and libraries: Articles on and by E.P. Joslin.

Oxford Historical Commission Report.

The Oxford Reconnaissance Report 2007.

Personal correspondence: Dr Donna Younger, Dr Donald M Barnett,

Matthew Brown, Jeff Mifflin, Mr Henry F Scannell, Cara Marcus, Cathleen Sullivan.

Index of names